Effects of Selenium and Other Micronutrient Intake on Human Health

Effects of Selenium and Other Micronutrient Intake on Human Health

Guest Editor

Shuang-Qing Zhang

MDPI

Basel • Beijing • Wuhan • Barcelona • Belgrade • Novi Sad • Cluj • Manchester

Guest Editor
Shuang-Qing Zhang
Department of Nutrition
and Metabolism
National Institute for
Nutrition and Health
Beijing
China

Editorial Office
MDPI AG
Grosspeteranlage 5
4052 Basel, Switzerland

This is a reprint of the Special Issue, published open access by the journal *Nutrients* (ISSN 2072-6643), freely accessible at: https://www.mdpi.com/journal/nutrients/special_issues/91QJ12NOOA.

For citation purposes, cite each article independently as indicated on the article page online and as indicated below:

Lastname, A.A.; Lastname, B.B. Article Title. *Journal Name* **Year**, *Volume Number*, Page Range.

ISBN 978-3-7258-5045-7 (Hbk)
ISBN 978-3-7258-5046-4 (PDF)
https://doi.org/10.3390/books978-3-7258-5046-4

Contents

About the Editor

Shuang-Qing Zhang

Shuang-Qing Zhang is a professor at the Department of Nutrition and Metabolism, National Institute for Nutrition and Health, Chinese Center for Disease Control and Prevention, Beijing, China. His areas of expertise include pharmaceutics, pharmacokinetics, bioanalysis, trace element nutrition, and nutritional toxicology. Dr. Zhang is internationally recognized for his studies on selenium's role in cognitive function, publishing extensively on selenium intake, pharmacokinetics, and its neuroprotective effects in animals and populations. His research group investigates fabrication and mechanism of osteoblast-targeted biomimetic nanoparticles for postmenopausal osteoporosis. Prof. Zhang has authored over 120 first- or corresponding-authored articles, 8 books and 4 book chapters.

nutrients

MDPI

Editorial

Effects of Selenium and Other Micronutrient Intake on Human Health

Shuang-Qing Zhang

National Institute for Nutrition and Health, Chinese Center for Disease Control and Prevention, 27 Nanwei Road, Beijing 100050, China; zhangsq@ninh.chinacdc.cn; Tel.: +86-10-66237226

Since its discovery in 1817, selenium had long been considered toxic, until 1957, when the element was demonstrated to protect vitamin E-deficient rats against liver necrosis and recognized as an essential micronutrient. So far, a total of 25 human selenoprotein genes have been reported since the first mammalian selenoprotein (glutathione peroxidase 1) was identified in 1973. By virtue of selenoproteins, selenium plays physiological roles in the maintenance of homeostasis, regulation of transcription factors and apoptosis, control of the cellular redox state, development of the central nervous system, and immune and reproductive functions. Recently, selenium has obtained special attention in human diseases, such as cancers, diabetes mellitus, neurodegenerative dysfunctions, and aging [1]. Due to the narrow safe dose range of selenium intake and significantly different bioavailability of various selenium species, both selenium deficiency and selenium excess result in adverse effects [2]. A sufficient amount of proteins and amino acids, especially of serine, influences selenium status and selenoprotein biosynthesis [3]. This Special Issue of *Nutrients* explores the impact of selenium and the intake of other micronutrients on human health, providing a comprehensive understanding of selenium and other micronutrients in aspects of cells, animals, and humans.

Bai et al. found that the total selenium intake was the major factor in the blood selenium concentration in American adults besides gender, race, education status, income, body mass index, smoking, and alcohol status (Contribution 1). Animal studies have disclosed that selenium reinforces erythrocytes by decreasing osmotic fragility, that chromium harms erythrocytes by forming reactive oxygen species, and that manganese is highly related to erythrocytes via the modulation of iron metabolism. By analyzing American adults from the National Health and Nutrition Examination Survey 2015–2020, Costal et al. firstly found that selenium and manganese were positively associated with human erythrocytes, and that chromium was negatively correlated with human erythrocytes (Contribution 2). Sodium selenite and its nanoparticles showed contrasting effects on the skeletal muscle development of adolescent rats via the insulin signaling pathway, consistent with adipose tissue, indicating the potential therapeutic effects of selenite on muscle growth, including muscular dystrophies, cachexia, or sarcopenia (Contribution 3). The synergistic effect of selenium with coenzyme Q was found in mice with metabolic dysfunction-associated steatohepatitis from the reduction in oxidative stress and lipid peroxidation, as well as the suppression of ferroptosis, demonstrating the therapeutic potential of combined selenium and coenzyme Q for steatohepatitis and liver injury (Contribution 4). Selol (a mixture of selenitriglicerides) significantly increased the antioxidant enzyme activity in healthy mice and influenced the morphology of tumor cells in prostate tumor-bearing mice (Contribution 5). In their systematic review and meta-analysis, Costescu et al. found that Crohn's disease patients had significantly lower serum magnesium levels and exhibited a lower magnesium intake; therefore, magnesium supplementation showed potential in alleviating Crohn's disease by enhancing remission rates and sleep quality (Contribution 6). The cross-sectional study conducted in Romania implied the preventive potential of vitamin D against respiratory infections among preschool children, and supported the establishment of a public health strategy to recommend vitamin D supplementation for children without adequate exposure to sunlight (Contribution 7). Zhao et al. summarized the renal-protective effects and mechanisms of micronutrients from botanicals with medicine–food homology, and proposed botanical ingredients for the prevention and management of kidney diseases (Contribution 8). In summary, these studies shed light on the beneficial or detrimental effects of selenium and other micronutrients on human health, and provide reliable and convincing evidence for their research and development in future.

In my opinion, regarding selenium, special emphasis should be placed on the definite elucidation of the biological functions of poorly understood selenoproteins and the wide expansion of the well-defined biofunctions of selenoproteins. More novel selenium compounds and selenoproteins should be synthesized for human diseases such as cancers and neurological disorders.

Conflicts of Interest: The author declares no conflicts of interest.

List of Contributions:

1. Bai, Y.Z.; Gao, Y.X.; Zhang, S.Q. Identification of Factors on Blood Selenium Levels in the US Adults: A Cross-Sectional Study. *Nutrients* **2024**, *16*, 1734. https://doi.org/10.3390/nu16111734.
2. Costa, A.M.; Sias, R.J.; Fuchs, S.C. Effect of Whole Blood Dietary Mineral Concentrations on Erythrocytes: Selenium, Manganese, and Chromium: NHANES Data. *Nutrients* **2024**, *16*, 3653. https://doi.org/10.3390/nu16213653.
3. Nogales, F.; Pajuelo, E.; Gallego-Lopez, M.D.C.; Romero-Herrera, I.; Mer-chan, F.; Carreras, O.; Ojeda, M.L. Dissimilar Effects of Selenite and Selenium Nano-particles on Skeletal Muscle Development Unrelated to GPx1 Activity During Adoles-cence in Rats. *Nutrients* **2025**, *17*, 1841. https://doi.org/10.3390/nu17111841.
4. Choi, H.; Choi, J.; Go, Y.; Chung, J. Coenzyme Q and Selenium Co-Supplementation Alleviate Methionine Choline-Deficient Diet-Induced Metabolic Dysfunction-Associated Steatohepatitis in Mice. *Nutrients* **2025**, *17*, 229. https://doi.org/10.3390/nu17020229.
5. Sochacka, M.; Hoser, G.; Remiszewska, M.; Suchocki, P.; Sikora, K.; Giebultowicz, J. Effect of Selol on Tumor Morphology and Biochemical Parameters Associated with Oxidative Stress in a Prostate Tumor-Bearing Mice Model. *Nutrients* **2024**, *16*, 2860. https://doi.org/10.3390/nu16172860.
6. Costescu, S.; Bratosin, F.; Popa, Z.L.; Hrubaru, I.; Citu, C. Does Magnesium Provide a Protective Effect in Crohn's Disease Remission? A Systematic Review of the Literature. *Nutrients* **2024**, *16*, 1662. https://doi.org/10.3390/nu16111662.
7. Sarau, O.S.; Rachabattuni, H.C.; Gadde, S.T.; Daruvuri, S.P.; Marusca, L.M.; Horhat, F.G.; Fildan, A.P.; Tanase, E.; Prodan-Barbulescu, C.; Horhat, D.I. Exploring the Preventive Potential of Vitamin D against Respiratory Infections in Preschool-Age Children: A Cross-Sectional Study. *Nutrients* **2024**, *16*, 1595. https://doi.org/10.3390/nu16111595.
8. Zhao, Y.; Song, J.Y.; Feng, R.; Hu, J.C.; Xu, H.; Ye, M.L.; Jiang, J.D.; Chen, L.M.; Wang, Y. Renal Health Through Medicine-Food Homology: A Comprehensive Review of Botanical Micronutrients and Their Mechanisms. *Nutrients* **2024**, *16*, 3530. https://doi.org/10.3390/nu16203530.

References

1. Bai, Y.Z.; Zhang, S.Q. Do selenium-enriched foods provide cognitive benefit? *Metab. Brain Dis.* **2023**, *38*, 1501–1502. [CrossRef] [PubMed]

2. Zhang, S.Q.; Shen, S.; Zhang, Y. Comparison of Bioavailability, Pharmacokinetics, and Biotransformation of Selenium-Enriched Yeast and Sodium Selenite in Rats Using Plasma Selenium and Selenomethionine. *Biol. Trace Elem. Res.* **2020**, *196*, 512–516. [CrossRef]
3. Zhang, S.Q.; Bai, Y.Z. Strategies for enhancing beneficial effects of selenium on cognitive function. *Metab. Brain Dis.* **2023**, *38*, 1857–1858. [CrossRef]

nutrients

MDPI

Article

Identification of Factors on Blood Selenium Levels in the US Adults: A Cross-Sectional Study

Ya-Zhi Bai †, Yi-Xiong Gao † and Shuang-Qing Zhang *

National Institute for Nutrition and Health, Chinese Center for Disease Control and Prevention, 27 Nanwei Road, Beijing 100050, China; yzbaichinacdc@163.com (Y.-Z.B.); gaoyx@ninh.chinacdc.cn (Y.-X.G.)

* Correspondence: zhangsq@ninh.chinacdc.cn or zhangshq@hotmail.com; Tel.: +86-10-66237226

† These authors contributed equally to this work.

Abstract: Selenium (Se) is an essential trace element for humans and its low or high concentration in vivo is associated with the high risk of many diseases. It is important to identify influential factors of Se status. The present study aimed to explore the association between several factors (Se intake, gender, age, race, education, body mass index (BMI), income, smoking and alcohol status) and blood Se concentration using the National Health and Nutrition Examination Survey 2017–2020 data. Demographic characteristics, physical examination, health interviews and diets were compared among quartiles of blood Se concentration using the Rao-Scott χ^2 test. Se levels were compared between the different groups of factors studied, measuring the strength of their association. A total of 6205 participants were finally included. The normal reference ranges of blood Se concentration were 142.3 (2.5th percentile) and 240.8 μg/L (97.5th percentile), respectively. The mean values of dietary Se intake, total Se intake and blood Se concentration of the participants were 111.5 μg/day, 122.7 μg/day and 188.7 μg/L, respectively, indicating they were in the normal range. Total Se intake was the most important contributor of blood Se concentration. Gender, race, education status, income, BMI, smoking and alcohol status were associated with blood Se concentration.

Keywords: Se intake; blood Se; factors; American adults; National Health and Nutrition Examination Survey

1. Introduction

Selenium (Se) as a crucial trace mineral for humans exerts substantial biological functions, such as the endoplasmic reticulum homeostasis, immune response, regulation of transcription factors and apoptosis, control of the cellular redox state and development of the central nervous system through selenoproteins [1]. Humans obtain Se mainly through foods and supplements, whereby the Se contents depend on the varied soil Se contents. Approximately 80% of the population in the world are deficient in Se (less than 55 μg/day) due to insufficient Se consumption [2].

Unfortunately, owing to a narrow safe range of Se, low or high Se status is found to be associated with the increased high risk of many diseases. Low Se levels increase the risk of Keshan disease, cretinism, immune dysfunction and cognitive impairment, whereas high Se levels elevate the occurrence of cancer, type 2 diabetes mellitus, neurological diseases such as amyotrophic lateral sclerosis, and endocrine diseases [3]. In addition, excessive Se intake or selenosis leads to some acute reactions, including garlic odor and metallic taste in mouth, hair or nail loss, nausea, diarrhea, skin rashes and irritability [4]. Because blood Se concentration is recognized as the reflection of Se intake [5], it is important to identify influential factors of Se status for the maintenance of a safe blood Se range to decrease those risks.

To our knowledge, there are few studies to simultaneously evaluate the effects of several factors (Se intake, gender, age, race, education, body mass index (BMI), income, smoking and alcohol status) on blood Se. Based on the controllability and practical significance of most of these factors, i.e., some factors are influenced by self-development and lifestyles of participants, we hypothesize that blood Se levels in the US adult population are normal and that there is an association between blood Se and diet, gender, age, race, socioeconomic status, BMI and lifestyle. Therefore, the present study aimed to explore the association between those factors and blood Se concentration among American adults.

2. Materials and Methods

2.1. Study Design and Participants

The national cross-sectional National Health and Nutrition Examination Survey (NHANES) conducted by the US Centers for Disease Control and Prevention National Center for Health Statistics (NCHS) used a complex multistage sampling method to obtain representative samples with a combination of interviews and examinations for the assessment of the health and nutritional status of children and adults in the USA. All the participants provided informed consent. Initially, questionnaires including demographic, health-related history and cigarette use were carried out among the participants aged 18 years or older via household interview by trained interviewers. After the at-home interview, the participants meeting all the inclusion criteria were invited to continue participation in the survey by coming to a mobile examination center (MEC) two to four weeks later. At the MEC, the first dietary recall interview was collected in-person followed by the alcohol data collection, and the second interview was collected by telephone 3 to 10 days later. During the MEC, body measure data and blood samples were collected for further testing.

The National Health and Nutrition Examination Survey (NHANES) suspended field operations due to the coronavirus disease 2019 pandemic, resulting in an incomplete cycle for the NHANES 2019–2020; therefore, the data of the NHANES 2019–2020 must be combined with NHANES 2017–2018 for analysis. The present study was based on the NHANES 2017–March 2020 with a total of 15,560 individuals, and following exclusion criteria as shown in Figure 1, 6205 participants were finally included. The NHANES was carried out in accordance with the principles of the Declaration of Helsinki and its ethics was approved by the Institutional Review Committee of the NCHS. Due to the present study being based on the secondary analysis, it did not need additional ethics approval.

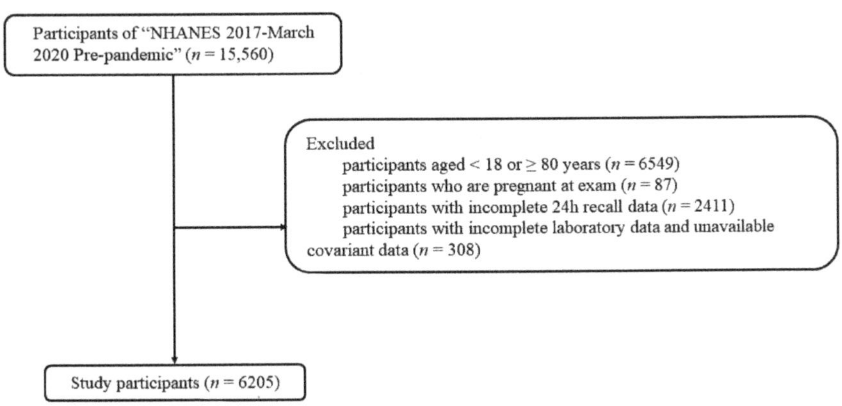

Figure 1. The selection process of study participants.

Gender, age and race were self-reported demographic information. Among these, race was categorized into Mexican American, other Hispanic, Non-Hispanic White, Non-Hispanic Black and other race. Education was defined by the question "What is the highest grade or level of school completed or the highest degree received?" and categorized into three levels: <high school, high school and >high school. The ratio of family income to poverty (PIR, <1.3 (low), 1.3–4.0 (medium), >4.0 (high)) [6] was a measure of household income and calculated by dividing total annual family (or individual) income by the poverty guidelines specific to the survey year. The lower PIR, the poorer participants [6]. The BMI data were calculated as weight in kilograms divided by height in meters squared and classified <18.5 (underweight), 18.5–25.0 (normal weight), 25.0–30.0 (overweight), ≥30.0 (obese). Smoking status was assessed via the question "Do you now smoke cigarettes?" and grouped as every day, somedays and never. Alcohol information was based on the self-report of the participants to the question "Ever have 4/5 or more drinks every day?" (yes/no).

2.2. Dietary and Supplemental Se Intakes, and Blood Se Concentration

Dietary data were acquired via two 24 h recalls. Total Se intake consisted of dietary and supplemental Se intakes obtained by averaging two respective 24 h recall data. Inadequate and excessive Se intakes were defined as less than the recommended dietary allowance (RDA) of 55 μg Se/day and more than the tolerable upper intake level of 400 μg Se/day for adults, respectively [7]. Blood Se concentration was detected by triple quadrupole inductively coupled plasma mass spectrometry. According to the previous study [4], the normal ranges of blood Se concentration were defined as the 2.5th and 97.5th percentiles for the overall US population. More experimental method details were described in the NHANES web at https://www.cdc.gov/nchs/nhanes/index.htm (accessed on 1 November 2021).

2.3. Statistical Analysis

Blood Se concentration was divided into quartiles based on the weighted population distribution. Demographic characteristics, physical examination, health interviews and diets were compared among quartiles of blood Se concentration using the Rao-Scott χ^2 test. The LSD (least significant difference) test was used to compare the differences in Se intake and Se level between different groups of factors. Weighted linear regression was conducted to evaluate the association between several factors (Se intake, gender, age, race, education, BMI, PIR, smoking and alcohol status) and blood Se concentration. A $p < 0.05$ was considered statistically significant. Statistical analyses were conducted by SAS 9.4 version (SAS Institute Inc., Cary, NC, USA).

3. Results

3.1. Population Characteristics for Blood Se Concentration

Table 1 shows characteristics of the population categorized by quartiles of blood Se concentration. The percentage values of males and females were 48.7% and 51.3%, respectively. The age of the participants varied from 18 to 79 years old. More than half the participants had a degree of more than high school level. Additionally, the percentage values of the participants with hypertension, diabetes and stroke history were 31.0%, 11.0% and 3.5%, respectively. The weighted mean values of dietary Se intake, total Se intake and blood Se concentration of participants were 111.5 μg/day, 122.7 μg/day and 188.7 μg/L, respectively. The numbers of the participants with inadequate and excessive Se intakes were 602 and 17, respectively. The normal reference ranges of blood Se concentration were 142.3 (2.5th percentile) and 240.8 μg/L (97.5th percentile), respectively. There were 155 (only 2%) persons with blood Se deficiency and 155 (also only 2%) participants with Se toxicity. The percentage of participants taking Se supplements was 18.7% (1162 participants). For gender, race and education, statistically significant differences were observed among quartiles of blood Se concentration. There was no significant difference for age, BMI, PIR, smoking status, alcohol status, dietary Se intake, total Se intake, hypertension history, diabetes history and stroke history between quartiles of blood Se concentration.

Table 1. Study population characteristics categorized by blood Se concentration in the NHANES 2017–2020.

Characteristic	**Overall *n* Weighted % (95% CI)**	**Blood Se Concentration (µg/L) Q1 (85.15–169.34)**	**Q2 (169.35–183.94)**	**Q3 (183.95–200.76)**	**Q4 (200.77–526.40)**	***p*-Value**
		n Weighted% (95% CI)				
	6205	1551 21.3 (18.3, 24.3)	1552 24.4 (22.8, 25.9)	1551 27.1 (24.4, 29.7)	1551 27.2 (24.4, 30.0)	
Gender						<0.05
Male	2988 48.7 (46.3, 51.0)	655 19.2 (15.6, 22.7)	728 22.9 (20.2, 25.7)	768 26.5 (22.5, 30.5)	837 31.4 (27.7, 35.1)	
Female	3217 51.3 (49.0, 53.6)	896 23.4 (20.0, 26.8)	824 25.7 (23.2, 28.2)	783 27.6 (24.9, 30.3)	714 23.3 (20.0, 26.5)	
Age						0.14
18–39	2134 38.9 (36.0, 41.8)	531 19.9 (15.7, 24.2)	553 27.2 (23.7, 30.8)	538 26.7 (23.5, 29.8)	512 26.2 (23.1, 29.3)	
40–59	2118 34.8 (32.4, 37.1)	492 21.9 (17.8, 26.1)	523 21.5 (19.2, 23.9)	553 29.2 (25.7, 32.6)	512 26.2 (23.1, 29.3)	
60–79	1953 26.3 (23.1, 29.6)	528 22.6 (19.3, 25.9)	476 23.9 (20.3, 27.5)	460 24.9 (20.8, 29.0)	489 28.6 (23.6, 33.7)	
Race						<0.05
Mexican American	750 8.8 (6.1, 11.5)	136 17.1 (12.7, 21.5)	206 27.2 (22.1, 32.3)	206 27.0 (20.2, 33.9)	202 28.7 (22.9, 34.4)	
Other Hispanic	647 8.0 (6.3, 9.7)	181 27.4 (23.8, 31.1)	171 25.3 (20.5, 30.2)	145 26.5 (19.9, 33.2)	150 20.7 (15.9, 25.5)	
Non-Hispanic White	2121 61.8 (56.3, 67.4)	481 20.3 (16.3, 24.4)	512 24.1 (22.0, 26.1)	587 28.0 (23.9, 32.0)	541 27.6 (23.7, 31.5)	
Non-Hispanic Black	1734 11.4 (8.3, 14.4)	562 27.4 (23.0, 31.8)	467 27.0 (23.8, 30.1)	358 22.7 (19.4, 25.9)	347 23.0 (17.9, 28.0)	
Other Race	953 10.0 (8.1, 11.9)	191 19.5 (15.3, 23.7)	196 20.1 (15.0, 25.1)	255 26.8 (23.9, 29.8)	311 33.6 (28.0, 39.2)	
Education						<0.05
<High school	940 9.2 (8.0, 10.4)	266 28.0 (23.2, 32.9)	243 25.1 (20.4, 29.8)	219 24.1 (18.5, 29.6)	212 22.9 (17.2, 28.5)	
High school	1391 26.8 (24.3, 29.3)	388 24.3 (19.8, 28.8)	361 26.4 (22.4, 30.5)	311 23.0 (18.6, 27.4)	331 26.3 (21.8, 30.7)	
>High school	3577 64.0 (61.0, 67.0)	841 19.4 (15.9, 22.9)	863 23.3 (21.6, 25.0)	950 29.3 (26.4, 32.2)	923 28.0 (24.5, 31.6)	
PIR						0.22
<1.3	1585 19.7 (17.5, 21.8)	485 25.1 (21.5, 28.8)	385 21.9 (19.2, 24.6)	380 28.6 (24.9, 32.4)	335 24.3 (19.9, 28.7)	
1.3–4.0	2378 39.4 (35.7, 43.1)	548 20.1 (16.3, 23.9)	589 24.4 (21.8, 27.0)	591 26.3 (23.0, 29.6)	650 29.2 (25.1, 33.3)	
>4.0	1520 40.9 (37.2, 44.7)	332 20.1 (15.9, 24.3)	379 24.8 (21.7, 27.9)	414 28.1 (23.2, 33.0)	395 27.0 (22.6, 31,4)	
BMI						0.64
<18.5	93 1.3 (0.8, 1.8)	29 30.0 (15.2, 44.8)	25 28.3 (11.2, 45.4)	10 20.1 (6.7, 33.5)	19 21.7 (6.6, 36.7)	
18.5–25.0	1459 24.8 (22.5, 27.0)	404 23.1 (18.7, 27.5)	369 25.1 (21.9, 28.2)	366 26.5 (21.8, 31.2)	320 25.3 (21.1, 29.6)	
25.0–30.0	1863 31.4 (29.2, 33.7)	410 19.5 (15.8, 23.3)	461 24.7 (22.2, 27.3)	463 26.1 (20.5, 31.7)	529 29.6 (25.0, 34.3)	
≥30.0	2742 42.5 (39.5, 45.5)	686 21.2 (17.4, 24.9)	688 23.6 (21.6, 25.7)	693 28.4 (24.4, 32.3)	675 26.8 (23.2, 30.4)	
Smoking status						0.32
Every day	866 30.5 (27.6, 33.5)	264 24.9 (20.5, 29.2)	215 26.6 (21.5, 31.8)	203 26.1 (21.9, 30.4)	184 22.3 (16.8, 27.9)	
Somedays	260 10.1 (7.6, 12.6)	73 19.3 (10.4, 28.3)	71 32.2 (19.0, 45.4)	57 25.7 (16.0, 35.4)	59 22.7 (12.2, 33.2)	
Not at all	1384 59.3 (55.5, 63.2)	328 21.5 (16.7, 26.3)	334 23.7 (19.4, 28.0)	343 25.2 (21.1, 29.3)	379 29.6 (24.5, 34.7)	

Table 1. *Cont.*

	Overall *n* Weighted % (95% CI)	Blood Se Concentration (μg/L) Q1 (85.15–169.34)	Q2 (169.35–183.94)	Q3 (183.95–200.76)	Q4 (200.77–526.40)	*p*-Value
Alcohol use						0.68
Yes	840	241	192	218	189	
	14.3 (12.6, 16.0)	21.9 (17.2, 26.6)	21.9 (17.9, 25.9)	28.9 (21.9, 35.8)	27.3 (20.6, 34.1)	
No	4672	1128	1202	1165	1177	
Dietary Se (μg/d)						0.52
6.70–73.84	1551	422	381	361	387	
	22.8 (20.8, 24.8)	20.5 (17.3, 23.7)	25.5 (22.8, 28.1)	27.7 (23.5, 31.9)	26.4 (22.6, 30.1)	
73.85–101.29	1551	417	384	386	364	
	25.4 (23.8, 27.0)	24.9 (21.0, 28.7)	24.3 (21.0, 27.6)	25.8 (20.7, 30.9)	25.0 (19.2, 30.9)	
101.30–135.74	1550	362	410	391	387	
	26.3 (24.5, 28.0)	19.0 (14.1, 23.9)	24.5 (21.6, 27.3)	28.4 (24.5, 32.2)	28.2 (23.1, 33.2)	
135.75–780.20	1553	350	377	413	413	
	25.6 (24.1, 27.0)	21.0 (16.4, 25.6)	23.4 (20.5, 26.3)	26.4 (22.0, 30.8)	29.2 (24.4, 34.0)	
Total Se (μg/d)						0.27
6.70–77.69	1549	422	398	350	379	
	22.2 (20.1, 24.3)	21,6 (17.5, 25.8)	26.3 (23.0, 29.6)	24.5 (20.8, 28.1)	27.6 (23.2, 31.9)	
77.70–107.64	1553	436	402	372	343	
	25.8 (24.1, 27.5)	24.4 (20.6, 28.2)	25.5 (21.0, 29.9)	26.6 (20.5, 32.8)	23.5 (17.7, 29.4)	
107.65–147.89	1551	377	386	386	402	
	25.8 (24.1, 27.5)	20.8 (15.0, 26.6)	24.5 (20.5, 28.6)	27.5 (22.9, 32.0)	27.2 (22.0, 32.3)	
147.90–830.20	1552	316	366	443	427	
	26.2 (24.3, 28.0)	18.6 (14.7, 22.5)	21.5 (18.9, 24.2)	29.3 (23.5, 35.1)	30.6 (25.9, 35.3)	
Hypertension history						
Yes	2252	583	546	535	588	0.42
	31.0 (28.5, 33.6)	21.6 (18.6, 24.6)	22.6 (19.7, 25.5)	26.5 (23.1, 30.0)	29.2 (25.1, 33.4)	
No	3947	966	1006	1015	960	
	68.9 (66.3, 71.5)	21.2 (17.6, 24.8)	25.2 (22.6, 27.8)	27.3 (24.1, 30.5)	26.3 (23.5, 29.1)	
Diabetes history						
Yes	883	235	202	196	250	0.23
	11.0 (10.1, 11.9)	22.9 (18.8, 26.9)	22.3 (16.4, 28.1)	23.4 (18.9, 28.0)	31.5 (25.6, 37.3)	
No	5144	1276	1306	1310	1252	
	86.7 (85.5, 87.9)	21.1 (18.0, 24.3)	24.7 (22.7, 26.7)	27.5 (24.6, 30.3)	26.7 (23.7, 29.7)	
Stroke history						
Yes	272	92	61	59	60	0.38
	3.5 (2.8, 4.3)	24.5 (16.6, 32.3)	19.3 (13.2, 25.3)	30.9 (25.6, 36.2)	25.3 (16.3, 34.4)	
No	5630	1402	1404	1419	1405	
	96.4 (95.6, 97.1)	21.4 (18.3, 24.5)	24.5 (22.8, 26.1)	26.9 (24.3, 29.6)	27.2 (24.2, 30.1)	

p value was tested by Rao-Scott χ^2 test. BMI: body mass index. PIR: poverty income ratio. Se: selenium.

3.2. Comparison of Se Intake and Se Level between Different Groups of Factors

Table 2 shows the Se intake and Se level between different groups of factors. Males had higher Se intake and blood Se than females. The participants aged 40–59 years had higher Se intake, but no difference in blood concentration was found among the three age groups. As for race, Mexican American, Non-Hispanic Whites and other races had greater Se intakes than Non-Hispanic Blacks and Non-Hispanic Whites, and Non-Hispanic Blacks had lower Se levels compared to other races. Additionally, Non-Hispanic Whites had higher Se levels than Non-Hispanic Blacks. The participants with more than high school level education possessed higher Se intake and blood Se concentration than those with less than high school and equal to high school education. Blood Se level was higher in overweight participants than in underweight, normal and obese participants. The participants with the highest income possessed the highest Se intake and those with the lowest income presented with the lowest blood Se concentration. Smokers showed lower blood Se. Alcohol users had higher Se intakes but lower blood Se concentrations.

Table 2. Comparison of Se intake and Se level between different groups of factors in the NHANES 2017–2020.

Characteristic	Se Intake (μg/d)	Differences	Blood Se Concentration (μg/L)	Differences
Gender				
Male	140.1 (137.6, 142.6)	M > F ($p < 0.0001$)	188.5 (187.5, 189.4)	M > F ($p < 0.0001$)
Female	101.1 (99.5, 102.8)		184.2 (183.3, 185.1)	
Age				
18–39	119.1 (116.5, 121.7)		185.5 (184.4, 186.5)	
40–59	122.5 (119.7, 125.2)	40–59 > 60–79 ($p < 0.05$)	186.9 (185.8, 187.9)	
60–79	118.0 (115.2, 120.8)		186.5 (185.1, 187.8)	
Race				
Mexican American	125.3 (121.0, 129.6)	Mexican American > Other Hispanic ($p < 0.05$)	189.0 (187.2, 190.8)	Other Race > Non-Hispanic White > Other Hispanic > Non-Hispanic Black ($p < 0.05$)
Other Hispanic	116.4 (111.5, 121.2)	Mexican American > Non-Hispanic Black ($p < 0.05$)	183.8 (181.9, 185.7)	Mexican American > Other Hispanic ($p < 0.05$)
Non-Hispanic White	122.1 (119.4, 124.8)	Other Hispanic < Non-Hispanic White ($p < 0.05$)	188.1 (186.9, 189.3)	
Non-Hispanic Black	113.5 (110.7, 116.3)	Other Hispanic< Other Race ($p < 0.05$)	180.9 (179.7, 182.0)	
Other Race	124.9 (120.7, 129.0)	Non-Hispanic White> Non-Hispanic Black ($p < 0.05$)	191.5 (189.8, 193.1)	
		Non-Hispanic Black < Other Race ($p < 0.05$)		
Education				
<High school	111.2 (107.6, 114.9)	"<High school" < ">High school"	183.8 (182.2, 185.4)	"<High school" < ">High school"
High school	116.1 (112.8, 119.4)	"High school" < ">High school"	184.4 (183.0, 185.8)	"High school" < ">High school"
>High school	124.4 (122.3, 126.5)		187.5 (186.6, 188.4)	
BMI				
Underweight	117.2 (104.5, 130.0)	Overweight > Obese ($p < 0.05$)	181.4 (175.5, 187.2)	Underweight < Overweight ($p < 0.05$)
Normal weight	121.2 (117.9, 124.4)		184.4 (183.1, 185.6)	Normal weight < Overweight ($p < 0.05$)
Overweight	121.7 (118.8, 124.7)		188.8 (187.6, 190.1)	Overweight > Obese ($p < 0.05$)
Obese	117.9 (115.6, 120.2)		185.9 (184.9, 186.9)	
PIR				
Low	111.4 (108.5, 114.2)	Low < Medium < High ($p < 0.05$)	182.7 (181.5, 184.0)	Low < Medium ($p < 0.05$)
Medium	120.3 (117.8, 122.7)		187.7 (186.6, 188.3)	Low < High ($p < 0.05$)
High	128.2 (124.7, 131.6)		188.4 (187.0, 189.7)	
Smoking status				
Every day	115.2 (111.2, 119.2)	Every day < Somedays ($p < 0.05$)	182.1 (180.4, 183.7)	Every day < Not at all ($p < 0.05$)
Somedays	127.5 (119.0, 135.9)	Every day < Not at all ($p < 0.05$)	183.3 (180.3, 186.2)	Somedays< Not at all ($p < 0.05$)
Not at all	125.6 (122.1, 129.1)		187.8 (186.4, 189.3)	
Alcohol use				
Yes	131.9 (127.4, 136.4)	Yes > No ($p < 0.0001$)	183.9 (182.0, 185.7)	Yes < No ($p < 0.05$)
No	119.6 (117.9, 121.4)		186.5 (185.7, 187.2)	

BMI: body mass index. PIR: poverty income ratio. Se: selenium.

3.3. Association between Factors and Blood Se Concentration

The association between all the factors and blood Se concentration is presented in Table 2. Total Se intake was the most important determinant of blood Se concentration (Table 3). Males tended to have higher blood Se concentration than females. The participants with greater educational levels appeared to have higher blood Se concentrations. The Non-Hispanic Blacks had lower blood Se concentration. Smokers had lower blood Se concentrations than nonsmokers (Table 3).

Table 3. Weighted linear regression analyses of the association between several factors (Se intake, gender, age, race, education, BMI, income, smoking and alcohol status) and blood Se concentration in the NHANES 2017–2020.

Factors	β (95% CI)	p-Value
Dietary Se (μg/day)	0.03 (0.01, 0.04)	<0.05
Total Se (μg/day)	0.05 (0.04, 0.07)	<0.001
Female (vs. male)	−2.66 (−5.26, −0.06)	<0.05
Age (y)	0.03 (−0.06, 0.11)	0.52
Race (vs. other race)		
Mexican American	−1.14 (−5.64, 3.36)	0.61
Other Hispanic	−6.59 (−11.2, −1.97)	<0.05
Non-Hispanic White	−1.98 (−5.16, 1.20)	0.21
Non-Hispanic Black	−6.65 (−10.8, 2.51)	<0.05
Educational status (vs. <high school)		
High school	−0.51 (−3.93, 2.91)	0.76
>High school	2.73 (−0.94, 6.40)	0.14
PIR (vs. low)		
Medium	1.49 (−0.84, 3.83)	0.20
High	0.07 (−2.56, 2.70)	0.96
BMI (vs. underweight)		
Normal weight	5.76 (−0.65, 12.17)	0.08
Overweight	8.52 (2.25, 14.79)	<0.05
Obese	7.33 (1.17, 13.49)	<0.05
Smoking status (vs. not at all)		
Everyday	−2.65 (−6.12, 0.81)	0.13
Somedays	−3.44 (−9.54, 2.66)	0.26
Alcohol use (vs. yes)	1.59 (−0.97, 4.16)	0.21

BMI: body mass index. PIR: poverty income ratio. Se: selenium.

4. Discussion

In this study, the NHANES 2017–2020 data were used to explore several factors affecting blood Se level. Males aged 40–59 years, some races (Mexican American, Non-Hispanic White and other race) and highest educated population had higher Se consumption. Overweight participants, highest educated Non-Hispanic White and Non-Hispanic Black had higher blood Se levels. Smokers and alcohol users showed lower Se levels.

The average total Se intake and blood Se concentration were 122.7 μg/day and 188.7 μg/L, respectively, which were lower than those (174 μg/day and 253 μg/L) in the American seleniferous areas [8]. However, Se intake and blood Se concentration in this study were higher than those reported in other countries worldwide [9,10], with Se intake of approximately 95% of the participants above 55 μg/day, suggesting sufficient soil Se content in the USA. The Se-rich foods include Brazil nuts, crab meat, shrimp, allium vegetables, brown rice, whole wheat bread and skimmed milk. Se intake and blood Se vary globally. In Finland, Se fertilization increased average dietary intake from 40.0 μg Se/day to 80.0 μg Se/day [10]. In the low Se area of China, mean daily Se intake was 8.8 μg/day, resulting in the very low serum Se (24 μg/L) in that population [9]. In the present study, only 17 participants (only 0.3%) had excessive Se intake (>400 μg/day), nevertheless, considering that excessive Se intake led to acute side effects and chronic Se exposure increased the risks of nervous system abnormalities, it was very vital to maintain a safe Se intake range to reduce Se toxicity.

In the present study, there was a significantly positive association between dietary Se/total Se intakes and blood Se concentration, especially, total Se was the most important contributor for blood Se. Similarly, a previous study conducted in the American seleniferous area also found a strong correlation between Se intake and blood Se concentration [8]. A dose-response analysis found a non-linear relationship between Se intake and plasma Se concentration, and the predicted coefficients below and above such a cut-off of 70.0 μg/day were 1.25 and 0.43, respectively [11]. The aforementioned different results might be attributed to the sample size and source, Se species in foods and supplements consumed by the participants (organic Se mainly in foods and inorganic Se mainly in supplements), Se bioavailability (organic Se > inorganic Se) and analysis methods [12]. Additionally, some metals such as lead and mercury could interact with Se [13–15]; unfortunately, the intake information for those metals were not available in the NHANES.

In the present study, males had higher blood Se than females, which was consistent with the results of previous studies [6,16,17], partly due to the apparent sexual dimorphism related to sex hormones [18]. The trans-selenation pathway was regulated by sex hormones, suggesting selenomethionine metabolism and selenocysteine formation and the availability for selenoprotein synthesis are not the same in both sexes [18]. Given the sex difference in Se intake and blood Se concentration, establishing gender-based Se reference intakes should be considered in future Se RDA revisions [3].

In our study, age was not significantly associated with blood Se concentration, which coincided with the findings of other studies in the USA [8,19]. There was no significant difference in blood Se concentration among the three age groups (18–39, 40–59, 60–79), although the participants aged 40–59 years had higher Se intake than those aged 60–79. However, the results of some previous studies were inconsistent, i.e., decreased blood Se [20] with age and increased serum Se [21] with age, partly because of changed absorption and excretion efficiency. Elevated Se concentration was demonstrated to improve cognitive functions [6,22], which was beneficial to the amelioration of cognitive decline in the elderly.

In the USA, the mean blood Se concentration was higher in white subjects compared to black subjects, which might be attributed to different geographical areas with varied soil Se content, differences in food choices and genetic differences in Se pharmacokinetics [17]. The participants with the education status of more than high school possessed prominently higher blood Se concentration, which was in line with the findings of the NHANES 2011–2014 [6,23], possibly because they cared more about dietary quality and had access to Se-enriched foods to enhance Se intake. The participants with low income had lower blood Se concentration than those with high income, which was similar to the previous report [24]. Interestingly, in our study, Se intake was higher in the high-income participants than those low-income participants. Moreover, participants with underweight were found to have a lower blood Se level than overweight participants, partly due to their lesser Se intake. Our study showed higher blood Se concentration in overweight participants compared to that in obese participants, and the previous result found reduced serum Se level in obese female patients [25]. There was an inverse association between smoking and blood Se. Smokers, especially those smoking every day, had significantly lower Se intake than non-smokers, which was in agreement with previous findings in the USA [8]. Notably, drinkers with more Se intake showed lower blood Se concentration compared to non-drinkers with less Se intake, which was caused by changes in hepatic structure and function induced by alcohol [26]

The strengths of the present study included a large representative sample for the reduction in sampling error, high-quality NHANES datasets and the weighted liner regression because of a complex survey design. The results could direct health-related policy decisions in the field of health and disease in the future.

However, there were several limitations in the present study. Firstly, owing to NHANES data based on a cross-sectional study, dietary Se data were self-reported with two 24 h recalls with inevitable recall bias and it only reflected short-term Se intake not long-term Se intake status. Therefore, a longitudinal study might be reasonable. Additionally, dietary data plus occupational exposure data more truly evaluated Se level in the human body. Secondly, Se species in foods and supplements were not available in the NHANES 2017–2020. Thirdly, alcohol information in the present study was not an optimal reflection of alcohol consumption levels of the participants.

5. Conclusions

The present results showed that the majority of US adults were in the safe range of blood Se concentrations and few participants were at risk of selenosis. Taken together, Se intake was the most primary determinant of blood Se. Gender, race, education status, income, BMI, smoking and alcohol status were associated with blood Se concentration. Considering the effects of Se status on certain chronic diseases shown in epidemiological studies, this study can provide baseline information for future health-related research and revision of guidance values.

Author Contributions: Original draft preparation; generation, collection, assembly, analysis and interpretation of data, Y.-Z.B.; data analysis and review, Y.-X.G.; conceptualization, supervision, review and editing, S.-Q.Z. All authors have read and agreed to the published version of the manuscript.

Funding: This research received no external funding.

Institutional Review Board Statement: The NHANES was approved by the Institutional Review Committee of the National Centre for Health Statistics. Due to the present study based on the secondary analysis, additional ethics approval was not required.

Informed Consent Statement: Written informed consent was obtained from all subjects involved in the study.

Data Availability Statement: The datasets generated and analyzed in the present study are available on the website of NHANES datasets 2017–2020 (https://www.cdc.gov/nchs/nhanes/index.htm (accessed in 2022)).

Conflicts of Interest: The authors declare no conflicts of interest.

References

1. Bai, Y.Z.; Zhang, S.Q. Do selenium-enriched foods provide cognitive benefit? *Metab. Brain Dis.* **2023**, *38*, 1501–1502. [CrossRef] [PubMed]
2. Wang, M.; Li, B.; Li, S.; Song, Z.; Kong, F.; Zhang, X. Selenium in Wheat from Farming to Food. *J. Agric. Food Chem.* **2021**, *69*, 15458–15467. [CrossRef] [PubMed]
3. Bai, Y.Z.; Zhang, S.Q. Evidence-based proposal for lowering Chinese tolerable upper intake level for selenium. *Nutr. Res.* **2024**, *123*, 53–54. [CrossRef]
4. Jain, R.B.; Choi, Y.S. Normal reference ranges for and variability in the levels of blood manganese and selenium by gender, age, and race/ethnicity for general U.S. population. *J. Trace Elem. Med. Biol.* **2015**, *30*, 142–152. [CrossRef] [PubMed]
5. Zhang, S.Q.; Shen, S.; Zhang, Y. Comparison of Bioavailability, Pharmacokinetics, and Biotransformation of Selenium-Enriched Yeast and Sodium Selenite in Rats Using Plasma Selenium and Selenomethionine. *Biol. Trace Elem. Res.* **2020**, *196*, 512–516. [CrossRef] [PubMed]
6. Yan, X.; Liu, K.; Sun, X.; Qin, S.; Wu, M.; Qin, L.; Wang, Y.; Li, Z.; Zhong, X.; Wei, X. A cross-sectional study of blood selenium concentration and cognitive function in elderly Americans: National Health and Nutrition Examination Survey 2011–2014. *Ann. Hum. Biol.* **2020**, *47*, 610–619. [CrossRef] [PubMed]
7. Institute of Medicine (US) Panel on Dietary Antioxidants and Related Compounds. *Dietary Reference Intakes for Vitamin C, Vitamin E, Selenium, and Carotenoids*; Institute of Medicine, The National Academies Press: Washington, DC, USA, 2000.
8. Swanson, C.A.; Longnecker, M.P.; Veillon, C.; Howe, M.; Levander, O.A.; Taylor, P.R.; McAdam, P.A.; Brown, C.C.; Stampfer, M.J.; Willett, W.C. Selenium intake, age, gender, and smoking in relation to indices of selenium status of adults residing in a seleniferous area. *Am. J. Clin. Nutr.* **1990**, *52*, 858–862. [CrossRef] [PubMed]
9. Luo, X.M.; Wei, H.J.; Yang, C.L.; Xing, J.; Qiao, C.H.; Feng, Y.M.; Liu, J.; Liu, Z.; Wu, Q.; Liu, Y.X.; et al. Selenium intake and metabolic balance of 10 men from a low selenium area of China. *Am. J. Clin. Nutr.* **1985**, *42*, 31–37. [CrossRef] [PubMed]
10. Alfthan, G.; Eurola, M.; Ekholm, P.; Venäläinen, E.R.; Root, T.; Korkalainen, K.; Hartikainen, H.; Salminen, P.; Hietaniemi, V.; Aspila, P.; et al. Effects of nationwide addition of selenium to fertilizers on foods, and animal and human health in Finland: From deficiency to optimal selenium status of the population. *J. Trace Elem. Med. Biol.* **2015**, *31*, 142–147. [CrossRef]
11. Turck, D.; Bohn, T.; Castenmiller, J.; de Henauw, S.; Hirsch-Ernst, K.I.; Knutsen, H.K.; Maciuk, A.; Mangelsdorf, I.; McArdle, H.J.; Peláez, C.; et al. Scientific opinion on the tolerable upper intake level for selenium. *Efsa J.* **2023**, *21*, e07704.
12. Zhang, S.Q.; Bai, Y.Z. Strategies for enhancing beneficial effects of selenium on cognitive function. *Metab. Brain Dis.* **2023**, *38*, 1857–1858. [CrossRef] [PubMed]
13. Naderi, M.; Puar, P.; Zonouzi-Marand, M.; Chivers, D.P.; Niyogi, S.; Kwong, R.W.M. A comprehensive review on the neuropathophysiology of selenium. *Sci. Total Environ.* **2021**, *767*, 144329. [CrossRef]

14. Adams, W.J.; Duguay, A. Selenium-mercury interactions and relationship to aquatic toxicity: A review. *Integr. Environ. Assess. Manag.* 2024, *preprint*. [CrossRef]
15. Tian, C.; Qiu, Y.; Zhao, Y.; Fu, L.; Xia, D.; Ying, J. Selenium protects against Pb-induced renal oxidative injury in weaning rats and human renal tubular epithelial cells through activating NRF2. *J. Trace Elem. Med. Biol.* **2024**, *83*, 127420. [CrossRef]
16. Pei, J.; Yan, L.; Wu, Y.; Zhang, X.; Jia, H.; Li, H. Association between low blood selenium concentrations and poor hand grip strength in United States adults participating in NHANES (2011–2014). *Appl. Physiol. Nutr. Metab.* **2023**, *48*, 526–534. [CrossRef] [PubMed]
17. Hu, X.F.; Chan, H.M. Factors associated with the blood and urinary selenium concentrations in the Canadian population: Results of the Canadian Health Measures Survey (2007–2011). *Int. J. Hyg. Environ. Health* **2018**, *221*, 1023–1031. [CrossRef]
18. Seale, L.A.; Ogawa-Wong, A.N.; Berry, M.J. Sexual dimorphism in selenium metabolism and selenoproteins. *Free Radic Biol. Med.* **2018**, *127*, 198–205. [CrossRef]
19. McAdam, P.A.; Smith, D.K.; Feldman, E.B.; Hames, C. Effect of age, sex, and race on selenium status of healthy residents of Augusta, Georgia. *Biol. Trace Elem. Res.* **1984**, *6*, 3–9. [CrossRef] [PubMed]
20. Dickson, R.C.; Tomlinson, R.H. Selenium in blood and human tissues. *Clin. Chim. Acta* **1967**, *16*, 311–321. [CrossRef]
21. Fernández-Banares, F.; Dolz, C.; Mingorance, M.D.; Cabré, E.; Lachica, M.; Abad-Lacruz, A.; Gil, A.; Esteve, M.; Giné, J.J.; Gassull, M.A. Low serum selenium concentration in a healthy population resident in Catalunya: A preliminary report. *Eur. J. Clin. Nutr.* **1990**, *44*, 225–229.
22. Zhang, S.Q. Selenium and cognitive function. *Metab. Brain Dis.* **2023**, *38*, 221–222. [CrossRef] [PubMed]
23. Ghimire, S.; Baral, B.K.; Feng, D.; Sy, F.S.; Rodriguez, R. Is selenium intake associated with the presence of depressive symptoms among US adults? Findings from National Health and Nutrition Examination Survey (NHANES) 2011–2014. *Nutrition* **2019**, *62*, 169–176. [CrossRef] [PubMed]
24. Niskar, A.S.; Paschal, D.C.; Kieszak, S.M.; Flegal, K.M.; Bowman, B.; Gunter, E.W.; Pirkle, J.L.; Rubin, C.; Sampson, E.J.; McGeehin, M. Serum selenium levels in the US population: Third National Health and Nutrition Examination Survey, 1988–1994. *Biol. Trace Elem. Res.* **2003**, *91*, 1–10. [CrossRef] [PubMed]
25. Alasfar, F.; Ben-Nakhi, M.; Khoursheed, M.; Kehinde, E.O.; Alsaleh, M. Selenium is significantly depleted among morbidly obese female patients seeking bariatric surgery. *Obes. Surg.* **2011**, *21*, 1710–1713. [CrossRef]
26. Korpela, H.; Kumpulainen, J.; Luoma, P.V.; Arranto, A.J.; Sotaniemi, E.A. Decreased serum selenium in alcoholics as related to liver structure and function. *Am. J. Clin. Nutr.* **1985**, *42*, 147–151. [CrossRef]

nutrients

MDPI

Article

Effect of Whole Blood Dietary Mineral Concentrations on Erythrocytes: Selenium, Manganese, and Chromium: NHANES Data

Arthur M. Costa [1,2], Rebecca J. Sias [2] and Sandra C. Fuchs [3,*]

[1] Department of Chemistry, University of Chicago, Chicago, IL 60637, USA; arthurcosta@uchicago.edu
[2] Department of Biochemistry and Molecular Biology, University of Chicago, Chicago, IL 60637, USA; rjsias@uchicago.edu
[3] Postgraduate Program in Cardiology, School of Medicine, Universidade Federal do Rio Grande do Sul, Porto Alegre 90035-003, RS, Brazil
* Correspondence: author:sfuchs@hcpa.edu.br

Abstract: Background: Selenium (Se), Manganese (Mn), and Chromium (Cr) are dietary minerals ingested from specific grains, vegetables, and animal meats. Prior research showed that these minerals affect animal erythrocyte health but have unknown effects on human red blood cells (RBCs) and hematology. This study evaluated the effects of these dietary minerals on RBC count, hematocrit, and hemoglobin. Methods: We conducted a cross-sectional analysis of 23,844 American participants from the 2015–2016 and 2017–2020 National Health and Nutrition Examination Survey. We evaluated sex, age, ethnicity, education, income, and smoking status as covariates. Linear regression analyses were conducted to evaluate the effect of Cr, Se, and Mn on RBC count, hematocrit, and hemoglobin levels. We employed subpopulation-exclusion regressions further to explore the distinct effects of mineral elevation and deficiency. Additional analyses were performed to examine the relationship between Mn and RBC hemoglobin, RBC distribution width, transferrin receptor concentrations, transferrin saturation, and serum iron levels to support the interpretation of our findings. Optimizable ensemble machine learning models were used to corroborate regression results. Results: Adjusting for covariates, Cr was inversely associated with RBC count (Exp(b) = 0.954), hemoglobin (Exp(b) = 0.868), and hematocrit (Exp(b) = 0.668). Conversely, Se was positively associated with RBC count (Exp(b) = 1.003), hemoglobin (Exp(b) = 1.012), and hematocrit (Exp(b) = 1.032). Mn was positively associated with RBC count (Exp(b) = 1.020) but inversely associated with hemoglobin (Exp(b) = 0.945) and hematocrit (Exp(b) = 0.891). Conclusions: Cr was harmful to RBC health in all subpopulations, whereas Se was protective. Mn appears to contribute to the development of microcytic anemia, but only in subjects with clinically elevated Mn levels. Thus, excessive consumption of foods and supplements rich in Cr and Mn may harm human erythrocyte health and hematology.

Keywords: chromium; selenium; manganese; erythrocytes; hematocrit; hemoglobin

1. Introduction

Selenium (Se), manganese (Mn), and Chromium (Cr) are essential dietary minerals [1]. They act as important cofactors and bio-redox catalysts, but high concentrations of Cr, Se, and Mn are implicated in developing hemolytic anemia, selenosis, and manganism, respectively.

Chromium is a mineral in fruits, vegetables, and animal meats [2,3]. In erythrocytes, hexavalent chromium (Cr VI) is reduced and transported to the nuclear membrane, leading to genomic instability [4,5]. Selenium is an essential nutrient found in animal meats and is a residue in selenoproteins, which are responsible for reducing oxidized antioxidants such as glutathione peroxidase [6]. At low concentrations, Se seems to protect against stroke and cardiovascular disease. However, excessive Se can become incorporated into cysteine and methionine residues, leading to protein malformation [7–9]. Se daily consumption guidelines have recently been under scrutiny and are being lowered worldwide because of the risk of developing selenosis from excessive Se consumption [10]. Manganese is an essential nutrient found in vegetables and grains [11]. It serves as a vital cofactor for enzymes involved in carbohydrate and lipid metabolism [12], as well as for the enzyme manganese superoxide dismutase 2 (SOD2), which is a scavenger of reactive oxygen species (ROS) located in the mitochondria [13]. Exposure to excess Mn causes neurotoxicity and widespread cytotoxicity, primarily attributed to excessive Mn absorption by the mitochondria, leading to ROS accumulation and calcium uptake [14,15].

Animal studies provide evidence that Cr can hurt erythrocytes by forming ROS, but limited research has been conducted on humans [16]. Conversely, animal studies have shown that Se enhances and reinforces erythrocytes at low concentrations, decreasing osmotic fragility [17]. The effects of Mn on human and animal erythrocytes are largely unknown [18] but are worth investigating since Mn is known to modulate iron metabolism, which is highly relevant to erythrocytes [18,19]. The scarcity of human studies on the influence of these vital dietary minerals on red blood cells underscores a gap in our understanding of the relationship between nutrition and human biochemistry. This study, therefore, aims to investigate the effects of dietary exposure to Cr, Se, and Mn on erythrocytes in a representative population-based sample.

2. Methodology

We performed a comprehensive analysis using data obtained from the National Health and Nutrition Examination Survey (NHANES) conducted by the Center for Disease Control and Prevention (CDC) in 2015–2016 and 2017–2020 [20,21]. Our study focused on 23,844 American participants aged 18 years and older. All statistical tests, analyses, and descriptions (other than optimizable ensemble analyses) were performed using IBM's Statistical Package for Social Sciences (SPSS, version 29.0.1.0, Chicago, IL, USA). Optimizable ensemble analyses were performed using MathWorks' MATLAB (version 24.2.0, Natick, MA, USA).

Participants were interviewed at home to collect demographic, socioeconomic, and smoking data through surveys conducted from 2015 to 2020. Additionally, laboratory data collected from the CDC mobile examination center were analyzed, including hematological parameters and blood concentrations of Cr (in nmol/L), Se (in umol/L), and Mn (in nmol/L) levels. The data on Cr were only collected from participants aged 40 and above, a limitation of the NHANES sample that cannot be overcome. The information included sex, age, ethnicity (categorized as Mexican, Hispanic-non-Mexican, Non-Hispanic white, Non-Hispanic black, Non-Hispanic Asian, Multiracial or other), level of education (classified as less than 9th grade, 9–12th grade, high school graduate or GED, some college or AA degree, college graduate or above, and unknown), income (ratio of family income to poverty), and smoking (lifetime consumption of at least 100 cigarettes). Participants present in all analyses provided complete survey information and underwent blood tests to obtain Cr, Se, Mn, RBC, hematocrit, and hemoglobin levels. Participants with missing information for one or more variables were only excluded from analyses that required that parameter. Levels of normality for hematological parameters were obtained from the Mayo Clinic [22] and were used to describe the population. Weights were recalculated according to NHANES weighting procedures to ensure our analyses accurately represented the American population [23]. When describing the population, the sampling weights were normalized to have an average value of 1.00, as a standard practice previously employed in NHANES-based analyses [24].

Characteristics of the studied population are displayed as absolute numbers and percentages. The analysis tested for collinearity between the dietary minerals and hematocrit; hemoglobin, RBC, and residuals were analyzed for normality. We also performed collinearity tests between Cr, Mn, and Se themselves. All analyses were conducted using the entire study population.

Additional regression analyses were performed on sub-populations to test specific hypotheses. Regression analyses excluded participants with deficiencies in each trace element to isolate the effects of elevated levels from those of deficiency. Similarly, regressions were then performed excluding participants with elevated trace element levels to further distinguish between the effects of elevation and deficiency. The analyses used linear regressions with RBC count, hematocrit, and hemoglobin as dependent variables. Each regression analysis investigated the relationship between one trace element (Cr, Se, or Mn) and these hematological parameters.

Finally, to more precisely investigate how Mn impacted RBCs, we conducted further regression analyses between Mn levels and RBC hemoglobin, transferrin receptor levels (TfR), serum iron (Fe), and transferrin binding capacity. We also conducted a binary logistic regression between Mn levels and the incidence of recent anemia treatment to better understand the relationship between Mn levels and the incidence of anemia.

Additionally, simple linear regression models were used to explore the potential influence of sex, age, ethnicity, education, income, and smoking as confounding factors, setting the significance level at $p < 0.2$. Subsequently, we performed multiple regression analyses, accounting for confounding factors. Additionally, a term for the interaction between income and education was introduced because these confounders may be correlated with dietary mineral intake patterns. To overcome some degree of heteroskedasticity, we adopted heteroskedasticity-robust standard errors for calculating significance and effect sizes, enhancing the reliability and accuracy of our findings. To ensure the accuracy of our findings when considering non-linear relationships between mineral levels and hematological outcomes, we conducted optimizable ensemble (OE) machine learning analyses. In these analyses, we trained models to predict changes in hematological parameters using all metals and covariates simultaneously, which provided the highest predictive validity as measured by root mean squared error and R^2. We did not consider sample weights due to limitations in the capability of even modern OE technology. However, the lack of weighting is not an issue because we used OE to evaluate the accuracy of our regression findings based on our sample data rather than using the OE to make broader claims about the effect of minerals on hematological parameters across the entire American population.

3. Results

3.1. Description of the Population

The NHANES sampling enrolled 23,844 individuals who provided information in the 2015–2016 or 2017–2020 surveys and a subset of 14,088 participants who also provided blood samples to assess whole blood hematological parameters.

Table 1 shows the characteristics of the weighted sample based on sex. There was an even distribution of sex, with participants averaging 48.27 ± 17.33 years old. Additionally, almost two-thirds of the participants were identified as non-Hispanic whites, which closely mirrors the demographic composition of the United States. Furthermore, most participants had completed at least a high school education and were non-smokers.

Table 1. Characteristics of the studied population according to sex [*n* (%)].

		Total	Men	Women	*p* Value *
Age (years)	20–29	2701 (18.4)	1352 (19.1)	1349 (17.7)	<0.001
	30–39	2603 (17.7)	1283 (18.1)	1320 (17.3)	
	40–49	2458 (16.7)	1212 (17.1)	1246 (16.3)	
	50–59	2641 (18)	1273 (18.0)	1368 (17.9)	
	60–69	2263 (15.4)	1072 (15.2)	1191 (15.6)	
	70–79	1350 (9.2)	607 (8.6)	743 (9.7)	
	≥80	684 (4.7)	273 (3.9)	411 (5.4)	

Table 1. *Cont.*

		Total	Men	Women	*p* Value *
Ethnicity	Mexican	1244 (8.5)	631 (8.9)	613 (8.0)	<0.001
	Hispanic-non-Mexican	1072 (7.3)	515 (7.3)	557 (7.3)	
	Non-Hispanic white	9256 (63)	4466 (63.2)	4790 (62.8)	
	Non-Hispanic black	1681 (11.4)	751 (10.6)	930 (12.2)	
	Non-Hispanic Asian	870 (5.9)	401 (5.7)	469 (6.2)	
	Multiracial or other	577 (3.9)	308 (4.4)	269 (3.5)	
Education	<9th grade	657 (4.5)	323 (4.6)	334 (4.4)	<0.001
	9–12th grade	1123 (7.6)	597 (8.5)	526 (6.9)	
	High school graduate or GED	3678 (25)	1861 (26.3)	1817 (23.8)	
	Some college or AA degree	4566 (31.1)	2088 (29.5)	2478 (32.5)	
	College graduate or above	4666 (31.7)	2199 (31.1)	2467 (32.4)	
Smoked ≥100 cigarettes in lifetime	Yes	6297 (42.8)	3571 (50.5)	2726 (35.8)	<0.001
	No	8395 (57.1)	3496 (49.5)	4899 (64.2)	

* Chi-square test.

Table 2 shows that most participants had Cr deficiency, and none had clinically elevated levels. Most participants had normal Mn levels and elevated Se levels. Regardless of sex, most participants had average RBC counts, hemoglobin, and hematocrit levels. However, men experienced higher rates of elevation in each hematological parameter, while women showed higher rates of deficiency.

Table 2. Whole blood characteristics of the sample population [*n* (%)].

	Normal Range	Total *n*	Deficient *n*	Elevated *n*
Chromium	0.7–28 µg/L	9040	8377 (92.7)	0 (0.0)
Manganese	4–15 µg/L	11,915	68 (0.6)	792 (6.6)
Selenium	120–160 µg/L	11,915	17 (0.1)	10,688 (89.7)
RBC count (male)	4.35–5.65 million cells/mcl	6728	483 (7.2)	367 (5.5)
RBC count (female)	3.92–5.13 million cells/mcl	7320	389 (5.3)	388 (5.3)
Hemoglobin (male)	13.2–16.6 g/dL	6728	408 (6.1)	440 (6.5)
Hemoglobin (female)	11.6–15 g/dL	7320	476 (6.5)	461 (6.3)
Hematocrit (male)	38.3–48.6%	6768	294 (4.3)	590 (8.7)
Hematocrit (female)	35.5–44.9%	7320	538 (7.3)	389 (5.3)

3.2. Regression Analysis Between Minerals and Blood Parameters

Table 3 presents the results of both unadjusted and adjusted linear regression models investigating the association between Cr, Mn, Se, and RBC count. Higher Cr levels were associated with a lower RBC count in the unadjusted model. After accounting for confounding variables and the interaction between income and education, the negative association between Cr and RBC count remained, although it was slightly attenuated. For each unit increase in Cr, the odds of having a higher RBC count decreased by approximately 4.6%, and after adjusting for covariates, this decrease was reduced to 3.7%.

Conversely, exposure to Mn was found to have a small positive association with RBC count. There was a 0.9% increase in the likelihood of a higher RBC count for each unit increase in Mn. This positive association became even stronger after accounting for confounding factors and the interaction between income and education, with the likelihood of having a higher RBC count increasing by 2.0% per unit increase in Mn. Se levels were positively associated with RBC count; for each unit increase in Se, the odds of the RBC count increased by 0.3%. The control for confounding factors did not significantly affect this association.

The analysis considered the potential interdependence between the dietary minerals Cr, Mn, and Se by using regression models to address multicollinearity. The collinearity diagnostics showed minimal multicollinearity between the independent variables (VIF < 1.400

and collinearity tolerance > 0.750). The highest collinearity was observed between income (VIF = 1.306) and education (VIF = 1.331). Still, the VIF values were low, indicating that multicollinearity was not significant enough to warrant excluding either variable as a covariate, especially considering the use of robust standard errors.

Table 3. Effect of dietary minerals: Chromium, Manganese, and Selenium on RBC count.

	n	Unstandardized Beta	Error	Exp(B) (95%CI)	*p* Value
Chromium level (μg/L)	9066	−0.047	8.19×10^{-5}	0.954 (0.954–0.954)	<0.001
Adjusted chromium (μg/L) *	7918	−0.038	7.80×10^{-5}	0.963 (0.962–0.963)	<0.001
Manganese level (μg/L)	10,686	0.009	1.14×10^{-5}	1.009 (1.009–1.009)	<0.001
Adjusted manganese (μg/L) *	9315	0.02	1.20×10^{-5}	1.020 (1.020–1.020)	<0.001
Selenium level (μg/L)	10,686	0.003	1.58×10^{-6}	1.003 (1.003–1.003)	<0.001
Adjusted selenium (μg/L) *	9315	0.003	1.47×10^{-6}	1.003 (1.003–1.003)	<0.001

Linear regression model with robust standard error. * Exp(B) 95%CI adjusted for age, sex, ethnicity, income, education, smoking, and income × education.

Table 4 presents the association between dietary minerals and hematocrit from unadjusted and adjusted linear regression models. The analyses for Cr showed a significant negative association with hematocrit, both in the unadjusted and adjusted analyses. In the former, it was found that for each unit increase in Cr, the odds of having a higher hematocrit decreased by approximately 33.2%. The negative association persisted after adjusting for confounders and the interaction term between income and education. However, the effect size was slightly attenuated, and it was observed that with each unit increase in Cr, the odds of having a higher hematocrit decreased by approximately 32.4%.

Table 4. Effect of dietary minerals: Chromium, Manganese, and Selenium on hematocrit.

	n	Unstandardized Beta	Error	Exp(B) (95%CI)	*p* Value
Chromium level (μg/L)	9066	−0.403	7.00×10^{-4}	0.668 (0.667–0.669)	<0.001
Adjusted chromium (μg/L) *	7918	−0.392	8.00×10^{-4}	0.676 (0.675–0.677)	<0.001
Manganese level (μg/L)	10,686	−0.116	1.00×10^{-4}	0.891 (0.891–0.891)	<0.001
Adjusted manganese (μg/L) *	9315	−0.026	1.00×10^{-4}	0.975 (0.975–0.975)	<0.001
Selenium level (μg/L)	10,686	0.032	1.29×10^{-5}	1.032 (1.032–1.032)	<0.001
Adjusted selenium (μg/L) *	9315	0.024	1.15×10^{-5}	1.024 (1.024–1.024)	<0.001

Linear regression model with robust standard error. * Exp(B) 95%CI adjusted for age, sex, ethnicity, income, education, smoking, and income × education.

In the unadjusted analysis, exposure to Mn exhibited a strong negative association with increased hematocrit, where higher Mn levels were linked to a 10.9% decrease in the odds of having a higher hematocrit. Adjusting for confounding factors substantially decreased the magnitude of this association, resulting in only a 2.5% decrease in hematocrit odds with increased Mn levels. This adjustment suggests that socioeconomic factors, along with other confounders, played an important role in modifying the relationship between Mn and hematocrit.

For each unit increase in Se, the odds of having a higher hematocrit increased by approximately 3.2%. After adjusting for confounding factors and the interaction term between income and education, the positive association remained statistically significant, although the effect size was slightly reduced. Specifically, for each unit increase in Se, the odds of having a higher hematocrit increased by about 2.4%.

Table 5 presents the outcomes from both unadjusted and adjusted linear regression models investigating the association between Cr, Mn, Se, and hemoglobin. It shows a robust inverse association between Cr and hemoglobin. Levels. It showed that for every unit increase in Cr, hemoglobin decreased by around 13.2%. After accounting for confounding factors and the interaction between income and education, the decrease in hemoglobin remained nearly the same at 13.3%. This suggests that socioeconomic factors did not significantly impact the relationship between Cr and hemoglobin. The association between Mn and hemoglobin level was found to be inverse. In the unadjusted analysis, it was observed that for each unit increase in Mn, hemoglobin decreased by about 5.5%. After adjusting for confounding factors and the interaction term between income and education, the association attenuated, and a unit increase in Mn was now associated with a 2.4% decrease in hemoglobin.

Table 5. Effect of dietary minerals: Chromium, Manganese, and Selenium on hemoglobin.

	n	Unstandardized Beta	Error	Exp(B) (95%CI)	*p* Value
Chromium level (μg/L)	9066	−0.141	3.00×10^{-4}	0.868 (0.868–0.869)	<0.001
Adjusted chromium (μg/L) *	7918	−0.142	3.00×10^{-4}	0.867 (0.867–0.868)	<0.001
Manganese level (μg/L)	10,686	−0.056	4.18×10^{-5}	0.945 (0.945–0.945)	<0.001
Adjusted manganese (μg/L) *	9315	−0.024	4.20×10^{-5}	0.976 (0.976–0.976)	<0.001
Selenium level (μg/L)	10,686	0.012	4.70×10^{-6}	1.012 (1.012–1.012)	<0.001
Adjusted selenium (μg/L) *	9315	0.009	4.10×10^{-6}	1.009 (1.009–1.009)	<0.001

Linear regression model with robust standard error. * Exp(B) 95%CI: adjusted for age, sex, ethnicity, income, education, smoking, and income × education.

Table 5 also shows a positive association between Se and hemoglobin levels. Higher Se levels were linked to slightly higher hemoglobin levels. After adjusting for confounding factors and including the interaction term between income and education, the Exp(Beta) decreased from 1.012 to 1.009. This indicates that for each unit increase in Se, hemoglobin, which initially increased by 1.2%, now increased by 0.9%. This slight decrease in the positive association suggests that other factors explained some of the variation, although Se still had a small positive effect on hemoglobin levels.

3.3. Basic Interpretation of Regression Results

Excluding participants with Cr deficiencies reduced the effect sizes ($|1 - \text{Exp(b)}|$) on RBC count, hematocrit, and hemoglobin outcomes. Still, the inverse relationship between Cr levels and each blood parameter remained consistent and significant (Supplementary Tables S1–S3). Considering that we observed no subjects with elevated Cr levels (Table 2), the reduced effect after excluding Cr-deficient subjects suggests that the negative association is most vital in subjects with normal Cr levels. There was, however, one unusual finding when deficient subjects were excluded: Cr showed a slight positive association with hematocrit when not accounting for covariates (Exp(b) = 1.007; $p < 0.001$). When covariates were considered, this association changed and more closely resembled the results in Table 4 (Exp(b) = 0.970; $p < 0.001$).

Both the models excluding Mn-deficient and those excluding elevated-Mn subjects had similar effects on RBC count, as reported in Table 3 (Tables S1 and S4). The fact that the association persisted despite removing deficient subjects suggests that increasing Mn levels, even within the normal range, continue to elevate RBC count. Similarly, models excluding Mn-deficient subjects did not show a significantly different effect on hematocrit or hemoglobin compared to the results in Tables 4 and 5 (Tables S2 and S3). However, the models that excluded subjects with elevated Mn levels showed significant positive associations between Mn and both hemoglobin and hematocrit (adjusted models: Exp(b) = 1.154, $p < 0.001$; Exp(b) = 1.044, $p < 0.001$), while Tables 4 and 5 reported negative associations between Mn and both hemoglobin and hematocrit (Tables S5 and S6). This finding suggests that Mn elevation may decrease hemoglobin and hematocrit levels. We considered that the simultaneous increase in RBC count alongside decreases in hemoglobin and hematocrit (in Mn-elevated subjects) suggests a reduction in RBC volume and conducted a further regression analysis between Mn and RBC volume, revealing a marked negative association (Exp(b) = 0.645, $p < 0.001$). Additionally, we performed another regression to analyze the effect of Mn on RBC distribution width, uncovering a significant positive association (Exp(b) = 1.125, $p < 0.001$).

Exploring the effects of Mn on TfR to explain how Mn could affect downstream hemoglobin and hematocrit levels, we conducted a further regression analysis between Mn and TfR levels, which showed a positive association (Exp(b) = 1.252, $p < 0.001$). Then, exploring the effect of Mn on iron metabolism as a mechanistic alternative, we conducted regression analyses between Mn and serum iron (Exp(b) = 0.175, $p < 0.001$), transferrin saturation, accounting for serum Fe as a covariate (Exp(b) = 0.452, $p < 0.001$), and RBC hemoglobin (Exp(b) = 0.834, $p < 0.001$), all of which showed significant negative associations. Finally, exploring the effect of Mn on the incidence of anemia, we found a significant positive association between Mn levels and being recently treated for anemia (Exp(b) = 1.095, $p < 0.001$).

Both models excluding Se deficient subjects (Tables S1–S3) and those excluding subjects with elevated Se (Tables S4–S6) showed similar effects on RBC count, hemoglobin, and hematocrit as those reported in Tables 3–5, but all models excluding subjects with elevated Se did have slightly higher effect sizes (Exp(b) range = 1.006–1.071) than those reported in Tables 3–5 (Exp(b) range = 1.003–1.032). Regardless, the positive associations remained significant even after excluding subjects with Se deficiency or elevation, indicating that the effects of Se on these hematological parameters are not due to clinical Se deficiency or elevation.

3.4. Optimizable Ensemble Machine Learning Analyses

The OE modeling analyzed the relationship between levels of each mineral and hematological outcomes and allowed us to plot partial dependence. The models effectively captured the nonlinear effects of minerals on hematological outcomes and showed moderate predictive significance (RBC counts $R^2 = 0.25$; hemoglobin $R^2 = 0.45$; hematocrit $R^2 = 0.44$). All R^2 values and partial dependence plots are from the testing (rather than training) data. Supplementary Figures S1–S9 show the partial dependence of RBC count, hemoglobin, and hematocrit on Cr, Mn, and Se. All partial dependence plots confirmed the general trends identified through our linear regression analyses. Chromium consistently showed negative associations with RBC count, hemoglobin, and hematocrit, which agrees with the regression results above (Figures S1, S4 and S7). Interestingly, beyond approximately 4 μg/L, further increases in Cr did not lead to additional decreases in RBC count, hemoglobin, or hematocrit in the sampled population. Manganese exhibited consistently positive associations with RBC count (Figure S2) and parabolic associations with hemoglobin and hematocrit, centered at approximately 12 μg/L, which is at the upper end of the normal range (4–15 μg/L) (Figures S5 and S8). These results agree with our regression results, which indicated a positive association between Mn and RBC count, a positive association with hemoglobin and hematocrit when subjects >15 μg/L Mn were excluded, and a negative association with hemoglobin and hematocrit when subjects >15 μg/L were included. Selenium consistently showed positive associations with RBC count, hemoglobin, and hematocrit, aligning with the regression results above (Figures S3, S6 and S9).

4. Discussion

The findings of negative associations between Cr and RBC, hematocrit, and hemoglobin are aligned with previous literature, which has demonstrated causative inverse relationships between blood Cr levels and hematocrit, hemoglobin, and RBC counts in animal studies [25,26]. In vitro studies show that Cr III does not permeate significantly into human erythrocytes, but Cr VI does [27]. After Cr VI enters erythrocytes, it binds to hemoglobin and peptides such as glutathione, forming stable complexes that sequester the Cr in the erythrocyte for an extended period [27]. Cr forming stable complexes with glutathione decreases RBC's antioxidant load. Furthermore, Cr VI is readily reduced to Cr V and then Cr III in erythrocytes [5]. This reduction pathway creates ROS byproducts. Cr being sequestered in erythrocytes for long periods, which decreases antioxidant capacity and directly generates ROS (leading to extensive damage), helps explain the negative associations between Cr and RBC count, hemoglobin, and hematocrit [5,28].

The Agency for Toxic Substances and Disease Registry has highlighted the potential adverse impact of Cr exposure on erythrocyte health, identifying it as a contributor to microcytic hypochromic anemia [29]. In accordance with this, our findings suggest that Cr may significantly negatively affect RBC health. However, the generalizability of these findings is limited because the analyzed population lacked blood Cr data for participants younger than 40 years. Furthermore, our population lacked any participants with a clinical excess in Cr, further limiting the generalizability of our findings. Thus, significant further investigation is needed into the mechanisms and effects of Cr on human erythrocytes and hematology.

The most plausible explanation for the positive associations we found between Se and RBC, hemoglobin, and hematocrit lies in the role of selenoproteins, which reduce hydroperoxides and ROS that can damage RBC cell membranes, hemoglobin, and membrane proteins [17,30,31]. Given that selenoproteins are needed to reduce hydroperoxide levels, lower Se (and thus selenoprotein) levels lead to hydroperoxide accumulation, leading to widespread damage (including RBCs and RBC progenitors). As the central role of Se is as a cofactor in selenoproteins, their antioxidizing properties are likely the most critical factors contributing to the positive association seen between Se and hemoglobin, hematocrit, and RBC counts. This finding aligns with existing animal studies, underscoring the importance of adequate Se concentrations for erythrocyte membrane health, hemoglobin levels, and the differentiation of hematopoietic stem cells into erythrocytes [17,31].

The positive relationship between Mn levels and RBC count we observed is likely due to the role of SOD2. SOD2 levels are inversely associated with ROS concentrations in RBC precursors; therefore, higher blood Mn levels may increase SOD2 levels, reducing oxidative stress on RBC progenitors and resulting in a more significant proportion of progenitors differentiating into mature erythrocytes [12,32,33]. However, our finding of negative associations between Mn and hemoglobin and hematocrit when subjects with clinical Mn elevation were included (despite the positive association between Mn and RBC) merited further mechanistic exploration. We first considered Mn's disruptive effect on Iron Regulatory Protein (IRP) activity [34]. IRPs bind to TfR mRNA sequences and other iron-responsive elements (IREs). Greater TfR mRNA stability afforded by IRP binding leads to more extensive TfR production and greater Fe uptake downstream because of TfR's central role in erythrocytic Fe uptake [5]. This idea is further supported by previous findings of a negative association between Mn and TfR levels [35]. Thus, we hypothesized that Mn interference with IRP activity could decrease TfR levels and, therefore, decrease Fe uptake, helping to explain the decreases in hemoglobin and hematocrit levels we associated with increased Mn levels. To test this, we conducted a regression analysis between Mn and blood TfR levels and found a positive relationship, rejecting our hypothesis.

We then considered the alternative hypothesis that Mn's effects on erythrocytes were primarily mediated by competitive inhibition of the divalent metal transporter (DMT1) [33,36]. DMT1 has a higher affinity for Mn than Fe, and in vitro models have shown that cellular incubation with Mn leads to decreased Fe uptake via DMT1 [33]. Furthermore, erythrocytes with mutated DMT1s have been shown to exhibit signs of microcytic anemia despite having adequate Fe levels in surrounding media, showing the importance of DMT1 to erythrocytic Fe uptake [33]. Mn-mediated competitive inhibition of DMT1 thus presents a plausible mechanism through which Mn would lead to decreased intracellular Fe levels and a subsequent decrease in hemoglobin and hematocrit.

Exploring these effects, we found a negative association between Mn and serum Fe consistent with the literature [33]. Investigating whether Mn was altering Fe uptake (as suggested by the DMT1 inhibition mechanism), we found negative associations between Mn and RBC hemoglobin and RBC volume, and a positive association between Mn and RBC distribution width. These findings (i.e., decreased RBC hemoglobin and volume with concurrently increased distribution width) are characteristic of microcytic anemia and are seen in patients with dysfunctional DMT1 [37–39]. To investigate the association between Mn and anemia, we conducted a regression between Mn and the incidence of recent anemia treatment (in the three weeks preceding data collection). We found a significant positive association, suggesting once more that Mn may contribute to the incidence of anemia. However, the generalizability of this finding is limited because it does not account for differential disposition to seeking treatment or socioeconomic conditions affecting treatment availability. Regardless, although Mn increases RBC count, it decreases hemoglobin and hematocrit levels and appears to be a potentially significant contributor to the onset of microcytic anemia because it inhibits DMT1-mediated Fe transport. Still, more research is needed to describe this association and its mechanism further.

These findings indicate that socioeconomic factors—income and education—may modify the impact of trace minerals, particularly Cr and Mn, on RBC count. While higher chromium levels were consistently associated with lower RBC count, Mn had a stronger positive association with RBC count. The positive association of Se with RBC count remained stable, with minimal impact from confounders.

The results also indicate that levels of trace minerals are associated with variations in hematocrit, and socioeconomic factors influence these relationships. Chromium and Mn showed a consistent negative association with hematocrit (when elevated subjects were included in Mn analyses), though the effect sizes were slightly reduced after adjusting for confounding factors. In contrast, Se maintained a positive association with hematocrit, and although the effect size decreased somewhat after adjustment, the relationship remained significant. These findings underscore the need to consider socioeconomic factors when evaluating the impact of dietary minerals on hematocrit levels.

After adjusting for confounding factors, the inverse and nearly unchanged association between Cr and hemoglobin suggests that socioeconomic factors had minimal influence. In contrast, the inverse association of Mn with hemoglobin (when elevated subjects were included) was halved after adjustment, indicating that socioeconomic factors may partly explain this relationship. The positive association of Se with hemoglobin decreased slightly, retaining a small positive effect on hemoglobin levels.

Our study has some limitations, which should be taken into account in the interpretation of the results. The absence of participants with clinically elevated Cr levels precluded analyzing the effects of overexposure. However, the NHANES provides a representative sample of the US population, and the lack of individuals with elevated Cr levels in a sample of over 23,000 reflects the real-world distribution of Cr exposure within the US. Although this limitation prevented us from assessing the effects of elevated Cr levels, the analysis remained robust for understanding its impact within low and normal ranges. Additionally, the sample included individuals with elevated levels of selenium and manganese, other essential minerals.

The data on Cr were only collected from participants aged 40 and above due to constraints in the NHANES lab sample. This limitation may restrict the generalizability of our findings to younger populations. While chromium may be involved in metabolic processes that could indirectly impact blood parameters, there is minimal direct evidence of its effect on RBC count, hematocrit, and hemoglobin in individuals under 40 with diabetes mellitus, cardiovascular diseases, and depression. Future research should include younger populations to understand age-related differences in dietary behaviors and exposure to chromium better.

The measurement of Cr had limited sensitivity, with some participants having levels below the detection limit. This has been addressed in the analysis. These values were set to the minimum detectable level and multiplied by $\sqrt{2}$, which required us to apply heteroskedasticity-robust standard errors in the regression models.

Similarly, only a few participants were clinically deficient in Se and Mn, limiting the extent to which our analyses could account for addressing the effect of deficiencies. Despite these limitations, we conducted analyses that provided insight into the impact of comparatively lower or higher dietary mineral levels on RBC count, hematocrit, and hemoglobin. We also performed subgroup analyses, allowing us to examine the effects of mineral deficiency and elevation. A final limitation is that our OE models are unweighted, preventing them from being provably reliable predictors for these effects in the general American population. This is not a problem, however, as they were used strictly to assess the reliability of our regression models by evaluating the isolated nonlinear effects of mineral levels on hematological outcomes in the sample population.

5. Conclusions

Our present findings suggest that excess Cr may adversely affect erythrocyte health, but further research with younger subjects and subjects with clinical Cr elevations is needed. The outcomes of our study also suggest that adequate Se levels may be an essential factor in maintaining erythrocyte health. Furthermore, our findings indicate that Mn deficiency may impede proper Fe metabolism. Moreover, we showed that Mn decreased RBC volume, RBC hemoglobin, and whole blood hemoglobin while increasing RBC distribution width, suggesting that it may be a significant contributing factor toward the development of microcytic anemia. Further in vitro and in vivo research is needed to understand the complete proteomic changes incurred to erythrocytes by exposure to these dietary minerals and the subsequent downstream effects of those changes.

Supplementary Materials: The following supporting information can be downloaded at: https://www.mdpi.com/article/10.3390/nu16213653/s1, Figure S1: Partial Dependence of RBC count on chromium; Figure S2. Partial Dependence of RBC count on manganese; Figure S3. Partial Dependence of RBC count on selenium; Figure S4. Partial Dependence of hemoglobin on chromium; Figure S5. Partial Dependence of hemoglobin on manganese; Figure S6. Partial Dependence of hemoglobin on selenium; Figure S7. Partial Dependence of hematocrit on chromium; Figure S8. Partial Dependence of hematocrit on manganese; Figure S9. Partial Dependence of hematocrit on selenium; Table S1: Effect of trace elements on elevated and normal subjects: Chromium, Manganese, and Selenium on RBC Count; Table S2: Effect of trace elements on elevated and normal subjects: Chromium, Manganese, and Selenium on Hematocrit; Table S3. Effect of trace elements on elevated and normal subjects: Chromium, Manganese, and Selenium on Hemoglobin; Table S4. Effect of trace elements on deficient and normal subjects: Chromium, Manganese, and Selenium on RBC Count; Table S5. Effect of trace elements on deficient and normal subjects: Chromium, Manganese, and Selenium on Hematocrit; Table S6. Effect of trace elements on deficient and normal subjects: Chromium, Manganese, and Selenium on Hemoglobin.

Author Contributions: Conceptualization was performed by A.M.C., S.C.F. and R.J.S. A.M.C., R.J.S. and S.C.F. completed the methodology, investigation, and formal analysis. S.C.F. completed the data curation. The first draft of the manuscript was written by A.M.C. and was edited by all authors. All authors have read and agreed to the published version of the manuscript.

Funding: This study was partially supported by FIPE-HCPA (Research Incentive Fund, Hospital de Clinicas de Porto Alegre). Sandra C. Fuchs was supported by a Fellowship from the National Council for Scientific and Technological Development (CNPq), ref. number 309023/2015-7 and later, number 316802/2021-2. The sponsors had no participation in the design and conduct of the study, preparation and approval of the manuscript.

Institutional Review Board Statement: The NHANES database is available publicly. This is a retrospective study, so no ethical approval is required by law or national ethical guidelines in the United States.

Informed Consent Statement: All participants in NHANES provided written informed consent.

Data Availability Statement: The datasets analyzed in this study are available in the 2015–2016 and 2017–2020 NHANES repositories, https://wwwn.cdc.gov/nchs/nhanes/continuousnhanes/default.aspx?BeginYear=2015, accessed on 25 September 2024 and https://wwwn.cdc.gov/nchs/nhanes/continuousnhanes/default.aspx?Cycle=2017-2020, accessed on 25 September 2024.

Conflicts of Interest: The authors declare no conflicts of interest.

References

1. Cannas, D.; Loi, E.; Serra, M.; Firinu, D.; Valera, P.; Zavattari, P. Relevance of Essential Dietary minerals in Nutrition and Drinking Water for Human Health and Autoimmune Disease Risk. *Nutrients* **2020**, *12*, 2074. [CrossRef] [PubMed]
2. Vincent, J.B. New Evidence against Chromium as an Essential Trace Element. *J. Nutr.* **2017**, *147*, 2212–2219. [CrossRef] [PubMed]
3. Shadreck, M.; Mugadza, T. Chromium, an essential nutrient and pollutant: A review. *Afr. J. Pure Appl. Chem.* **2013**, *7*, 310–317.
4. Zhang, Z.; Xie, B.; Zhong, Q.; Dai, C.; Xu, X.; Huo, X. Abnormal erythrocyte-related parameters in children with Pb, Cr, Cu and Zn exposure. *Biometals* **2024**. *online ahead of print*.
5. Ray, R.R. Adverse hematological effects of hexavalent chromium: An overview. *Interdiscip. Toxicol.* **2016**, *9*, 55–65. [CrossRef] [PubMed]
6. Andrade, I.G.A.; Suano-Souza, F.I.; Fonseca, F.L.A.; Lago, C.S.A.; Sarni, R.O.S. Selenium levels and glutathione peroxidase activity in patients with ataxia-telangiectasia: Association with oxidative stress and lipid status biomarkers. *Orphanet J. Rare Dis.* **2021**, *16*, 83. [CrossRef]
7. Johansson, A.L.; Collins, R.; Arnér, E.S.J.; Brzezinski, P.; Högbom, M. Biochemical Discrimination between Selenium and Sulfur 2: Mechanistic Investigation of the Selenium Specificity of Human Selenocysteine Lyase. Kobe B, editor. *PLoS ONE* **2012**, *7*, e30528. [CrossRef]
8. Lazard, M.; Dauplais, M.; Blanquet, S.; Plateau, P. Recent advances in the mechanism of selenoamino acids toxicity in eukaryotic cells. *Biomol. Concepts* **2017**, *8*, 93–104. [CrossRef]
9. Zhao, K.; Zhang, Y.; Sui, W. Association Between Blood Selenium Levels and Stroke: A Study Based on the NHANES (2011–2018). *Biol. Trace Elem. Res.* **2024**, *202*, 25–33. Available online: https://pubmed.ncbi.nlm.nih.gov/37004705/ (accessed on 30 July 2024). [CrossRef]
10. Li, J.M.; Bai, Y.Z.; Zhang, S.Q. Considerations for Chinese tolerable upper intake level for selenium. *Metab. Brain Dis.* **2024**, *39*, 485–486. [CrossRef]
11. Buchman, A.R. Manganese. In *Modern Nutrition in Health and Disease*, 11th ed.; Ross, A.C., Cousins, R.J., Tucker, K.L., Ziegler, T.R., Eds.; Lippincott Williams & Wilkins: Baltimore, MD, USA, 2014; pp. 238–244.
12. Li, L.; Yang, X. The Essential Element Manganese, Oxidative Stress, and Metabolic Diseases: Links and Interactions. *Oxidative Med. Cell. Longev.* **2018**, *2018*, 1–11. Available online: https://www.hindawi.com/journals/omcl/2018/7580707/ (accessed on 8 February 2020). [CrossRef]
13. Holley, A.K.; Bakthavatchalu, V.; Velez-Roman, J.M.; St Clair, D.K. Manganese Superoxide Dismutase: Guardian of the Powerhouse. *Int. J. Mol. Sci.* **2011**, *12*, 7114–7162. [CrossRef] [PubMed]
14. Deng, X.; Guo, Y.; Jin, X.; Si, H.; Dai, K.; Deng, M.; He, J.; Hao, C.; Yao, W. Manganese accumulation in red blood cells as a biomarker of manganese exposure and neurotoxicity. *NeuroToxicology* **2024**, *102*, 1–11. Available online: https://www.sciencedirect.com/science/article/pii/S0161813X24000238?via=ihub (accessed on 23 October 2024). [CrossRef] [PubMed]
15. Evans, G.R.; Masullo, L.N. *Manganese Toxicity*; StatPearls Publishing: Treasure Island, FL, USA, 2021. Available online: https://www.ncbi.nlm.nih.gov/books/NBK560903/ (accessed on 4 May 2024).
16. Shaheen, T.; Akhtar, T. Assessment of chromium toxicity in Cyprinus carpio through hematological and biochemical blood markers. *Turk. J. Zool.* **2012**, *36*, 682–690. [CrossRef]
17. Duan, S.; Chen, S.; Liang, W.; Chen, M.; Chen, Y.; Guo, M. Dietary Selenium Deficiency Facilitated Reduced Stomatin and Phosphatidylserine Externalization, Increasing Erythrocyte Osmotic Fragility in Mice. *Biol. Trace Elem. Res.* **2020**, *199*, 594–603. [CrossRef] [PubMed]

18. Zheng, W.; Fu, S.; Dydak, U.; Cowan, D.M. Biomarkers of manganese intoxication. *Neurotoxicology* **2011**, *32*, 1–8. [CrossRef]
19. Chandel, M.; Jain, G.C. Manganese induced hematological alteration in Wistar rats. *J. Environ. Occup. Sci.* **2016**, *5*, 77. [CrossRef]
20. P_DEMO [Internet]. 2018. Available online: https://wwwn.cdc.gov/Nchs/Nhanes/2017-2018/P_DEMO.htm#SDDSRVYR (accessed on 30 July 2024).
21. Laboratory Data—Continuous NHANES [Internet]. Available online: https://wwwn.cdc.gov/Nchs/Nhanes/search/datapage.aspx?Component=Laboratory (accessed on 30 July 2024).
22. Mayo Clinic. Complete Blood Count (CBC) [Internet]. *Mayo Clinic*. 2023. Available online: https://www.mayoclinic.org/tests-procedures/complete-blood-count/about/pac-20384919 (accessed on 4 May 2024).
23. NHANES Survey Methods and Analytic Guidelines [Internet]. Available online: https://wwwn.cdc.gov/nchs/nhanes/analyticguidelines.aspx#estimation-and-weighting-procedures (accessed on 4 May 2024).
24. Chen, J.; Kan, M.; Ratnasekera, P.; Deol, L.K.; Thakkar, V.; Davison, K.M. Blood Chromium Levels and Their Association with Cardiovascular Diseases, Diabetes, and Depression: National Health and Nutrition Examination Survey (NHANES) 2015–2016. *Nutrients* **2022**, *14*, 2687. [CrossRef]
25. Islam, S.M.M.; Rohani, M.F.; Zabed, S.A.; Islam, M.T.; Jannat, R.; Akter, Y.; Shahjahan, M. Acute effects of chromium on hemato-biochemical parameters and morphology of erythrocytes in striped catfish Pangasianodon hypophthalmus. *Toxicol. Rep.* **2020**, *7*, 664–670. [CrossRef]
26. Thatheyus, A.J. Effect of Nickel and Hexavalent Chromium on the Haematology of the Common carp, Cyprinus carpio. *Int. J. Hematol. Blood Disord.* **2018**, *3*, 1–3. [CrossRef]
27. Devoy, J.; Géhin, A.; Müller, S.; Melczer, M.; Remy, A.; Antoine, G.; Sponne, I. Evaluation of chromium in red blood cells as an indicator of exposure to hexavalent chromium: An in vitro study. *Toxicol. Lett.* **2016**, *255*, 63–70. [CrossRef]
28. Wise, J.P.; Young, J.L.; Cai, J.; Cai, L. Current understanding of hexavalent chromium [Cr(VI)] neurotoxicity and new perspectives. *Environ. Int.* **2022**, *158*, 106877. [CrossRef] [PubMed]
29. Wilbur, S.; Abadin, H.; Fay, M.; Yu, D.; Tencza, B.; Ingerman, L.; Klotzbach, J.; James, S. *Toxicological Profile for Chromium*; Agency for Toxic Substances and Disease Registry (US): Atlanta, GA, USA, 2012. Available online: https://www.ncbi.nlm.nih.gov/books/NBK158855/ (accessed on 18 December 2019).
30. Zhang, F.; Li, X.; Wei, Y. Selenium and Selenoproteins in Health. *Biomolecules* **2023**, *13*, 799. [CrossRef] [PubMed]
31. Weaver, K.; Skouta, R. The Selenoprotein Glutathione Peroxidase 4: From Molecular Mechanisms to Novel Therapeutic Opportunities. *Biomedicines* **2022**, *10*, 891. [CrossRef] [PubMed]
32. Case, A.J.; Madsen, J.; Motto, D.G.; Meyerholz, D.K.; Domann, F.E. Manganese superoxide dismutase depletion in murine hematopoietic stem cells perturbs iron homeostasis, globin switching, and epigenetic control in erythrocyte precursorcells. *Free Radic. Biol. Med.* **2013**, *56*, 17–27. [CrossRef] [PubMed]
33. Bjørklund, G.; Aaseth, J.; Skalny, A.V.; Suliburska, J.; Skalnaya, M.G.; Nikonorov, A.A.; Tinkov, A.A. Interactions of iron with manganese, zinc, chromium, and selenium as related to prophylaxis and treatment of iron deficiency. *J. Diet. Miner. Med. Biol.* **2017**, *41*, 41–53. [CrossRef]
34. Kwik-Uribe, C.L.; Reaney, S.; Zhu, Z.; Smith, D. Alterations in cellular IRP-dependent iron regulation by in vitro manganese exposure in undifferentiated PC12 cells. *Brain Res.* **2003**, *973*, 1–15. [CrossRef]
35. Ponka, P.; Lok, C.N. The transferrin receptor: Role in health and disease. *Int. J. Biochem. Cell Biol.* **1999**, *31*, 1111–1137. [CrossRef]
36. Roth, J.A.; Garrick, M.D. Iron interactions and other biological reactions mediating the physiological and toxic actions of manganese. *Biochem. Pharmacol.* **2003**, *66*, 1–13. [CrossRef]
37. Shawki, A.; Knight, P.; Maliken, B.D.; Niespodzany, E.; Mackenzie, B. H+-Coupled Divalent Metal-Ion Transporter-1. *Curr. Top. Membr.* **2012**, *70*, 169–214.
38. Chaudhry, H.S.; Kasarla, M.R. *Microcytic Hypochromic Anemia*; StatPearls Publishing: Treasure Island, FL, USA, 2019. Available online: https://www.ncbi.nlm.nih.gov/books/NBK470252/ (accessed on September 25 2024).
39. Flynn, M.M.; Reppun, T.S.; Bhagavan, N.V. Limitations of Red Blood Cell Distribution Width (RDW) in Evaluation of Microcytosis. *Am. J. Clin. Pathol.* **1986**, *85*, 445–449. [CrossRef]

nutrients

MDPI

Article

Dissimilar Effects of Selenite and Selenium Nanoparticles on Skeletal Muscle Development Unrelated to GPx1 Activity During Adolescence in Rats

Fátima Nogales [1], Eloísa Pajuelo [2,*], María del Carmen Gallego-López [1], Inés Romero-Herrera [1], Francisco Merchán [2], Olimpia Carreras [1] and María Luisa Ojeda [1]

[1] Departamento de Fisiología, Facultad de Farmacia, Universidad de Sevilla, 41012 Sevilla, Spain; fnogales@us.es (F.N.); mgallego3@us.es (M.d.C.G.-L.); iromero3@us.es (I.R.-H.); olimpia@us.es (O.C.); ojedamuri11@us.es (M.L.O.)

[2] Departamento de Microbiología y Parasitología, Facultad de Farmacia, Universidad de Sevilla, 41012 Sevilla, Spain; fmerchan@us.es

* Correspondence: epajuelo@us.es; Tel.: +34-954556767

Abstract: Background/Objectives: During adolescence, the critical growth period, the antioxidant selenium (Se), either as sodium selenite or selenium nanoparticles (SeNPs), has shown contrasting effects on adipose tissue (AT) in rats, due to its role in insulin signaling. Since skeletal muscle (SKM) is also a key insulin-target tissue, this study aimed to assess whether a similar effect occurs in this tissue. **Methods**: Three groups of male adolescent rats (n = 18) were used: control (C), selenite supplemented (S), and SeNPs supplemented (NS). Low doses of Se were administered via drinking water in both supplemented groups. AT was utilized for transcriptomic analyses, while SKM was analyzed for oxidative balance, insulin-induced anabolic effects, and proteolysis. Myokine levels in serum were also determined. **Results**: SeNPs administration decreased SKM mass and protein content, increased serum creatinine, and decreased insulin levels, indicating impaired SKM development. Both supplemented groups upregulated genes related to creatine metabolism and muscle contraction. However, only the NS group showed upregulation of genes associated with glycogenolysis and glycolysis. Despite unchanged GPx1 expression, NS rats presented lower oxidation and insulin–pmTOR activation, and higher expression of proteins related to proteolysis (pAMPK, SIRT1, ULK1, FOXO3a, and MaFbx) and a myokine profile compatible to muscle atrophy, fatty acid oxidation, and impaired myoblast proliferation. Ultimately, the selenite group impaired SKM catabolism mainly by increasing insulin–pmTOR activation. **Conclusions**: Once again, the form of Se administration exerts opposing effects on metabolism tissues, suggests a potential therapeutic role for selenite in disorders that compromise muscle growth, such as muscular dystrophies, cachexia, or sarcopenia.

Keywords: selenite; nanoparticles; skeletal muscle; glutathione peroxidase

1. Introduction

Adolescence is a critical life period of growth and endocrine changes, marked by rapid physical, hormonal, and neurodevelopmental transformations that significantly influence body weight and composition [1]. These shifts are clearly manifested in the development of adipose tissue (AT) and skeletal muscle (SKM) mass. When this stage of growth and endocrine maturation is disrupted, obesity and insulin resistance (IR) could appear [2]; conversely, anorexia nervosa may also develop [3]. Lately, the prevalence of these disorders is dramatically increasing during adolescence [2,3]. Moreover, these pathologies share the common fact that insulin-target tissues—adipose tissue (AT), skeletal muscle (SKM), and liver—are affected, compromising health during this critical developmental period [4,5].

Selenium (Se) is a vital trace element known for its antioxidant and anti-inflammatory properties, which are largely mediated by selenoproteins like glutathione peroxidases (GPx) [6]. Beyond its antioxidant role, Se is increasingly recognized as a key regulator of the endocrine system, influencing hypothalamic–pituitary–peripheral feedback circuits, the thyroid hormone axis, glucoregulatory and adrenal hormones, the gonads in both sexes, the musculoskeletal system, and the skin [7]. The 25 identified selenoproteins intricately regulate the endocrine system and intracellular signaling, including GPx1, GPx3, GPx4, thioredoxin reductases (TXNRDs), Deiodinases (DIO 1–3), endoplasmic reticulum-resident SELS or SELW, and the hepatokine SELP [8]. Selenium regulates cell growth, metabolism and the endocrine function, since a proper oxidative balance is essential for the endocrine signaling and for cell proliferation/differentiation [9].

Our research group has focused on the study of Se supplementation on white adipose tissue (WAT) function, insulin secretion, and related molecular mechanisms in adolescent male rats [10–12]. Our approach consisted of employing two different forms of Se supplementation, soluble selenite or selenium nanoparticles (SeNPs), administered at the same concentration.

Our studies have demonstrated the contrasting effects of selenite and Se NPs supplementation on AT. In fact, selenite supplementation was shown to promote adipogenesis via the insulin signaling pathway in WAT (Figure 1). Conversely, SeNP administration prevented fat accumulation in WAT by decreasing insulin signaling and promoting FOXO3a-mediated autophagy, a cellular recycling process, leading to reduced inflammation [10]. Notably, these effects were independent of GPx1 expression or activity. This selenoprotein has the lowest Se hierarchy, being highly sensitive to Se status; therefore, it is usually used to evaluate tissue Se levels [13]. The similar GPx1 values found in both groups confirm that both treatments used the same dose of Se, and that alternative mechanisms are involved [10]. In this regard, the possibility of an implication of the microbiota–liver–bile salt axis as a novel mechanism underlying the divergent effects of selenite and SeNPs on adipose tissue development was investigated. Selenite primarily affected the liver, decreasing the farnesoid X receptor (FXR) activity, and leading to bile salt accumulation, to an increased Firmicutes/Bacteroidetes ratio in the gut microbiota, and to a greater secretion of GLP-1. In contrast, SeNPs primarily impacted the gut microbiota, shifting it towards a more Gram-negative profile enriched in *Akkermansia* and *Muribaculaceae*, and decreasing the Firmicutes/Bacteroidetes ratio [11]. This microbial profile was associated with lower WAT mass, and SeNPs did not alter the pool of circulating bile salts. Transcriptomics of the WAT have shed some light on the mechanisms underlying the differential effects of selenite and SeNPs on gene expression in WAT [12]. SeNP supplementation led to a greater number of differentially expressed genes and impacted more cellular processes than selenite. Specifically, SeNPs upregulated genes associated with the immune system, catabolism, the mitochondrial function, and the oxidative balance. Gene ontology and KEGG pathway enrichment analyses revealed increased catabolic activity and decreased growth signaling in the SeNP group, contributing to a reduced WAT mass. Despite increased antioxidant enzyme activity, SeNP-treated rats also showed elevated H_2O_2 and malondialdehyde levels, indicating a complex interplay with oxidative stress (OS) [12]. These findings suggested a potential role for SeNPs in WAT reduction and immune response modulation during adolescence.

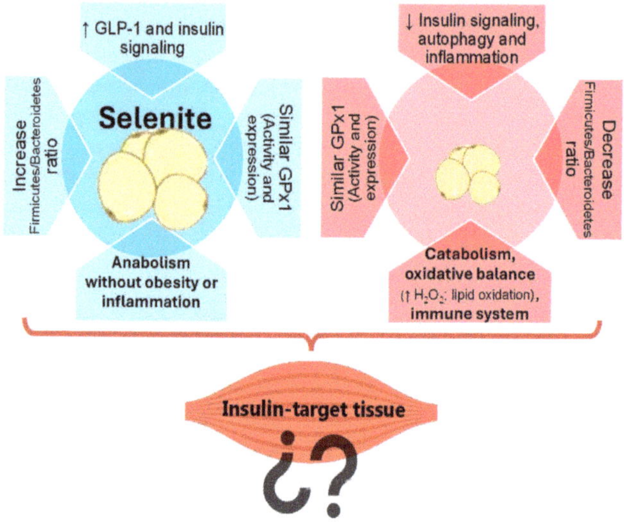

Figure 1. Contrasting effects of selenite and SeNPs on white adipose tissue: Exploring the implications for skeletal muscle.

The transcriptomic analysis also revealed that, after Se treatments, a great number of genes related specifically to SKM function were differentially affected. SKM development is critical during adolescence [14] and is deeply related to the endocrine function and metabolism. Apart from its well-known contractile function and representing the 50% of the total human mass, this insulin-target tissue is the primary site for glucose disposal in response to insulin and the major reservoir of amino acids in the body [15]. Moreover, it is a secretory organ, synthesizing several myokines, which exert important paracrine, autocrine, and endocrine functions necessary for maintaining the general metabolic homeostasis [16,17]; interestingly, not all myokines are synthesized exclusively in this tissue. In addition, SKM contents nearly half of the total Se from the body, acting as a reservoir when there are deficiencies [18]. In the SKM, Se regulates various physiological functions; it has antioxidant, anti-inflammatory and anti-apoptotic properties [19]. Furthermore, Se has broader biological effects on SKM, being involved in energy balance and serving as a crucial regulator of myogenesis [18]. These roles highlight Se as a promising target for future therapies aimed at protecting and promoting SKM development.

Due to the fact that both WAT and SKM are tissues specially developed during adolescence and insulin-target tissues; and that transcriptomic analysis in WAT revealed that genes related to the SKM function were affected. In this work we will investigate whether the supplementation with either selenite or SeNPs can also have contrasting effects on the physiology of the SKM of adolescent rats, as happens in their WAT. Firstly, we will analyze specific genes related to the muscle tissue function, differently affected in WAT. Secondly, we will study different SKM parameters, such as mass, protein content, OS, the insulin signaling process, protein homeostasis, and myokine secretion.

2. Materials and Methods

2.1. Animals

In the present study, 18 adolescent male Wistar rats from Animal Production and Experimentation Centre of Vice-Rectorate for Scientific Research, of the University of Seville were used. At 21 days of age, they were brought in and kept in pairs with environmental enrichment for a one-week acclimation period. The experiment lasted three weeks, from postnatal day (PND) 28 to 47, corresponding to adolescence in Wistar rats [20]. The animals were kept in a climate-controlled room (22–23 °C) and 12:12 h light/dark cycle (light on 9:00 a.m.). All animal procedures were conducted in accordance with ethical standards and received prior approval from the Ethics Committee of the University of Seville (Approval Code: CEEA-US2019-4; Date: 27 February 2019) and the Andalusian Regional Authority (Approval Code: 05-04-2019-065; Date: 9 April 2019). The study complied with the guidelines set forth in European Union Directive 2010/63/EU and Spanish legislation as detailed in Royal Decree 53/2013 (BOE 34/11370).

At PND 28, experimental animals (n = 6/group; weight = 49.8 ± 3.3 g) were randomly distributed into the three following groups: control (C) (rats that received standard diet and water ad libitum); Selenite (S) (rats that received standard diet and selenite supplementation in water ad libitum); and SeNPs (NS) (standard diet and selenium nanoparticles supplementation in water ad libitum). This number of experimental units was carefully determined to minimize pain and distress, in accordance with the principles of replacement, reduction, and refinement.

Three groups had ad libitum access to a standard pellet diet (LASQCdiet® Rod14-R, Märkische, Germani) which contained 0.2 ppm of Se provided as sodium selenite. The Se supplemented groups (S and NS) received an extra 0.14 ppm of Se through their drinking water throughout the experimental period. This supplementation was administered either as anhydrous sodium selenite (Panreac, Barcelona, Spain) or as SeNPs (developed at the Department of Organic and Medicinal Chemistry, Faculty of Pharmacy, University of Seville, Spain) [10].

2.2. *Morphological and Biochemical Parameters, Samples*

Throughout the experimental period, daily records were kept of the rats' body weight as well as their intake of liquids and solids. Se consumption was estimated by multiplying the concentration of Se in food and water by the amount of food and water ingested daily. All measurements were taken at 9:00 a.m. to avoid changes due to circadian rhythm.

After a 12 h fasting period at the end of the experimental period, adolescent rats were weighed to record the final body weight and then subsequently anesthetized with an i.p. injection of 28% *w/v* urethane (0.5 mL/100 g body weight). Blood samples were collected through cardiac puncture and transferred into tubes for serum separation by centrifugation at 1300× g for 15 min. A midline abdominal incision was performed to obtain tissues. Retroperitoneal WAT and the gastrocnemius SKM from the right hindlimb were excised, weighed, frozen in liquid nitrogen and stored at −80 °C until later biochemical analyses were performed. The somatic index of SKM (SKMSI) was calculated as the ratio of muscle weight to body weight.

Creatinine and insulin levels were measured in the serum of adolescent rats using an automated analyzer (Technicon RA-1000, Bayer Diagnostics, Leverkusen, Germany).

The SKM homogenate was prepared in phosphate buffer (50 mM K_2HPO_4, 50 mM KH_2PO_4, 0.01 mM EDTA (Sigma-Aldrich, Madrid, Spain), pH 7.0) with a protease inhibitor at a 1:10 ratio (Complete Protease Inhibitor Cocktail Tablets, ROCHE, Madrid, Spain), using a Fisherbrand™ 850 homogenizer (Thermo Fisher Scientific Inc., Waltham, MA, USA) in an ice bath. Total protein levels in the SKM homogenate were determined using the Lowry method [21].

2.3. *Transcriptomic Analysis*

Total RNA was extracted from WAT samples from the corresponding experimental group (C, S, and NS) using the RNeasy Lipid Tissue Mini Kit (QIAGEN, Barcelona, Spain), following the manufacturer's instructions [12]. RNA quality was analyzed by electrophoresis on a 1% agarose gel, and the presence of intact 18 S and 28 S ribosomal bands, along with a sufficient RNA quantity, was considered an indication of good RNA quality. All RNA samples were stored at −80 °C.

Messenger RNA was isolated from total RNA using oligo(dT)-coupled magnetic beads. Following fragmentation, first-strand cDNA synthesis was carried out using random hexamer primers, followed by second-strand synthesis employing dTTP, and generating a non-stranded cDNA library. The sequencing library was constructed through end repair, A-tailing, adapter ligation, size selection, PCR amplification, and purification, using a paired-end 150 bp protocol. Library quality control was performed using Qubit, real-time PCR, and a bioanalyzer prior to sequencing on the Illumina NovaSeq platform (Novogene, Cambridge, UK). Adapter sequences and low-quality reads were removed using the fastp software (v0.24.1) [22,23].

Reads were aligned to the *Rattus norvegicus* reference genome using HISAT2 (v2.0.5). The assembly was performed with StringTie (v1.3.3b), applying a genome-guide strategy. Read counts per gene were obtained using FeatureCounts (v1.5.0-p3), and expression values were reported in FPKM (Fragments Per Kilobase of transcript per Million mapped reads).

These expression levels were statistically analyzed using DESeq2 (v1.20.0), which identifies significantly and differentially expressed genes based on a negative binomial model. p-values were adjusted using the Benjamini–Hochberg method, considering genes with adjusted $p \leq 0.05$ as differentially expressed. The analysis was conducted on two biological samples with 12 million high-quality paired end reads, showing high intra-sample correlation (mean: 93.8%). Gene expression changes were evaluated using the log2 fold change. Genes with $|\log2(FC)| \geq 1.5$ were considered significantly differentially expressed.

2.4. Oxidative Balance Analysis in SKM

To determine the oxidative balance in SKM, endogenous enzymes antioxidant activity, lipid and protein oxidation, levels of H_2O_2, and GPx1 and NOX4 expressions were assessed. The activity of superoxide dismutase (SOD), catalase (CAT), and glutathione peroxidase (GPx) was measured following the methods previously described [12,24]. Lipid oxidation in SKM was measured by quantifying malondialdehyde (MDA) levels (mol/mg protein) using the method of Draper and Hadley [25], and protein oxidation was assessed using the method of Reznick and Packer [26], which analyzes the carbonyl group levels in the sample (nmol/mg protein) through a reaction with 2,4-dinitrophenylhydrazine. H_2O_2 levels, as an indication of reactive oxygen species in this tissue, were measured using the Hydrogen Peroxide Colorimetric Detection Kit (Abnova, Taipei, Taiwan).

Finally, GPx1 and NOX4 proteins were analyzed by the Western blot technique according to the protocols used in our laboratory [24]. Specific primary antibodies were used at the following dilutions: GPx1:1:1000 (sc-133160; Santa Cruz Biotechnology, Santa Cruz, CA, USA); and NOX4:1:1000 (sc-518092; Santa Cruz Biotechnology, Santa Cruz, CA, USA). As secondary antibody Goat Anti-Mouse IgG (H + L) Horseradish Peroxidase Conjugate (catalog number 170-6516, BioRad, Hercules, CA, USA) was used in a 1:2500 dilution; as loading control, monoclonal mouse anti GAPDH (sc-32233, Santa Cruz Biotechnology, Santa Cruz, CA, USA) was used in a 1:1000 dilution.

2.5. Myokines

The serum levels of the myokines interleukin 6 (IL-6), myostatin, interleukin 15 (IL-15), fractalkine (CX3CL1), fibroblast growth factor 21 (FGF21), irisin, brain-derived neurotrophic factor (BDNF), follistatin-like protein 1 (FSTL-1) and fatty acid binding protein 3 (FABP-3), were quantified using the MILLIPLEX® Rat Myokine Panel (Millipore Corp., St. Charles, MO, USA), utilizing xMAP technology (Luminex Corp., Austin, TX, USA) [27]. This multiplex immunoassay allows the simultaneous detection and quantification of multiple analytes in a single small-volume sample.

The samples, reagents, and standards were prepared according to Luminex xMAP protocol, using 25 µL of serum. Serum samples were incubated with magnetic beads pre-coated with analyte-specific capture antibodies. Following a series of washing steps to remove unbound material, biotinylated detection antibodies and streptavidin-phycoerythrin were added to generate a fluorescent signal. The intensity of the fluorescence was measured using a LABScan 100 analyzer (Luminex Corporation, Austin, TX, USA) with xPONENT software (v3.0) for data acquisition. Serum myokine levels were determined by comparing the mean fluorescence intensity of each duplicate sample against the corresponding assay's standard calibration curve.

2.6. Statistical Analysis

The results related to morphology, nutrition, serum and SKM samples were presented as mean values with their corresponding standard error (±SEM). Statistical evaluations were performed using GraphPad Prism software (version 8.0.2; San Diego, CA, USA). Each experimental group consisted of six samples. A p value < 0.05 was considered statistically significant and assessed using one-way analysis of variance (ANOVA). When ANOVA indicated significant differences, post hoc analyses were conducted using the Tukey–Kramer test.

3. Results

Selenite or SeNPs treatments doubled Se intake ($p < 0.001$) in the S and NS rat groups, demonstrating that both supplementations were similar (Table 1). However, the muscle organosomatic index and total protein levels were significantly lower in SeNP-treated rats compared to the C group ($p < 0.01$ and $p < 0.001$, respectively) and the S group ($p < 0.001$ vs. C; $p < 0.05$ vs. CSe), although body weight gain was similar in all groups. These results suggested that SeNPs treatment provoked muscle degradation, as indicated by elevated creatinine levels in these rats compared with the rest of the groups ($p < 0.001$). In these SeNPs treated rats, it is also observed that there is a decrease in insulin levels compared to the C and S group ($p < 0.05$ and $p < 0.01$, respectively). By contrast, S group had higher insulin serum levels than C group ($p < 0.05$).

Table 1. Nutritional and Morphological Parameters in Adolescent Rats Following Treatment with Selenite or SeNPs.

	C	S	NS
Increased body weight (g/d)	6.01 ± 0.1	6.07 ± 0.2	5.98 ± 0.2
Total Se intake (µg/d)	3.48 ± 0.08	6.81 ± 0.14 ccc	6.59 ± 0.09 ccc
SKMSI (%)	0.67 ± 0.016	0.70 ± 0.022	0.58 ± 0.013 cc, sss
SKM protein (mg/g WT)	67.1 ± 2	63.7 ± 1.5	56.5 ± 1.3 ccc, s
Creatinine (mg/dL)	0.45 ± 0.005	0.43 ± 0.006	0.49 ± 0.006 ccc, sss
Insulin (mU/L)	0.019 ± 0.001	0.028 ± 0.004 c	0.013 ± 0.001 c, ss

The results were expressed as means ± SEMs and analyzed using a multifactorial one-way ANOVA followed by Tukey's test. The number of animals used in each group is $n = 6$. Experimental groups: C, control group; S, selenite group; NS, SeNP group. Significance: vs. C; c $p < 0.05$; cc $p < 0.01$; ccc $p < 0.001$; vs. S; s $p < 0.05$; ss $p < 0.01$; sss $p < 0.001$. SKMSI: Skeletal muscle somatic index.

Table 2 shows the list of differently expressed genes in adipocytes related specifically or preferably to SKM. Some of these genes can be expressed also in the cardiac muscle, but not in the smooth tissue, so the expression level of these genes cannot be assigned to the smooth muscle of the blood vessels of the adipose tissue. Thus, when analyzing the gene expression profile in adolescent S rats, five genes were identified as significantly upregulated compared to C rats. These genes were involved in creatine metabolism (*Ckm*) and muscle contraction (*Acta1, Myh1, Myh7* and *Mylpf*) and presented changes in their expression levels ranging from 2.3- to 6.7-fold change (log_2FC). The gene *Ckm* exhibited the highest upregulation.

Table 2. List of statistically significant differentially regulated genes (Log_2 fold change) related specifically to SKM after Selenite and SeNPs treatments in adipocytes.

Status	Gene_Symbol	Related Function	Log_2FC
UPREGULATED by Selenite vs. Control	*Ckm*	Creatine metabolism	6.7
	Acta1	Muscle contraction	4.9
	Myh1	Muscle contraction fast fibers	4.8
	Myh7	Muscle contraction slow fibers	3.7
	Mylpf	Muscle contraction fast fibers	2.3
UPREGULATED by SeNPs vs. Control	*Ckm*	Creatine metabolism	10.9
	Acta1	Muscle contraction	9.1
	Myh1	Muscle contraction fast fibers	9.7
	Myh7	Muscle contraction slow fibers	8.5
	Mylpf	Muscle contraction fast fibers	6.9
	Pgam2	Glycolysis	2.7
	Casq1	Ca^{2+} channel transport	2.5
	Eno3	Glycolysis	1.9
	Pygm	Glycogen metabolism	1.8
DOWN REGU-LATED by Selenite vs. SeNPs	*Myh1*	Muscle contraction fast fibers	−4.8
	Myh7	Muscle contraction slow fibers	−4.8
	Mylpf	Muscle contraction fast fibers	−4.7
	Acta1	Muscle contraction	−4.1
	Ckm	Creatine metabolism	−4.2
	Pgam2	Glycolysis	−2.6
	Casq1	Ca^{2+} channel transport	−1.6

Compared to the control, SeNPs treatment resulted in the significant upregulation of nine genes. These genes were involved not only in creatine metabolism (*Ckm*) and muscle contraction (*Acta1, Myh1, Myh7* and *Mylpf*) but also in the glycolysis pathway (*Pgam2, Eno3*), glycogen metabolism (*Pygm*), and Ca^{2+} transport (*Casq1*). All of them exhibited expression level changes ranging from 1.8 to 10.9 log_2 fold change (log_2FC). SeNPs treatment presented the highest log_2FC values among the groups' comparison. *Ckm* showed the highest upregulation.

However, the comparison between selenite and SeNPs treatments resulted in the downregulation of seven genes related to SKM function. In this comparison, genes involved in muscle contraction (*Acta1, Myh1, Myh7* and *Mylpf*) exhibited the greatest repression, very closely followed by those associated with creatine metabolism (*Ckm*), and then by those related to glycolysis (*Pgam2*) and calcium transport (*Casq1*).

Relative to oxidative balance in SKM (Figure 2), selenite treatment increases SOD ($p < 0.05$), GPx1 ($p < 0.05$) activities, and GPx1 ($p < 0.05$) and NOX4 ($p < 0.01$) protein expressions, without affecting lipid or protein oxidation. SeNPs also showed an increase in GPx1 ($p < 0.05$) activity, GPx1 ($p < 0.05$), and NOX4 ($p < 0.01$) expressions. Nevertheless, SeNPs decreased SOD and CAT activities ($p < 0.001$ vs. C and S), MDA ($p < 0.001$ vs. C and S), PC ($p < 0.01$ vs. C, $p < 0.001$ vs. S), and H_2O_2 ($p < 0.05$ vs. C, $p < 0.01$ vs. S) levels in SKM.

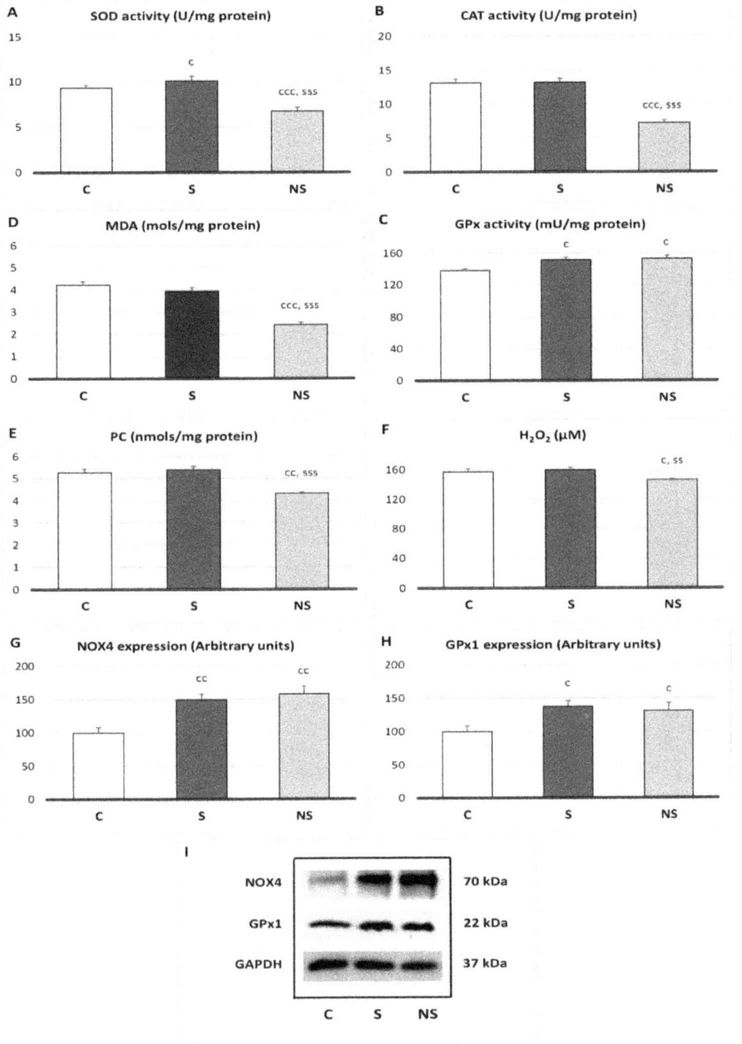

Figure 2. Oxidative balance in skeletal muscle of adolescent rats after treatment with selenite or SeNPs. (**A**) Superoxide dismutase (SOD) activity; (**B**) catalase (CAT) activity; (**C**) glutathione peroxidase (GPx) activity; (**D**) malondialdehyde levels (MDA), showing lipid peroxidation; (**E**) protein carbonyl group (PC), showing protein oxidation; (**F**) hydrogen peroxide (H_2O_2) concentration, a reactive oxygen species (ROS); (**G**) NADPH oxidase 4 (NOX4) expression; (**H**) glutathione peroxidase 1 expression; and (**I**) Western blot expression images with GAPDH as load control. The results were expressed as means ± SEMs and analyzed using a multifactorial one-way ANOVA followed by Tukey's test. The number of animals used in each group is $n = 6$. Experimental groups: C, control group; S, selenite group; NS, SeNP group. Significance: vs. C, c $p < 0.05$, cc $p < 0.01$, ccc $p < 0.001$; vs. S, ss $p < 0.01$, sss $p < 0.001$.

Both experimental groups, S and NS, increased IRS-1 expression in SKM ($p < 0.01$). However, selenite significantly increased *p*-mTOR expression ($p < 0.001$ vs. C and NS), and SeNPs treatment increased mTOR expression ($p < 0.001$ vs. C, $p < 0.05$ vs. S) and decreased *p*-MTOR expression ($p < 0.05$ vs. C) (Figure 3).

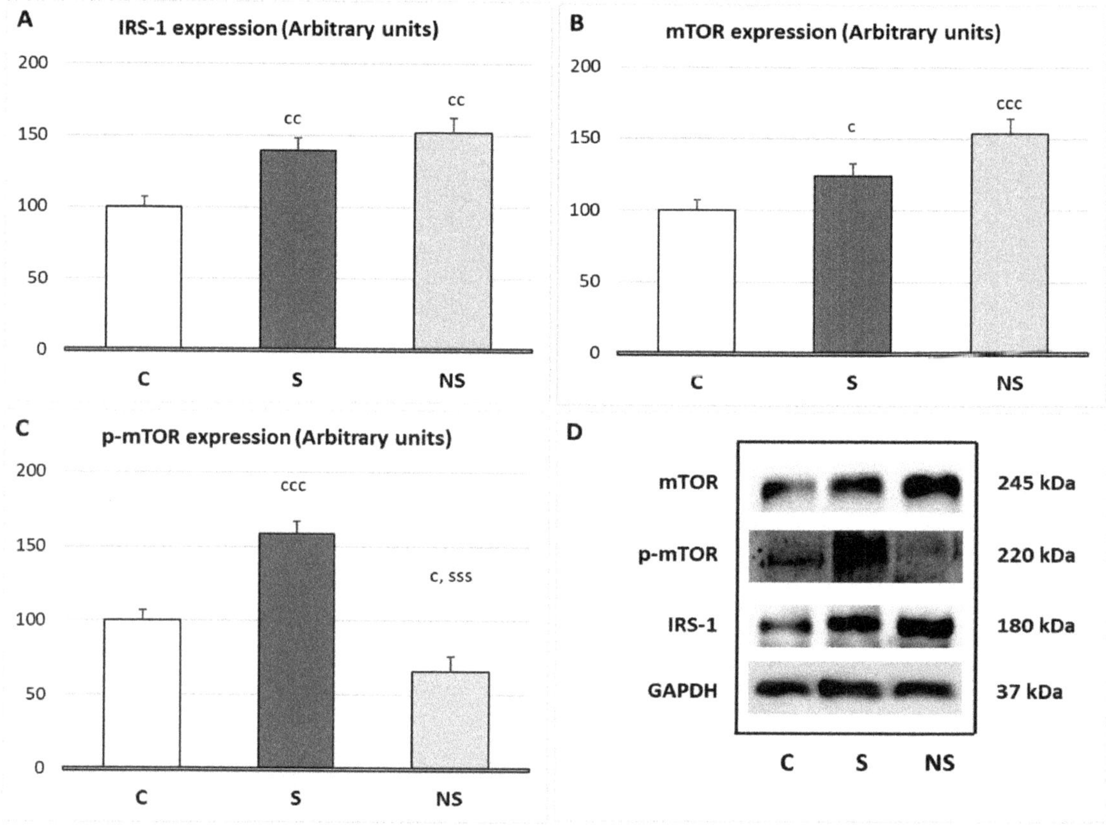

Figure 3. (**A**) Expression of the proteins Insulin receptor substrate 1 (IRS-1); (**B**) mammalian target of rapamycin (mTOR); (**C**) phospho-mTOR (Ser2448) (*p*-mTOR) after treatment with selenite or SeNPs in SKM; and (**D**) Western blot expression images with GAPDH as a loading control. The results were expressed as means ± SEMs and analyzed using a multifactorial one-way ANOVA followed by Tukey's test. The number of animals used in each group is $n = 6$. Experimental groups: C, control group; S, selenite group; NS, SeNP group. Significance: vs. C, c $p < 0.05$, cc $p < 0.01$, ccc $p < 0.001$; vs. S, sss $p < 0.001$.

Regarding protein degradation in SKM (Figure 4), selenite only increased the expression of *p*-AMPK ($p < 0.05$ vs. C); however, the ratio *p*-AMPK/AMPK was unaltered. By contrast, SeNPs enhanced the expression of *p*-AMPK ($p < 0.001$ vs. C, $p < 0.01$ vs. S) and its ratio ($p < 0.001$ vs. C), and the expression of SIRT-1 ($p < 0.01$ vs. C, $p < 0.001$ vs. S), FOXO3a ($p < 0.001$ vs. C and S), MaFbx ($p < 0.001$ vs. C and S) and ULK1 ($p < 0.01$ vs. C and S).

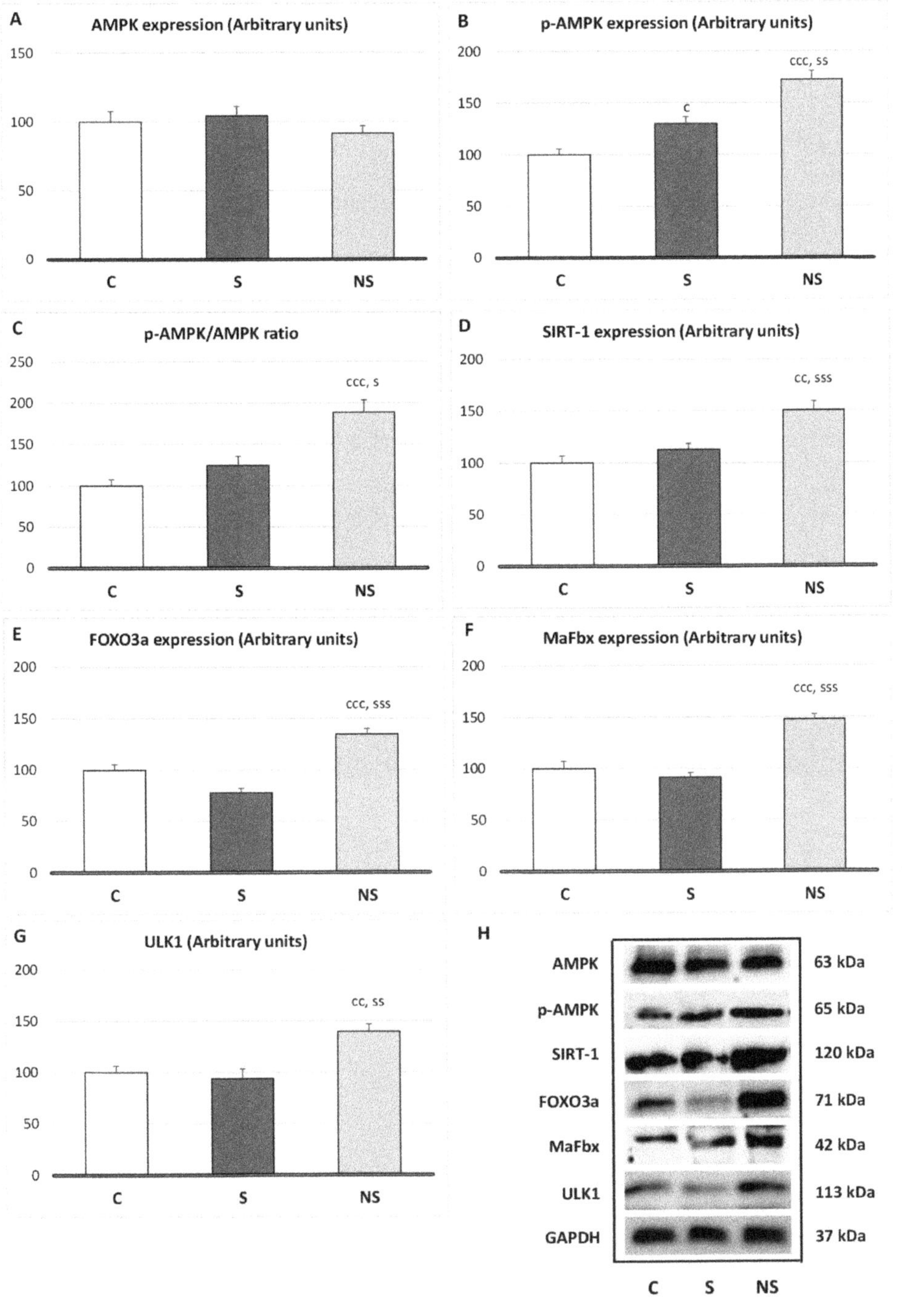

Figure 4. (**A**) Expression of total AMPK; (**B**) *p*-AMPK; (**C**) the *p*-AMPK/AMPK ratio; (**D**) additional expressions of SIRT-1; (**E**) FOXO3a; (**F**) MaFbx; and (**G**) ULK following treatment with selenite or SeNPs; and (**H**) Western blot images show protein expression with GAPDH as a loading control. The results were expressed as means ± SEMs and analyzed using a multifactorial one-way ANOVA followed by Tukey's test. The number of animals used in each group is $n = 6$. Experimental groups: C, control group; S, selenite group; NS, SeNP group. Significance: vs. C, c $p < 0.05$, cc $p < 0.01$, ccc $p < 0.001$; vs. S, s $p < 0.05$, ss $p < 0.01$, sss $p < 0.001$.

Relative to myokines secretion (Table 3), both treatments SNPs and selenite led to an increase in Il-6 ($p < 0.05$), and a decrease in LIF (S: $p < 0.001$; NS: $p < 0.01$), Apelin ($p < 0.001$) and SPARC ($p < 0.01$) serum levels vs. control rats. S adolescent animals showed an enhancement in FGF21 ($p < 0.001$), FSTL-1 ($p < 0.01$) and FABP3 ($p < 0.01$ vs. C; $p < 0.001$ vs. NS) levels. NS rats presented higher levels of serum IL-15 vs. C ones ($p < 0.05$), and BDNF vs. C ($p < 0.01$) and vs. S ($p < 0.05$) animals.

Table 3. Serum myokines levels in adolescent rats after treatment with selenite or SeNPs.

Myokine (pg/mL)	C	S	NP	Secretory Tissue
IL-6	0.31 ± 0.006	0.42 ± 0.03 c	0.42 ± 0.01 c	Muscle, AT, Liver, and Immune system
MYOSTATIN	393.2 ± 2.9	390 ± 4.4	401 ± 3.6	Muscle
LIF	7.2 ± 0.3	4.5 ± 0.4 ccc	5.4 ± 0.4 cc	Muscle
IL-15	1.09 ± 0.04	1.31 ± 0.06	1.39 ± 0.08 c	Muscle
FGF21	3.5 ± 0.15	14.85 ± 0.7 ccc	4.03 ± 0.1 sss	Muscle, AT and Liver
IRISIN	205 ± 5	199 ± 6	202 ± 1	Muscle
BDNF	3527 ± 135	3797 ± 240	4548 ± 123 cc, s	Muscle and Brain
FSTL-1	2571 ± 71	4090 ± 245 cc	2696 ± 374 ss	Muscle and AT
Apelin	106.9 ± 1.6	92.1 ± 0.9 ccc	89.3 ± 0.8 ccc	Muscle
FABP3	9022 ± 340	12,988 ± 846 cc	6543 ± 663 sss	Muscle, Kidney, Lung and Brain
Osteonectin (SPARC)	4.4 ± 0.2	3.04 ± 0.6 cc	3.07 ± 0.1 cc	Muscle and AT

The results were expressed as means ± SEMs and analyzed using a multifactorial one-way ANOVA followed by Tukey's test. The number of animals used in each group is $n = 6$. Experimental groups: C, control group; S, selenite group; NS, SeNP group. Significance: vs. C; c $p < 0.05$; cc $p < 0.01$; ccc $p < 0.001$; vs. S; s $p < 0.05$; ss $p < 0.01$; sss $p < 0.001$.

4. Discussion

4.1. Se Supplementation Modulates Genes Related to Muscle Function in Adipocytes by Upregulating Creatinine Kinase and Muscle Contraction Genes—These Effects Are Higher in SeNPs Treated Rats

Previously, we observed that in WAT either selenite or SeNPs supplementation had different effects on transcriptomic studies, mainly by SeNP's upregulation of genes implicated in the immune system, catabolism, the mitochondrial function, the oxidative balance, and even in muscle tissue function. Despite the fact that adipocytes are not contractile cells, they can express genes related to SKM contraction. This can happen because mesenchymal cells, from which adipocytes, myocytes, osteocytes, and chondrocytes are derived, have high cellular plasticity and the capacity to differentiate into different types of cells depending on external factors, such as hormones [28,29]. The adipocyte gene expression related to SKM contraction, such as actin or myosin, is a clear example of how adipocytes can adapt and response to external signals [30].

In this study, we have found that Se supplementation, regardless of its form of administration (either selenite or SeNPs), enhanced the expression of the *Ckm* gene, which encodes creatine phosphokinase (CPK), the predominant in skeletal muscle (SKM) in adipocytes. This enzyme is essential for rapidly regenerating ATP, by transferring a phosphate group from phosphocreatine (PCr) to ADP, being the energy source the PCr. It is extremely important for explosive, high-intensity activities since ATP is generated in 10–15 s [31]. These data indirectly indicate that Se provides a rapid energy supply in SKM, which is greater when administered as SeNPs. Se supplementation in both forms also upregulates the genes which encode the proteins related to SKM contraction: alpha-actin of SKM, a key structural protein in muscle contraction (gen *Acta1*); myosin heavy chain 1 of SKM, one of the myosin isoforms responsible for muscle contraction in fast fibers (gen *Myh1*); myosin heavy chain 7 of SKM, one of the myosin isoforms responsible for muscle contraction in slow fibers (gen *Myh7*); and myosin light chain specific to fast SKM, which regulates myosin activity in muscle contraction (gen *Mylpf*) [32,33]. In all cases, the upregulation of these genes was significantly greater after SeNPs-treatment. These results indicate that Se enhances SKM contraction process, especially in the form of SeNPs.

Moreover, SeNPs also enhanced specific genes from SKM related to glycolysis (*Pgam* and *Eno3*), to glycogen degradation (*Pygm*), and to calcium transport (*Casq1*). These genes are involved in anaerobic glycolysis, which converts glucose into pyruvate, providing ATP quickly, but leading to muscle fatigue due to lactate accumulation if oxygen is insufficient. This process generates ATP in 30 s to 2 min [34]. In this context, *Pgam* encodes the enzyme phosphoglycerate mutase (PGAM), which catalyzes the conversion of 3-phosphoglycerate to 2-phosphoglycerate, and *Eno3* encodes beta-enolase (ENO3), another glycolytic enzyme that converts 2-phosphoglycerate to phosphoenolpyruvate, contributing to ATP generation in SKM for muscle contraction. Finally, *Pygm* encodes glycogen phosphorylase, an enzyme that breaks down glycogen into glucose-1-phosphate, providing fuel for glycolysis in SKM, and therefore for PGAM and ENO3. These proteins together ensure a higher supply of ATP for SKM contraction in SeNPs treated animals. Moreover, *Casq1* encodes calsequestrin-1, a calcium-binding protein in the sarcoplasmic reticulum, which regulates calcium release for muscle contraction, contributing to a proper calcium excitation-contraction signaling. Together, these genes indicate that during SeNPs treatment, energy is supplied by generating ATP via PCr system and through anaerobic glycolysis. It is known that fast fibers have lower amount of mitochondria and usually activate PCr system and anaerobic glycolysis to obtain ATP [35]. In this study, the upregulation of *Myh1* and *Mylpf,* which encode for proteins responsible for muscle contraction in fast fibers, is in consonance with these results, indicating that SeNPs promote fast muscle fibers contraction.

Finally, the most efficient pathway generating ATP per glucose molecule in the SKM is the oxidative phosphorylation. It occurs in the mitochondria, uses oxygen, and is crucial for endurance activities, lasting its effects from minutes to hours. It is the main energy source of slow fibers, which also have a greater number of mitochondria than fast fibers [36]. Since SeNPs treatment increases genes related to slow fibers contraction (*Myh7*) in adipocytes approximately eightfold more than in C rats, this energy pathway should also be enhanced in these animals.

During oxidative phosphorylation, reactive oxygen species (ROS) are produced naturally as a byproduct of the electron transport chain. Although under physiological conditions this generation is discrete, under stress conditions, when mitochondrial activity is increased, these levels can reach excessive values, leading to OS and to cell damage. For this reason, the endogenous antioxidant systems, superoxide dismutase (SOD), catalase (CAT) and glutathione peroxidase (GPx), which neutralize ROS to minimize oxidative damage, should be balanced. Therefore, we will analyze the oxidative balance in SKM.

4.2. SeNPs Decreases H_2O_2 Generation in SKM, Coinciding with Lower SKM Mass

The main known function of Se is its antioxidant activity, since it is part of the catalytic center of the antioxidant enzyme GPx. Along with CAT and SOD, GPx is one of the three main antioxidant endogenous enzyme in the body to combat ROS, such as the superoxide anion and hydrogen peroxide (H_2O_2); consequently, they are essential for maintaining a correct oxidative balance. In SKM, oxidative balance plays a pivotal role in myogenic proliferation and differentiation. For proper proliferation from satellite cells to myoblasts, low H_2O_2 concentrations are necessary. However, for differentiation from myoblasts to myotube formation, certain levels of H_2O_2 are required [37]. Moreover, it has been described that specifically an upregulation of GPx activity during proliferation, combined with appropriate H_2O_2 levels, enhances myotube formation [38].

In terms of oxidative balance, selenite supplementation to adolescent rats slightly increased SOD activity as well as GPx1 activity and expression, without affecting H_2O_2 concentration or lipid or protein oxidation in SKM. This final effect occurred because GPx1 specifically converts the H_2O_2 generated by SOD into H_2O and O_2. Moreover, to prevent a significant decrease in H_2O_2 concentration, which is necessary for differentiation and growth, the pro-oxidant enzyme NOX4 is upregulated, generating physiological levels of H_2O_2. In fact, a physiological adaptive relationship among NOX4, GPx1 and H_2O_2 stability in SKM has been described [39]. For this reason, in selenite supplemented rats, SKM mass is physiologically developed. In previous papers, we have observed similar results in WAT mass of these animals [10].

Nevertheless, SeNPs supplementation, at the same dose as selenite, reduced the antioxidant activities of SOD and CAT. This decline in antioxidant activity was not associated with a higher oxidative profile, as lipid and protein oxidation remained below control values in SKM, indicating a decrease in ROS levels. Moreover, although GPx1 and NOX4 were enhanced, functioning together to maintain proper H_2O_2 levels, H_2O_2 SKM deposits were significantly reduced. This suggests the presence of an independent mechanism beyond GPx1 activity, which leads to this deep antioxidant effect. This mechanism should be likely related to lower ROS formation; for this reason, CAT and SOD activities were decreased.

Considering that mitochondria are highly abundant in SKM, especially in slow fibers, due to the high energy demand of muscle contraction [36], and that they serve as the main source of ROS in SKM [40], the transcriptional studies undertaken could provide further insights into this phenomenon. It is known that CPK, which is strongly upregulated in adipocytes treated with SeNPs, plays a crucial role not only in energy function but also in preventing mitochondria ROS generation through an ADP-recycling mechanism [41]. This mechanism could partially explain the strong antioxidant effect of SeNPs in SKM and the lower H_2O_2 levels detected in SeNPs-treated rats, which may impair a correct differentiation process, coinciding with a reduced SKM mass.

4.3. SeNPs Deeply Affect Proteosynthesis and Proteolysis Leading to Protein Loss

The regulation of SKM mass is mainly controlled by a fine balance between protein synthesis (proteosynthesis) and protein degradation (proteolysis). In this context, after selenite supplementation, the expression of IRS-1 in SKM was upregulated, similar to what we observed previously in WAT [10], leading to the activation of the IRS-1/Akt/mTOR pathway, the main regulator of proteosynthesis [42]. Since these rats also presented higher insulin serum levels, the activation of this pathway was ensured. It is well described that selenite acts as a secretagogue of insulin through various mechanisms [43], such as increasing the incretin GLP-1 [11]. However, these animals presented normal protein content in SKM, since, as it will be analyzed later, their myokine profile involves catabolic effects. Regarding proteolysis, despite the activation of IRS-1/Akt/mTOR pathway, which inhibits proteolytic processes by suppressing FOXO3 (responsible for autophagy and the ubiquitin–proteasome system) [44], selenite did not reduce any of the proteolytic routes studied, as these remained unaffected.

By contrast, despite SeNPs miocytes presenting higher IRS-1 expression than those treated with selenite, they did not activate the IRS-1/Akt/mTOR pathway. This could be due to two main reasons. First, these animals have lower serum insulin levels compared to physiological conditions. Second, H_2O_2 acts as a second messenger in the insulin pathway [39], and in this group of animals its levels are decreased. Since SeNPs reduced H_2O_2 levels in SKM, insulin sensitivity is compromised. These data are in consonance with the high activity found in fast fibers, since these fibers are less dependent on insulin and glucose uptake from blood, unlike slow fibers [45]. Fast fibers rely on PCr system and anaerobic glycolysis; in this context, in insulin-resistant individuals, a higher recruitment of fast fibers has been described [46].

Moreover, like in WAT, catabolic pathways related to proteolysis are increased following SeNPs exposure [10,12]. Both crucial cellular energy sensors, AMP-activated protein kinase (AMPK) and NAD^+-dependent deacetylase sirtuin-1 (SIRT1), which are activated when energy is necessary, were enhanced [47]. In fact, these sensors activate different catabolic routes to obtain energy, leading to proteolysis. These data align with the lower protein content and reduced SKM mass found in the SeNPs-treated group.

AMPK enhances its activity when ATP levels are required, and in order to obtain energy initiates different routes to avoid anabolism, for example, by inhibiting IRS-1/Akt/mTOR pathway [48], and activates catabolic routes such as ubiquitin–proteasome (UPS) route via MaFbx/atrogin-1 and the autophagic-lysosomal system by activating unc-51-like kinase 1(ULK1), increasing proteolysis [49].

Moreover, SeNPs enhanced SIRT1 expression, this energy sensor is also activated when energy is required and is intrinsically linked to cellular metabolism [50]. SIRT1 usually acts in coordination with AMPK, but it also exhibits its own properties. For instance, in SKM, SIRT1 promotes myogenic proliferation, while preventing differentiation by decreasing MyoD expression [51]. Additionally, it downregulates insulin signaling and enhances fatty acid oxidation and mitochondrial biogenesis by inducing PGC-1alfa and FOXO3a [52]. In this context, by activating FOXO3a, SIRT1 induces MaFbx expression and proteolysis via the UPS, and the autophagic–lysosomal system [53]. Finally, SIRT1, mainly by deacetylating various proteins, contributes to cellular antioxidant responses. For example, it deacetylates FOXO3 and PGC-1alfa, which contribute to induce the activity of antioxidant enzymes, and to the reduction in ROS generation [54,55]. The enhancement of SIRT1 and FOXO3a could be another point to take into consideration in the high antioxidant capacity observed after SeNPs-treatment in SKM.

It is evident that SeNPs, by decreasing H_2O_2 levels, affect myogenic differentiation and IRS-1/Akt/mTOR activation, thereby avoiding proper protein synthesis and SKM mass development. Moreover, SeNPs increase catabolic process in SKM through different pathways (AMPK, SIRT1 and FOXO3a), which increase MaFbx and ULK1 expression, and therefore the UPS and autophagy system. These results align with the highest creatinine serum levels found in these animals.

Finally, SKM is a highly ductile organ, which has the capability to adapt to various physiological conditions by changing its size, composition, and metabolic properties. Therefore, to determine whether these catabolic changes have repercussions on the serum myokine profile, the main myokines were analyzed.

4.4. Different Myokine Secretion Pattern After Selenite or SeNPs Administration

Both treatments selenite and SeNPs alter the homeostasis of several myokines towards a catabolic profile (increased Il-6 and decreased LIF, Apelin and SPARC) which collaborate, among others, to muscle atrophy and fatty acid oxidation, impaired myoblast proliferation and compromised SKM repair and remodeling [56]. However, both treatments presented a different alternative mechanism to avoid muscle breakdown, being the strategy of the S group more potent, as shown in the results relative to SKM protein content, SKM mass and *p*-mTOR results (Figure 5).

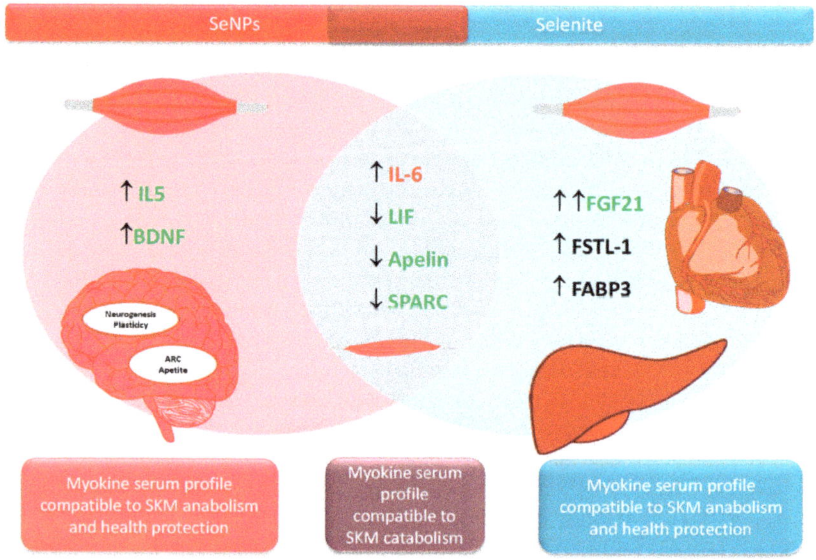

Figure 5. The Venn diagram shows the contrasting effects of Selenite and SeNPs supplementation on the levels of myokines. Whereas, some myokines such as IL-6, LIF, Apelin and SPARC showed similar behavior in both treatments, others such as FGF21, FSTL-1 and FABP3 are much induced in NS rats, and IL-15 together with BDNF are induced specifically in S rats. Other target organs for these contrasting myokines are indicated. An ↑ indicates an increase, an ↓ indicates a decrease. A double mark indicates a more significant change.

It is important to underline that some myokines, as shown in Table 3, are also secreted by other tissues such as the liver and AT (insulin-target tissues), indicating that the endocrine crosstalk among the liver, SKM and AT is greater than expected [57,58]. Therefore, selenite significantly enhanced FGF21 serum levels, which is related to higher muscle mass and mitochondria biogenesis by increasing Akt/mTOR pathway [56]. In fact, it could be established that selenite increases muscle protein synthesis, among others, by promoting FGF21 synthesis. This myokine also has important endocrine actions, such as enhancing insulin sensitivity [16], protecting against cardiac hypertrophy [59], and it also has important beneficial roles in the liver, reducing fat accumulation, inflammation and fibrosis [60]. Selenite supplementation to adolescent rats also increased serum levels of myokines with important endocrine functions, such as FSTL-1 and FABP-3. The first one contributes to increasing glucose uptake and to enhancing β-cell function by improving insulin sensitivity. This is the case in our S rats, where IRS-1 and *p*-mTOR expressions are increased. FSTL-1 also attenuates liver fibrosis, increases endothelial function and revascularization, and improves cardioprotection [16]. FABP-3 acts as a fatty acid carrier specialized in supplying energy to the heart, critical for maintaining the homeostatic function of skeletal and cardiac muscles [61]. In fact, selenite supplementation has been found to be a useful strategy to avoid SKM and cardiovascular damage [62].

SeNPs treatment developed another tactic to increase muscle mass; however, in terms of SKM mass development, this was less efficient. This treatment increases IL-15 and BNDF serum levels. IL-15 contributes to myoblast differentiation, increases fat metabolism preventing fat depots, and enhances antioxidant capacity in SKM [16]. It also has important endocrine functions, and decreases visceral fat by increasing fat metabolism, but also by enhancing energy expenditure and mitochondrial function [63], promoting lean body weight regulation [64]. These effects of SeNPs in adolescent rats are consistent with those found in previous studies, where SeNPs treatment influenced the gut microbiota, shifting it towards a more Gram-negative profile enriched in *Akkermansia* and *Muribaculaceae*, both important bacterial families linked to weight loss, while also decreasing the Firmicutes/Bacteroidetes ratio, associated with a leaner body composition [11].

SeNPs also increased serum BNDF levels, which contribute to muscle regeneration and, as IL-15, to fatty acid oxidation in SKM. This catabolic effect of SeNPs is in consonance with the catabolic status found in the SKM of the rats used in this work. BDNF plays a significant role in memory and plasticity by boosting hippocampal neurogenesis, clearly indicating that SeNPs improve neural function. Finally, BDNF acts in the arcuate nucleus and decreases appetite [64].

These results demonstrate that both Se supplementations modulate SKM and AT morphology, metabolism, and function, clearly highlighting their crosstalk, which may affect energy metabolism and muscle contractility.

5. Conclusions

This study demonstrates that Se supplementation, either in form of selenite or SeNPs, differentially affects the expression of several specific genes, related to SMK, in adipocytes, suggesting a stimulation of fibers. However, SeNPs present a stronger effect in ATP generation by PCr system and anaerobic glycolysis, mainly improving the function of fast fibers; nevertheless, slow fibers also seem to be stimulated. Direct studies on SKM reveal that selenite and SeNPs have different effects on SKM, reducing SeNPs SKM mass. This detriment is mainly due to the fact that SeNPs have a potent antioxidant activity, which decreases H_2O_2 SKM levels, potentially impairing muscle differentiation and an appropriate function of the IRS-1/Akt/mTOR pathway. These factors clearly hinder the proper growth and development of SKM mass. Moreover, SeNPs also activate catabolic routes through AMPK and SIRT1 upregulation, which are in consonance with the transcriptomic results related to higher muscle contraction founded. Finally, SeNPs alters the homeostasis of several myokines towards a catabolic profile, but increases serum IL-15 and BNDF levels, which contribute to muscle regeneration, and to fatty acid oxidation and neuronal plasticity, respectively. These effects of SeNPs on SKM are parallel to those in WAT mass. However, despite selenite treatment also altering some of the routes evaluated, its final effect was physiological, not affecting SKM mass. Further studies are needed to confirm these findings in humans and to clarify the long-term effects of Se supplementation. Selenite may be useful therapeutically in muscle-wasting conditions, such as muscular dystrophies or cachexia, while SeNPs, due to their stimulation of fast fibers and ATP production, could be relevant for enhancing muscle performance.

Limitations of the study. One of the main limitations of the present study is that the expression data for skeletal muscle-related genes were derived from transcriptomic analysis of WAT, rather than directly from SKM. Although adipocytes are not contractile cells, they can express genes related to SKM contraction. This can happen because mesenchymal stem cells, from which adipocytes, myocytes, osteocytes, and chondrocytes are derived, have high cellular plasticity and the ability to differentiate into various cell types in response to external factors, such as hormones. Moreover, it should be emphasized that all genes selected in this study are predominantly or exclusively expressed in SKM. Despite the fact that some of these genes can also be expressed in the cardiac muscle, none are expressed in smooth muscle; therefore, their expression in WAT cannot be attributed to the smooth muscle cells of blood vessels from WAT. The detection of these genes in WAT may instead reflect inter-organ communication mechanisms. Finally, to confirm and elucidate these findings, a comprehensive transcriptomic analysis using SKM is planned as the next step in this research.

Author Contributions: Conceptualization, E.P., O.C. and M.L.O.; data curation, F.N., E.P., M.d.C.G.-L., I.R.-H. and M.L.O., F.M.; formal analysis, F.N., E.P. and M.L.O.; funding acquisition, E.P. and F.M.; investigation, F.N., M.d.C.G.-L., I.R.-H. and M.L.O.; methodology, F.N., M.d.C.G.-L. and I.R.-H.; project administration, O.C. and F.M.; supervision, F.N., E.P. and O.C.; validation, O.C. and M.L.O.; visualization, E.P., M.d.C.G.-L., I.R.-H., O.C. and M.L.O.; writing—original draft, E.P. and M.L.O.; writing—review and editing, F.N., I.R.-H. and F.M. All authors have read and agreed to the published version of the manuscript.

Funding: This research was also funded by Junta de Andalucía, proyectos FEDER Andalucía, grant numbers: US-1380878; and for its support to CTS-193 research group. Funding was also received from Ministerio de Ciencia, Innovación y Universidades (grant number: PID2019-109371GB-I00).

Institutional Review Board Statement: The procedures and experimental protocols concerning the protection of experimental animals were in accordance with the guidelines of the European Union Council (Directive 2010/63/UE) and the Spanish Royal Decree (BOE 34/11370, 2013). The research protocol was approved by both the Ethics Committee of the University of Seville (CEEA-US2019-4) and the Junta de Andalucía (05-04-2019-065). The experimental protocols have been approved by the Ethic Committee of the University of Sevilla (Approval Code: CEEA-US2019-4; Date: 27 February 2019) and the Andalusian Regional Authority (Approval Code: 05-04-2019-065; Date: 9 April 2019). The study complied with the guidelines set forth under the European Union Directive 2010/63/EU and Spanish legislation as detailed in Royal Decree 53/2013 (BOE 34/11370).

Informed Consent Statement: Not applicable.

Data Availability Statement: The data are not publicly available due to the presence of a significant amount of unpublished information. However, they can become accessible to interested scientists upon request.

Acknowledgments: We thank Nobogene Company for their technical support.

Conflicts of Interest: The authors declare no conflicts of interest.

References

1. Nicolaou, M.; Toumba, M.; Kythreotis, A.; Daher, H.; Skordis, N. Obesogens in Adolescence: Challenging Aspects and Prevention Strategies. *Children* **2024**, *11*, 602. [CrossRef]
2. Jebeile, H.; Kelly, A.S.; O'Malley, G.; Baur, L.A. Obesity in Children and Adolescents: Epidemiology, Causes, Assessment, and Management. *Lancet Diabetes Endocrinol.* **2022**, *10*, 351–365. [CrossRef]
3. Tan, J.S.K.; Tan, L.E.S.; Davis, C.; Chew, C.S.E. Eating Disorders in Children and Adolescents. *Singap. Med. J.* **2022**, *63*, 294–298. [CrossRef] [PubMed]
4. Tong, Y.; Xu, S.; Huang, L.; Chen, C. Obesity and Insulin Resistance: Pathophysiology and Treatment. *Drug Discov. Today* **2022**, *27*, 822–830. [CrossRef]
5. Misra, M.; Klibanski, A. Endocrine Consequences of Anorexia Nervosa. *Lancet Diabetes Endocrinol.* **2014**, *2*, 581–592. [CrossRef]
6. Zoidis, E.; Seremelis, I.; Kontopoulos, N.; Danezis, G.; Zoidis, E.; Seremelis, I.; Kontopoulos, N.; Danezis, G.P. Selenium-Dependent Antioxidant Enzymes: Actions and Properties of Selenoproteins. *Antioxidants* **2018**, *7*, 66. [CrossRef]
7. Köhrle, J. Selenium in Endocrinology-Selenoprotein-Related Diseases, Population Studies, and Epidemiological Evidence. *Endocrinology* **2021**, *162*, bqaa228. [CrossRef] [PubMed]

8. Köhrle, J. The Selenoenzyme Family of Deiodinase Isozymes Controls Local Thyroid Hormone Availability. *Rev. Endocr. Metab. Disord.* **2000**, *1*, 49–58. [CrossRef]
9. Abo El-Magd, N.F.; Barbosa, P.O.; Nick, J.; Covalero, V.; Grignetti, G.; Bermano, G. Selenium, as Selenite, Prevents Adipogenesis by Modulating Selenoproteins Gene Expression and Oxidative Stress–Related Genes. *Nutrition* **2022**, *93*, 111424. [CrossRef]
10. Ojeda, M.L.; Nogales, F.; Carreras, O.; Pajuelo, E.; Gallego-López, M.d.C.; Romero-Herrera, I.; Begines, B.; Moreno-Fernández, J.; Díaz-Castro, J.; Alcudia, A. Different Effects of Low Selenite and Selenium-Nanoparticle Supplementation on Adipose Tissue Function and Insulin Secretion in Adolescent Male Rats. *Nutrients* **2022**, *14*, 3571. [CrossRef]
11. Ojeda, M.L.; Nogales, F.; Carrasco López, J.A.; Gallego-López, M.d.C.; Carreras, O.; Alcudia, A.; Pajuelo, E. Microbiota-Liver-Bile Salts Axis, a Novel Mechanism Involved in the Contrasting Effects of Sodium Selenite and Selenium-Nanoparticle Supplementation on Adipose Tissue Development in Adolescent Rats. *Antioxidants* **2023**, *12*, 1123. [CrossRef] [PubMed]
12. Nogales, F.; Pajuelo, E.; Romero-Herrera, I.; Carreras, O.; Merchán, F.; Carrasco López, J.A.; Ojeda, M.L. Uncovering the Role of Selenite and Selenium Nanoparticles (SeNPs) in Adolescent Rat Adipose Tissue beyond Oxidative Balance: Transcriptomic Analysis. *Antioxidants* **2024**, *13*, 750. [CrossRef]
13. Saedi, M.S.; Smith, C.G.; Frampton, J.; Chambers, I.; Harrison, P.R.; Sunde, R.A. Effect of Selenium Status on MRNA Levels for Glutathione Peroxidase in Rat Liver. *Biochem. Biophys. Res. Commun.* **1988**, *153*, 855–861. [CrossRef]
14. Yapici, H.; Gulu, M.; Yagin, F.H.; Eken, O.; Gabrys, T.; Knappova, V. Exploring the Relationship between Biological Maturation Level, Muscle Strength, and Muscle Power in Adolescents. *Biology* **2022**, *11*, 1722. [CrossRef]
15. Peifer-Weiß, L.; Al-Hasani, H.; Chadt, A. AMPK and Beyond: The Signaling Network Controlling RabGAPs and Contraction-Mediated Glucose Uptake in Skeletal Muscle. *Int. J. Mol. Sci.* **2024**, *25*, 1910. [CrossRef] [PubMed]
16. Chen, W.; Wang, L.; You, W.; Shan, T. Myokines Mediate the Cross Talk between Skeletal Muscle and Other Organs. *J. Cell. Physiol.* **2021**, *236*, 2393–2412. [CrossRef]
17. Mancinelli, R.; Checcaglini, F.; Coscia, F.; Gigliotti, P.; Fulle, S.; Fanò-Illic, G. Biological Aspects of Selected Myokines in Skeletal Muscle: Focus on Aging. *Int. J. Mol. Sci.* **2021**, *22*, 8520. [CrossRef] [PubMed]
18. Wesolowski, L.T.; Semanchik, P.L.; White-Springer, S.H. Beyond Antioxidants: Selenium and Skeletal Muscle Mitochondria. *Front. Vet. Sci.* **2022**, *9*, 1011159. [CrossRef]
19. Lee, S.C.; Lee, N.H.; Patel, K.D.; Jun, S.K.; Park, J.H.; Knowles, J.C.; Kim, H.W.; Lee, H.H.; Lee, J.H. A Study on Myogenesis by Regulation of Reactive Oxygen Species and Cytotoxic Activity by Selenium Nanoparticles. *Antioxidants* **2021**, *10*, 1727. [CrossRef]
20. Spear, L. Modeling Adolescent Development and Alcohol Use in Animals. *Alcohol Res. Health* **2000**, *24*, 115–123.
21. Lowry, O.H.; Rosebrough, N.J.; Farr, A.L.; Randal, R.J. Protein Measurement with the Folin Phenol Reagent. *J. Biol. Chem.* **1951**, *193*, 265–275. [CrossRef] [PubMed]
22. Chen, S. Ultrafast One-Pass FASTQ Data Preprocessing, Quality Control, and Deduplication Using Fastp. *iMeta* **2023**, *2*, e107. [CrossRef] [PubMed]
23. Chen, S.; Zhou, Y.; Chen, Y.; Gu, J. Fastp: An Ultra-Fast All-in-One FASTQ Preprocessor. *Bioinformatics* **2018**, *34*, i884–i890. [CrossRef]
24. Romero-Herrera, I.; Nogales, F.; Gallego-López, M.d.C.; Díaz-Castro, J.; Carreras, O.; Ojeda, M.L. Selenium Supplementation via Modulation of Selenoproteins Ameliorates Binge Drinking-Induced Oxidative, Energetic, Metabolic, and Endocrine Imbalance in Adolescent Rats' Skeletal Muscle. *Food Funct.* **2024**, *15*, 7988–8007. [CrossRef]
25. Draper, H.H.; Hadley, M. Malondialdehyde Determination as Index of Lipid Peroxidation. *Methods Enzymol.* **1990**, *186*, 421–431. [CrossRef]
26. Reznick, A.Z.; Packer, L. [38] Oxidative Damage to Proteins: Spectrophotometric Method for Carbonyl Assay. *Methods Enzymol.* **1994**, *233*, 357–363. [CrossRef] [PubMed]
27. Romero-Herrera, I.; Nogales, F.; Díaz-Castro, J.; Moreno-Fernandez, J.; Gallego-Lopez, M.C.; Ochoa, J.; Carreras, O.; Ojeda, M.L. Binge Drinking Leads to Oxidative and Metabolic Damage in Skeletal Muscle during Adolescence, Contributing to Insulin Resistance via Myokines. *J. Physiol. Biochem.* **2023**, *79*, 799–810. [CrossRef]
28. Gronthos, S.; Zannettino, A.C.W.; Hay, S.J.; Shi, S.; Graves, S.E.; Kortesidis, A.; Simmons, P.J. Molecular and Cellular Characterisation of Highly Purified Stromal Stem Cells Derived from Human Bone Marrow. *J. Cell Sci.* **2003**, *116*, 1827–1835. [CrossRef]
29. Phinney, D.G.; Prockop, D.J. Concise Review: Mesenchymal Stem/Multipotent Stromal Cells: The State of Transdifferentiation and Modes of Tissue Repair--Current Views. *Stem Cells* **2007**, *25*, 2896–2902. [CrossRef]
30. Byun, S.E.; Sim, C.; Chung, Y.; Kim, H.K.; Park, S.; Kim, D.K.; Cho, S.; Lee, S. Skeletal Muscle Regeneration by the Exosomes of Adipose Tissue-Derived Mesenchymal Stem Cells. *Curr. Issues Mol. Biol.* **2021**, *43*, 1473–1488. [CrossRef]
31. Hargreaves, M.; Spriet, L.L. Skeletal Muscle Energy Metabolism during Exercise. *Nat. Metab.* **2020**, *2*, 817–828. [CrossRef]
32. Long, K.; Su, D.; Li, X.; Li, H.; Zeng, S.; Zhang, Y.; Zhong, Z.; Lin, Y.; Li, X.; Lu, L.; et al. Identification of Enhancers Responsible for the Coordinated Expression of Myosin Heavy Chain Isoforms in Skeletal Muscle. *BMC Genom.* **2022**, *23*, 519. [CrossRef]
33. Khodabukus, A. Tissue-Engineered Skeletal Muscle Models to Study Muscle Function, Plasticity, and Disease. *Front. Physiol.* **2021**, *12*, 619710. [CrossRef]

34. Hargreaves, M.; Spriet, L.L. Exercise Metabolism: Fuels for the Fire. *Cold Spring Harb. Perspect. Med.* **2018**, *8*, a029744. [CrossRef] [PubMed]
35. Picard, M.; Hepple, R.T.; Burelle, Y. Mitochondrial Functional Specialization in Glycolytic and Oxidative Muscle Fibers: Tailoring the Organelle for Optimal Function. *Am. J. Physiol. Cell Physiol.* **2012**, *302*, C629–C641. [CrossRef]
36. Leduc-Gaudet, J.P.; Hussain, S.N.A.; Barreiro, E.; Gouspillou, G. Mitochondrial Dynamics and Mitophagy in Skeletal Muscle Health and Aging. *Int. J. Mol. Sci.* **2021**, *22*, 8179. [CrossRef]
37. Kozakowska, M.; Pietraszek-Gremplewicz, K.; Jozkowicz, A.; Dulak, J. The Role of Oxidative Stress in Skeletal Muscle Injury and Regeneration: Focus on Antioxidant Enzymes. *J. Muscle Res. Cell Motil.* **2015**, *36*, 377–393. [CrossRef] [PubMed]
38. Hidalgo, M.; Marchant, D.; Quidu, P.; Youcef-Ali, K.; Richalet, J.P.; Beaudry, M.; Besse, S.; Launay, T. Oxygen Modulates the Glutathione Peroxidase Activity during the L6 Myoblast Early Differentiation Process. *Cell. Physiol. Biochem.* **2014**, *33*, 67–77. [CrossRef]
39. Xirouchaki, C.E.; Jia, Y.; McGrath, M.J.; Greatorex, S.; Tran, M.; Merry, T.L.; Hong, D.; Eramo, M.J.; Broome, S.C.; Woodhead, J.S.T.; et al. Skeletal Muscle NOX4 Is Required for Adaptive Responses That Prevent Insulin Resistance. *Sci. Adv.* **2021**, *7*, eabl4988. [CrossRef]
40. Lamb, G.D.; Westerblad, H. Acute Effects of Reactive Oxygen and Nitrogen Species on the Contractile Function of Skeletal Muscle. *J. Physiol.* **2011**, *589*, 2119–2127. [CrossRef]
41. Meyer, L.E.; Machado, L.B.; Santiago, A.P.S.A.; Da-Silva, W.S.; De Felice, F.G.; Holub, O.; Oliveira, M.F.; Galina, A. Mitochondrial Creatine Kinase Activity Prevents Reactive Oxygen Species Generation: Antioxidant Role of Mitochondrial Kinase-Dependent ADP Re-Cycling Activity. *J. Biol. Chem.* **2006**, *281*, 37361–37371. [CrossRef] [PubMed]
42. Solsona, R.; Pavlin, L.; Bernardi, H.; Sanchez, A.M.J. Molecular Regulation of Skeletal Muscle Growth and Organelle Biosynthesis: Practical Recommendations for Exercise Training. *Int. J. Mol. Sci.* **2021**, *22*, 2741. [CrossRef]
43. Wang, X.; Sui, H.; Su, Y.; Zhao, S. Protective Effects of Sodium Selenite on Insulin Secretion and Diabetic Retinopathy in Rats with Type 1 Diabetes Mellitus. *Pak. J. Pharm. Sci.* **2021**, *34*, 1729–1735. [CrossRef]
44. Ferreira, R.P.; Duarte, J.A. Protein Turnover in Skeletal Muscle: Looking at Molecular Regulation towards an Active Lifestyle. *Int. J. Sports Med.* **2023**, *44*, 763–777. [CrossRef] [PubMed]
45. Nolte, L.A.; Galuska, D.; Martin, I.K.; Zierath, J.R.; Wallberg-Henriksson, H. Elevated Free Fatty Acid Levels Inhibit Glucose Phosphorylation in Slow-Twitch Rat Skeletal Muscle. *Acta Physiol. Scand.* **1994**, *151*, 51–59. [CrossRef]
46. Zierath, J.R.; Hawley, J.A. Skeletal Muscle Fiber Type: Influence on Contractile and Metabolic Properties. *PLoS Biol.* **2004**, *2*, e348. [CrossRef]
47. Cantó, C.; Auwerx, J. PGC-1α, SIRT1 and AMPK, an Energy Sensing Network That Controls Energy Expenditure. *Curr. Opin. Lipidol.* **2009**, *20*, 98–105. [CrossRef]
48. Cetrullo, S.; D'Adamo, S.; Tantini, B.; Borzì, R.M.; Flamigni, F. MTOR, AMPK, and Sirt1: Key Players in Metabolic Stress Management. *Crit. Rev.™ Eukaryot. Gene Expr.* **2015**, *25*, 59–75. [CrossRef] [PubMed]
49. Sanchez, A.M.J.; Csibi, A.; Raibon, A.; Cornille, K.; Gay, S.; Bernardi, H.; Candau, R. AMPK Promotes Skeletal Muscle Autophagy through Activation of Forkhead FoxO3a and Interaction with Ulk1. *J. Cell. Biochem.* **2012**, *113*, 695–710. [CrossRef]
50. Chang, H.-C.; Guarente, L. SIRT1 and Other Sirtuins in Metabolism. *Trends Endocrinol. Metab.* **2014**, *25*, 138–145. [CrossRef]
51. Pardo, P.S.; Boriek, A.M. The Physiological Roles of Sirt1 in Skeletal Muscle. *Aging* **2011**, *3*, 430–437. [CrossRef] [PubMed]
52. Boutant, M.; Cantó, C. SIRT1 Metabolic Actions: Integrating Recent Advances from Mouse Models. *Mol. Metab.* **2014**, *3*, 5–18. [CrossRef] [PubMed]
53. Zhang, H.; Lin, F.; Zhao, J.; Wang, Z. Expression Regulation and Physiological Role of Transcription Factor FOXO3a During Ovarian Follicular Development. *Front. Physiol.* **2020**, *11*, 595086. [CrossRef]
54. Chen, J.; Wang, Q.; Li, R.; Li, Z.; Jiang, Q.; Yan, F.; Ye, J. The Role of Sirtuins in the Regulatin of Oxidative Stress during the Progress and Therapy of Type 2 Diabetes Mellitus. *Life Sci.* **2023**, *333*, 122187. [CrossRef]
55. Guan, G.; Chen, Y.; Dong, Y. Unraveling the AMPK-SIRT1-FOXO Pathway: The In-Depth Analysis and Breakthrough Prospects of Oxidative Stress-Induced Diseases. *Antioxidants* **2025**, *14*, 70. [CrossRef] [PubMed]
56. Lee, J.H.; Jun, H.S. Role of Myokines in Regulating Skeletal Muscle Mass and Function. *Front. Physiol.* **2019**, *10*, 42. [CrossRef]
57. Dos Santos, A.R.d.O.; Zanuso, B.d.O.; Miola, V.F.B.; Barbalho, S.M.; Santos Bueno, P.C.; Flato, U.A.P.; Detregiachi, C.R.P.; Buchaim, D.V.; Buchaim, R.L.; Tofano, R.J.; et al. Adipokines, Myokines, and Hepatokines: Crosstalk and Metabolic Repercussions. *Int. J. Mol. Sci.* **2021**, *22*, 2639. [CrossRef]
58. Raschke, S.; Eckel, J. Adipo-Myokines: Two Sides of the Same Coin—Mediators of Inflammation and Mediators of Exercise. *Mediat. Inflamm.* **2013**, *2013*, 320724. [CrossRef]
59. Itoh, N. FGF21 as a Hepatokine, Adipokine, and Myokine in Metabolism and Diseases. *Front. Endocrinol.* **2014**, *5*, 107. [CrossRef]
60. Maratos-Flier, E. Fatty Liver and FGF21 Physiology. *Exp. Cell Res.* **2017**, *360*, 2–5. [CrossRef]
61. Li, B.; Syed, M.H.; Khan, H.; Singh, K.K.; Qadura, M. The Role of Fatty Acid Binding Protein 3 in Cardiovascular Diseases. *Biomedicines* **2022**, *10*, 2283. [CrossRef] [PubMed]

62. Shimada, B.K.; Alfulaij, N.; Seale, L.A. The Impact of Selenium Deficiency on Cardiovascular Function. *Int. J. Mol. Sci.* **2021**, *22*, 10713. [CrossRef] [PubMed]
63. Putu, G.; Aryana, S.; Ayu, A.A.; Hapsari, R.; Ayu, R.; Kuswardhani, T. Myokine Regulation as Marker of Sarcopenia in Elderly. *Mol. Cell. Biomed. Sci.* **2018**, *2*, 38–47. [CrossRef]
64. Grannell, A.; Kokkinos, A.; le Roux, C.W. Myokines in Appetite Control and Energy Balance. *Muscles* **2022**, *1*, 26–47. [CrossRef]

approved by the Kyung Hee University Institutional Animal Care and Use Committee (#KHSASP-21-341).

2.2. Serum and Hepatic Biochemical Parameters

Serum aspartate aminotransferase (AST) and alanine aminotransferase (ALT) activities were measured using assay kits (#AM102-K and #AM103-K, respectively, Asan Pharmaceutical Co., Hwa-sung, Kyung-gi, Republic of Korea). Hepatic triglyceride (TG) and total cholesterol (TC) concentrations were measured using assay kits (#AM157S and #AM202, Asan Pharmaceutical Co.). Hepatic MDA contents were measured using an assay kit (#MAK085, Sigma-Aldrich®, Saint Louis, MO, USA). Hepatic non-heme iron contents were measured according to the method described by Choi et al. [16]. Hepatic glutathione (GSH) and oxidized glutathione (GSSG) contents, hepatic catalase (CAT), superoxide dismutase (SOD), and GPX activity were measured using commercially available kits (Cayman Chemical, Ann Arbor, MI, USA). All procedures were performed according to the manufacturer's protocols.

2.3. Histological Analysis

Fixed liver tissues, embedded in paraffin, were sliced into 5 μm thick slices and stained with hematoxylin and eosin (H&E) (KP&T Co., Ltd., Cheong-ju, Chung-buk, Republic of Korea). The MASLD activity score (MAS) score was evaluated by examining the degree of steatosis, lobular inflammation, and hepatocellular ballooning [16]. To assess liver fibrosis, Sirius Red staining was performed. Then, the area of the red part as a percentage of the total area was quantified using ImageJ software version 1.53 (NIH, Bethesda, MD, USA). The average of the five fields was calculated. All stained-liver sections were observed under an optical microscope (Olympus, Tokyo, Japan) at 200× magnification.

2.4. Quantitative Real Time RT-PCR

Total RNA was extracted from 25 mg of liver tissue using the RNAiso Plus reagent (Takara Bio Inc., Shiga, Japan). For cDNA synthesis, 100 ng of total RNA was reverse transcribed using the PrimeScript™ RT reagent Kit (Takara Bio Inc.). Real-time reverse transcription polymerase chain reaction (RT-PCR) was performed to amplify specific genes with the SYBR Premix Ex Taq kit (Takara Bio Inc.). mRNA expression levels were quantified relative to the control group using the $2^{-\Delta\Delta Ct}$ method.

2.5. Western Blot Analysis

Liver tissue (50 mg) was lysed in 200 μL of lysis buffer with protease inhibitors and centrifuged at 17,000 rpm for 15 min at 4 °C. Protein concentrations were measured using a Protein Quantification Kit (Thermo Fisher Scientific Inc., Waltham, MA, USA). Lysates were separated by Sodium Dodecyl Sulfate Polyacrylamide Gel Electrophoresis (SDS-PAGE), transferred to a Polyvinylidene Fluoride (PVDF) membrane, blocked, and incubated overnight at 4 °C with primary antibodies (anti-GPX4 (Abcam, Cambridge, UK), anti-4HNE (R&D systems, Minneapolis, MN, USA), anti-ferritin, anti-acyl-CoA synthetase long-chain family member 4 (ACSL4), anti-12-lipoxygenase (LOX), and anti-glyceraldehyde-3-phosphate dehydrogenase (GAPDH) (all from Santa Cruz Biotechnology, Dallas, TX, USA)). Membranes were incubated with a secondary antibody for 1 h and developed with Enhanced Chemiluminescence solution (Bio-Rad, Hercules, CA, USA). Bands were visualized using a ChemiScope (Clinx Science Instruments Co., Shanghai, China) and quantified.

2.6. Statistical Analysis

All data were analyzed using SAS 9.4 software and expressed as mean ± SEM. One-way Analysis of Variance (ANOVA) with post-hoc Duncan's multiple range test was performed to test the significant difference among groups. p-values less than 0.05 were considered statistically significant.

3. Results

3.1. CoQ and Se Alleviate Liver Injury in MASH Mice Induced by MCD Diet

In the histopathological analysis of H&E-stained liver sections, mice on the MCD diet exhibited a significant increase in both the size and number of fat droplets, along with pronounced inflammatory cell infiltration and ballooning degeneration, compared to those on the MCS diet control (Figure 1a). Conversely, treatments with CoQ, Se, or their combination markedly reduced hepatic steatosis, decreased inflammatory foci, and improved ballooning degeneration. The MAS scores were significantly lower in the CoQ, Se, and CoQ + Se groups compared to the MCD group, with the CoQ + Se group reaching the lowest scores among the four MCD diet-fed groups (Figure 1b). Serum levels of ALT and AST, which were significantly elevated in the MCD group relative to the MCS group, were notably reduced by treatments with CoQ, Se, or CoQ + Se (Figure 1c,d). Hepatic TG and TC concentrations were considerably higher in the MCD group than in the MCS group (Figure 1e,f). While there was a trend towards reduced hepatic TG and total cholesterol levels with CoQ or Se treatment alone, these changes were not statistically significant. However, the combination of CoQ and Se significantly lowered both hepatic TG and cholesterol concentrations compared to the MCD group.

3.2. CoQ and Se Alleviate Inflammation and Fibrosis in MASH Mice Induced by MCD Diet

The degree of fibrosis was evaluated using Sirius Red staining of liver sections. Collagen staining was much more pronounced in the MCD group compared to the MCS control group but was significantly reduced in the groups treated with CoQ, Se, or CoQ + Se (Figure 2a,b). The combination treatment further decreased collagen staining compared to treatment with CoQ or Se alone. The mRNA expression levels of Collagen 1α1, Collagen 3α1, and transforming growth factor-β (TGF-β), indicators of fibrosis, were significantly higher in the MCD group compared to the MCS group, and were substantially reduced following CoQ, Se, and CoQ + Se treatments (Figure 2c).

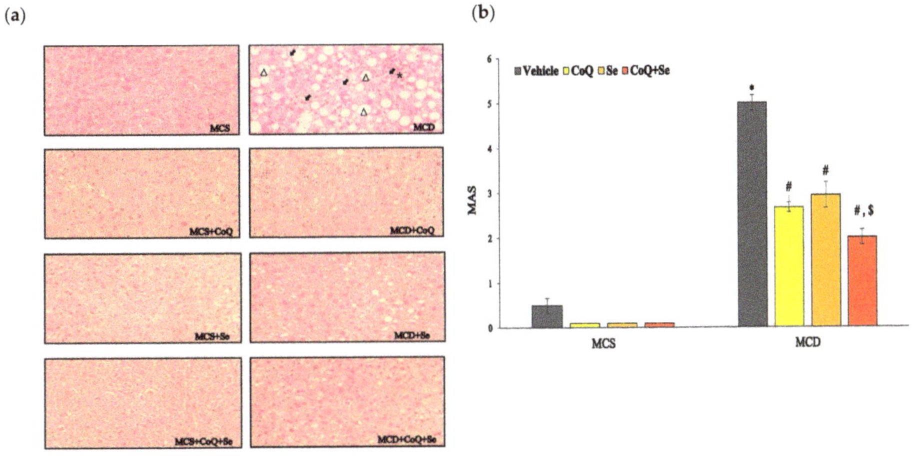

Figure 1. *Cont.*

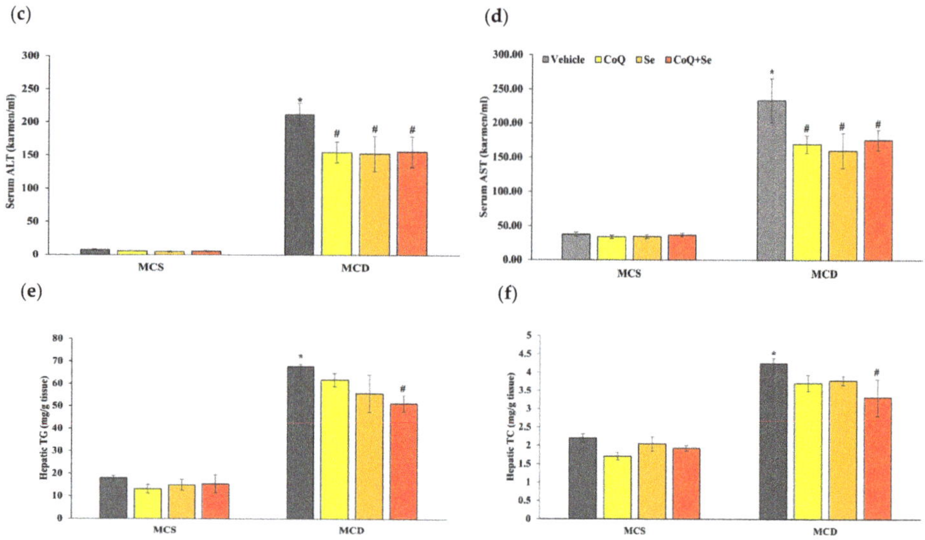

Figure 1. Effects of CoQ and Se treatment on liver injury in MCD diet-induced MASH mice. (**a**) Liver sections stained with H&E (steatosis (Δ), lobular inflammation (*), and ballooning degeneration (→)), (**b**) MAS score, (**c**) Serum ALT activity, (**d**) Serum AST activity, (**e**) Hepatic TG concentration, (**f**) Hepatic total cholesterol (TC) concentration. Data are shown as mean ± SEM. * $p < 0.05$ vs. MCS vehicle, # $p < 0.05$ vs. MCD vehicle, \$ $p < 0.05$ vs. MCD + CoQ.

In addition, the mRNA levels of pro-inflammatory cytokine related genes such as interleukin-1β (IL-1β) and interleukin-6 (IL-6) were significantly increased in the MCD group compared to the MCS group. In contrast, treatment with CoQ, Se, or CoQ + Se markedly downregulated both IL-1β and IL-6 mRNA levels. Moreover, the level of cyclooxygenase-2 (COX2) protein expression, which mediates inflammatory responses, was significantly increased in the MCD vehicle group. The combination of CoQ and Se treatment, but not CoQ or Se alone, significantly down-regulated COX2 protein expression compared to the MCD group.

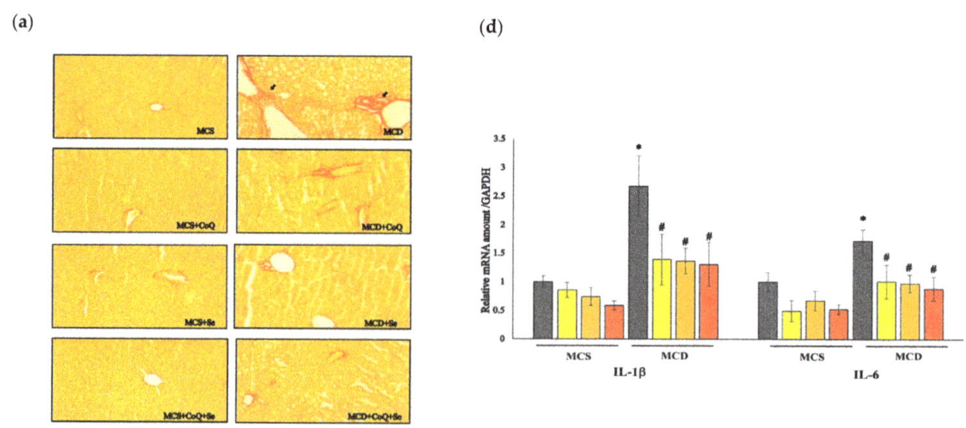

Figure 2. *Cont.*

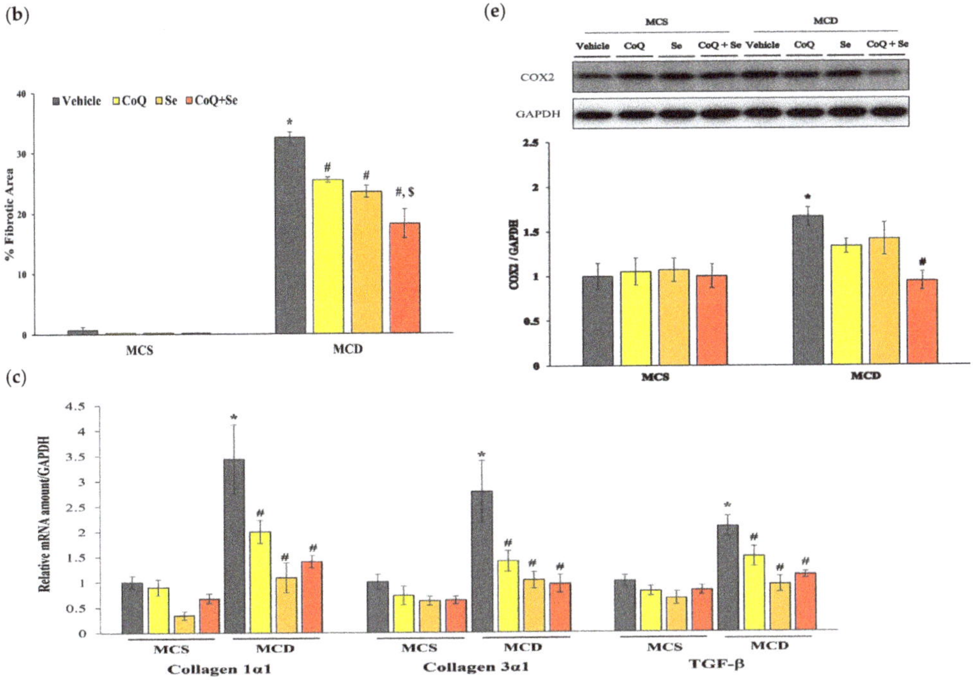

Figure 2. Effects of CoQ and Se treatment on hepatic inflammation and fibrosis in MCD diet-induced MASH mice. (**a**): Liver sections stained with Sirius Red staining (200× magnification); The arrow indicates collagen staining, (**b**) % Fibrotic area, (**c**) the mRNA levels of fibrotic markers, (**d**) Hepatic mRNA levels of pro-inflammatory cytokines, (**e**) Hepatic protein levels of COX2 with representative blot (upper panel). Data are shown as mean ± SEM. * $p < 0.05$ vs. MCS vehicle, # $p < 0.05$ vs. MCD vehicle, $ $p < 0.05$ vs. MCD + CoQ.

3.3. CoQ and Se Alleviate Hepatic Oxidative Stress in MCD Diet-Induced MASH Mice

Antioxidant enzymes such CAT, SOD, and GPX play crucial roles in defending against ROS. In this study, the MCD diet significantly reduced CAT and SOD activities compared to the MCS control group, indicating induced oxidative stress (Table 1). Although treatment with CoQ or Se alone showed a trend of increasing CAT and SOD activities, these changes were not statistically significant. However, the combination of CoQ and Se significantly enhanced both CAT and SOD activities, demonstrating a synergistic effect that effectively counteracts the oxidative stress from the MCD diet (Table 1). GPX activity was higher in the MCD group compared to the MCS control, as a response to increased oxidative stress. Administration of CoQ or Se alone further enhanced GPX activity, with their combination resulting in a statistically significant increase compared to the MCD group, highlighting their potent combined effect in enhancing the GSH antioxidant defense system.

Furthermore, the MCD diet significantly decreased the GSH/GSSG ratio, a key marker of cellular redox balance, but combined supplementation of CoQ and Se substantially improved this ratio to levels comparable to the MCS group, emphasizing their capacity to restore a favorable redox balance and mitigate oxidative damage.

Table 1. Effects of coenzyme Q (CoQ) and selenium (Se) on hepatic oxidative stress in MASH mice.

	MCS	MCD			
	Vehicle	Vehicle	CoQ	Se	CoQ + Se
CAT activity (U/mg protein)	1045.9 ± 197.5 [a]	355.1 ± 24.7 [c]	537.0 ± 54.6 [bc]	373.5 ± 23.8 [c]	649.2 ± 78.8 [b]
SOD activity (U/mg protein)	33.3 ± 1.1 [a]	20.4 ± 1.3 [c]	23.0 ± 2.3 [bc]	24.2 ± 0.8 [bc]	27.2 ± 0.8 [ab]
GPX activity (U/mg tissue)	0.1 ± 0.1 [d]	1.6 ± 0.3 [bc]	2.1 ± 0.4 [b]	2.1 ± 0.1 [b]	4.0 ± 0.5 [a]
GSH/GSSG	20.0 ± 5.4 [a]	4.9 ± 0.7 [c]	7.3 ± 1.5 [bc]	6.2 ± 2.2 [c]	16.4 ± 3.9 [ab]

Data are expressed as the mean ± SEM. Different superscripts represent statistical significance ($p < 0.05$). One-way ANOVA followed by Duncan's post-hoc test. CAT, catalase; SOD, superoxide dismutase; GPX, glutathione peroxidase; GSH, glutathione; GSSG, oxidized glutathione.

3.4. CoQ and Se Inhibit Hepatic Lipid Peroxidation in MCD Diet-Induced MASH Mice

The increase in hepatic lipid peroxidation is closely linked to the onset and progression of MASH. We investigated whether CoQ, Se, or their combination could mitigate these effects in MCD diet-induced MASH mice. The data showed that the MCD diet significantly increased hepatic MDA levels compared to the MCS control diet (Figure 3a). Levels of 4-HNE were also significantly elevated in the MCD group compared to the MCS group (Figure 3b). In contrast, treatment with CoQ, Se, or both significantly decreased hepatic MDA levels induced by the MCD diet. Additionally, the combination of CoQ and Se significantly reduced hepatic 4-HNE levels. As MDA and 4-HNE are key biomarkers of lipid peroxidation, these findings indicate that CoQ and Se treatments significantly ameliorated hepatic lipid peroxidation in MASH mice.

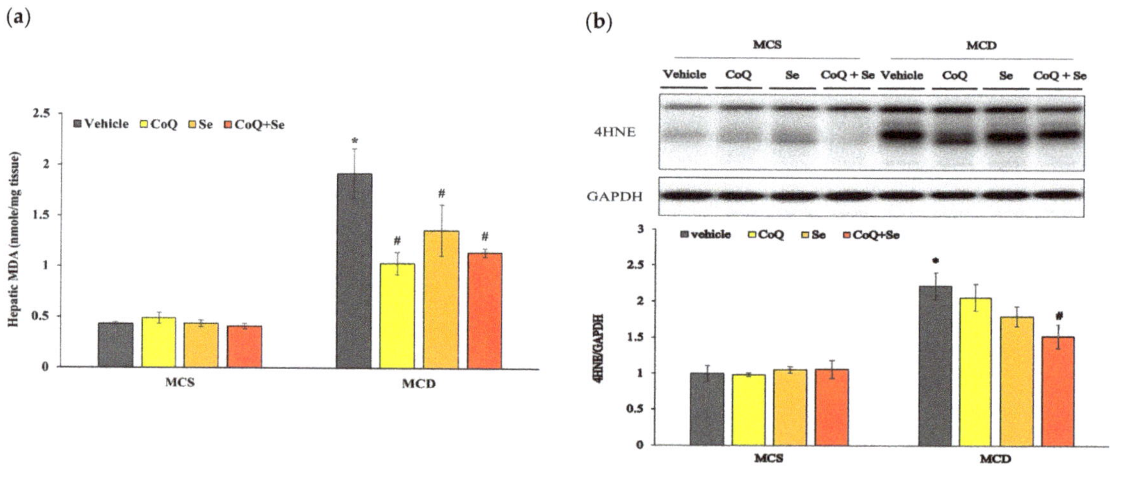

Figure 3. Effects of CoQ and Se treatment on hepatic lipid peroxidation in MCD diet-induced MASH mice. (**a**) Hepatic MDA concentration, (**b**) Hepatic protein levels of 4-HNE with representative blot (upper panel). Data are shown as mean ± SEM. * $p < 0.05$ vs. MCS vehicle, # $p < 0.05$ vs. MCD vehicle.

3.5. CoQ and Se Inhibit Changes in Ferroptosis Related Markers in the Liver of MCD Diet-Induced MASH Mice

Emerging evidence suggests that ferroptosis, a type of cell death characterized by iron-dependent lipid peroxidation, plays a critical role in the pathogenesis of MASH. To further investigate the molecular mechanisms underlying the effects of CoQ and Se in reducing lipid peroxidation and mitigating liver injury, we examined markers of ferroptosis in this study. The expression level of the ACSL4 protein was significantly increased in the MCD group compared to the MCS control group; however, treatment with CoQ, Se, or their combination (CoQ + Se) resulted in a significant decrease in ACSL4 protein expression (Figure 4a). Similarly, the expression of the LOX protein was markedly elevated in the MCD group compared to the MCS vehicle group. Notably, only the combination treatment of CoQ and Se led to a significant reduction in LOX protein expression (Figure 4b). Furthermore, the protein levels of GPX4 were increased in the MCD group compared to the MCS vehicle group. GPX4 expression was further elevated in the Se alone and CoQ + Se treatment groups compared to the MCD group (Figure 4c).

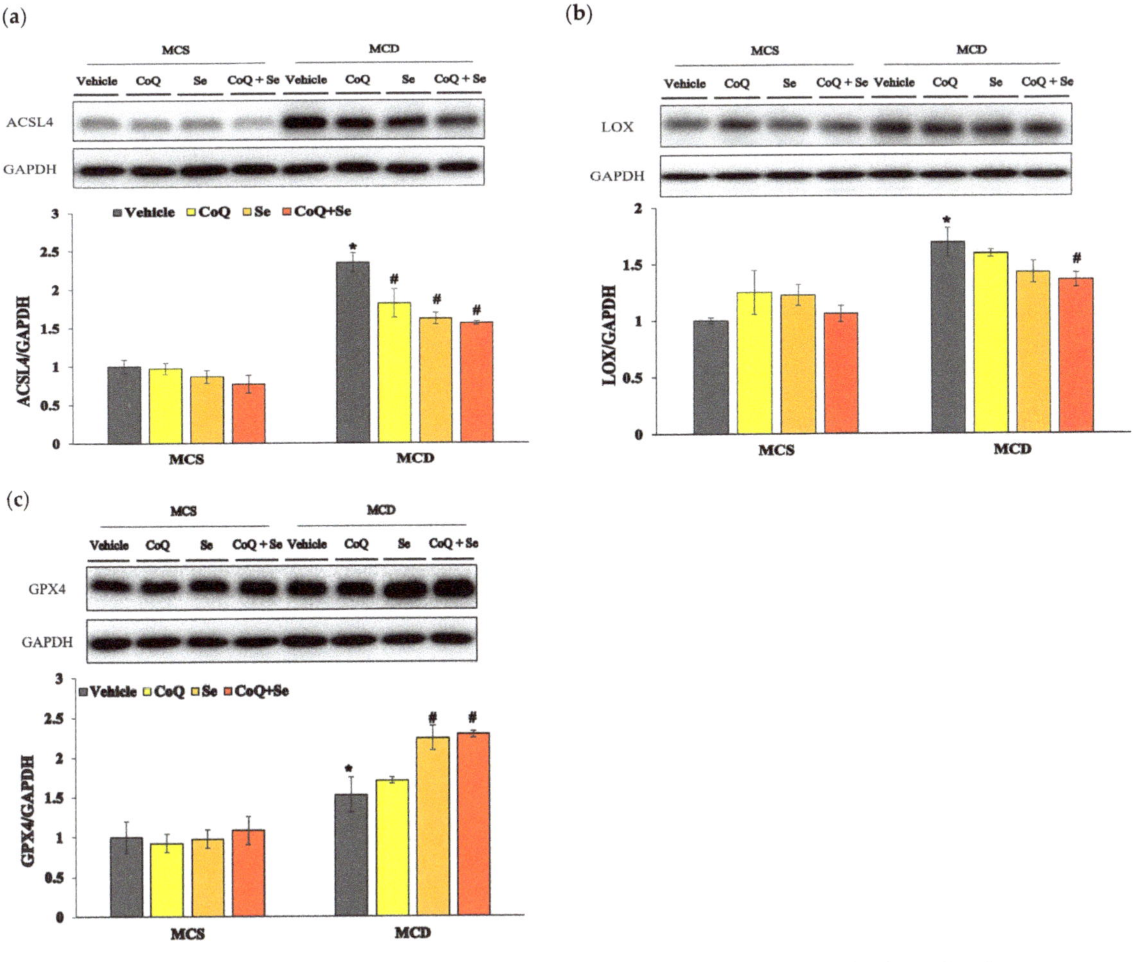

Figure 4. Effects of CoQ and Se treatment on hepatic ferroptosis markers in MCD diet-induced MASH mice. Hepatic protein levels of (**a**) ACSL4, (**b**) LOX, and (**c**) GPX4. Data are shown as mean ± SEM. * $p < 0.05$ vs. MCS vehicle, # $p < 0.05$ vs. MCD vehicle.

We also evaluated changes in hepatic iron content by measuring non-heme iron concentrations and ferritin levels, which is a cellular iron storage protein. The non-heme iron concentration was significantly higher in the MCD group compared to the MCS vehicle group, whereas treatment with CoQ + Se significantly reduced non-heme iron levels compared to the MCD group (Figure 5a). Among the groups fed the MCS diet, Se alone and CoQ + Se treatments resulted in significantly lower non-heme iron concentrations compared to the MCS vehicle group. Ferritin protein levels were significantly increased in the MCD diet groups compared to the MCS control group. In contrast, ferritin protein levels showed a significant decrease in the group treated with the combination of CoQ and Se compared to the MCD group (Figure 5b).

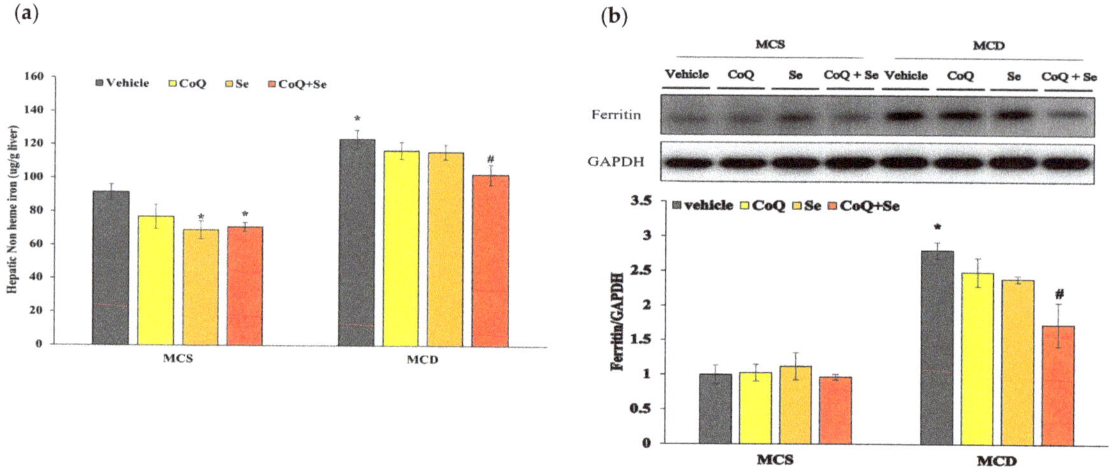

Figure 5. Effects of CoQ and Se treatment on hepatic non-heme iron concentrations and hepatic ferritin protein level in MCD diet-induced MASH mice. (**a**) Hepatic non-heme iron concentration, (**b**) Hepatic protein levels of ferritin. Data are shown as mean ± SEM. * $p < 0.05$ vs. MCS vehicle, # $p < 0.05$ vs. MCD vehicle.

4. Discussion

MASH, a severe form of MASLD, is a major global health concern due to its association with hepatic inflammation, fibrosis, and progression to cirrhosis or hepatocellular carcinoma. Despite its growing prevalence, effective therapeutic options remain limited. In this study, we provide compelling evidence that co-supplementation with CoQ and Se effectively ameliorates the progression of MASH induced by an MCD diet in mice. The combined treatment significantly alleviated hepatic steatosis, inflammation, and fibrosis. These effects were associated with the suppression of oxidative stress, lipid peroxidation, and markers of ferroptosis.

The pathogenesis of MASH is closely associated with increased oxidative stress [17]. Depletion of GSH and CoQ and decreases in the activity of certain antioxidant enzymes such as CAT and SOD were reported in patients with MASH, which were correlated with the severity of the disease [18]. One major consequence of oxidative stress is lipid peroxidation, where ROS attack polyunsaturated fatty acids in cell membrane phospholipids. This process produces toxic byproducts like MDA and 4-HNE, which can activate Kupffer and hepatic stellate cells, leading to inflammation and the onset of fibrogenesis. In this study, we observed a significant reduction in CAT and SOD activities, along with a decreased GSH/GSSG ratio, in the liver tissues of MCD-diet-fed mice compared to MCS controls. Hepatic levels of MDA and 4-HNE were also markedly elevated in the MCD group, indicating increased oxidative stress and lipid peroxidation due to MCD-diet feeding. Conversely, CoQ and Se co-supplementation significantly enhanced CAT and SOD activities, restored the GSH/GSSG ratio to levels comparable to those of the MCS controls, and significantly reduced MDA and 4-HNE levels, contributing to improvements in NAS, inflammation, and fibrosis. CoQ prevents both the initiation and propagation of lipid peroxidation [19]. Additionally, Se-dependent GPX4 is the major antioxidant enzyme known to catalyze the conversion of toxic lipid hydroperoxide into non-toxic lipid alcohols [20]. While CoQ and

Se have each been individually reported to exhibit hepatoprotective effects [8–10], their roles in MASH have not been well established. This study provides novel evidence of the synergistic effects of CoQ and Se co-supplementation in mitigating MASH progression.

Recent studies have emphasized the critical role of ferroptosis in the progression of MASH [11–13]. In line with this, our study demonstrated significant increases in hepatic expression of ferroptosis markers, including ACSL4 and LOX, in the MCD group compared to MCS controls. These changes were accompanied by elevated hepatic iron content and markedly increased levels of MDA and 4-HNE, key indicators of lipid peroxidation. Similar findings were reported by [7], who showed that iron and lipid ROS accumulation in the liver of MCD-diet-fed mice was alleviated by ferroptosis inhibitors, leading to reductions in inflammation, fibrosis, and liver injury. These observations suggest that ferroptosis contributes to MCD-diet-induced MASH progression, as corroborated by our findings.

To further elucidate the molecular mechanisms underlying the hepatoprotective effects of CoQ and Se against MASH progression, we investigated changes in ferroptotic markers. Notably, the combination of CoQ and Se significantly reduced hepatic LOX protein levels, accompanied by marked decreases in lipid peroxidation, as indicated by lower MDA and 4-HNE levels. In contrast, CoQ treatment alone did not significantly alter hepatic LOX protein or 4-HNE levels. Interestingly, treatment with Se or CoQ + Se induced a more than two-fold increase in hepatic GPX4 expression compared to MCS controls. GPX4, a pivotal enzyme for eliminating lipid peroxides, is essential for ferroptosis regulation; its deletion leads to lipid peroxide accumulation and ferroptosis, whereas its overexpression suppresses ferroptosis [20,21]. Se has been shown to transcriptionally upregulate selenoproteins, including GPX4, protecting cells from ferroptotic stimuli [13]. Additionally, Se treatment has been shown to increase GPX4 protein levels in palmitic acid-treated hepatocytes, preventing ferroptotic cell death and promoting cell survival [6]. In our study, the induction of GPX4 was associated with the suppression of ACSL4 and LOX expression, suggesting that CoQ and Se treatment mitigates MASH progression, at least in part, by suppressing ferroptosis.

Interestingly, Se treatment alone induced GPX4 expression to a level comparable to those achieved by CoQ + Se treatment; however, hepatic 4-HNE level was further decreased in the CoQ + Se treatment group compared to the Se-alone group. This suggests that CoQ may provide additional antioxidant activity beyond GPX4 induction mediated by Se. Alternatively, CoQ might suppress ferroptosis via a GPX4-independent pathway. The CoQ oxidoreductase FSP1, for example, has been shown to confer resistance to ferroptosis and acts in parallel to GPX4 in inhibiting ferroptosis [14,22]. Therefore, CoQ and Se may synergistically suppress ferroptosis through activation of FSP1- and GPX4-dependent pathways, respectively. Future studies are necessary to elucidate the dose-response relationships and further identify the optimal combinations of CoQ and Se supplementation to maximize therapeutic efficacy.

In this study, hepatic non-heme iron concentrations and hepatic ferritin levels were significantly increased in the MCD group compared to the MCS controls. Consistent with this finding, Palladini et al. [23] also reported an increase in iron levels in both serum and tissues during the progression from steatosis to steatohepatitis in an MCD-diet rat model. Excessive iron can induce oxidative stress through the Fenton reaction and has been shown to aggravate liver injury associated with MASLD [24,25]. In addition, iron has been suggested to enhance lipid peroxidation through the activation of enzymes such as LOX [26]. Moreover, the administration of deferoxamine (an iron-chelating agent) has been found to reduce MASH severity in MCD-fed mice [6], indicating that inhibiting iron accumulation may suppress disease progression and associated liver injury. In the current study, the co-treatment of CoQ and Se significantly decreased hepatic ferritin, an iron storage protein, and markers of hepatic iron content, suggesting that this combination is effective in reducing hepatic iron levels. Since synthetic compounds like deferoxamine have limitations such as low oral bioavailability and a short plasma half-life, our findings suggest that CoQ and Se could be alternatives to prevent iron-related diseases.

The mechanisms by which CoQ and Se treatment reduce hepatic iron levels are unclear. A recent study demonstrated that nobiletin, a flavonoid with antioxidant properties, alleviated myocardial ischemia-reperfusion injury by reducing the expression of nuclear receptor coactivator 4 (NCOA4) [27]. NCOA4 is integral to ferritinophagy, an autophagic pathway responsible for ferritin degradation and iron release. Interestingly, erastin, which generates lipid ROS, has been shown to decrease NCOA4 levels, disrupting ferritinophagy and resulting in iron accumulation and increased ferritin levels [28]. Whether CoQ or Se influences hepatic iron levels through modulation of NCOA4 expression or activity warrants further investigation in future studies.

In this study, we demonstrated that CoQ + Se treatment significantly reduced hepatic triglyceride and total cholesterol concentrations. Hepatic lipid accumulation is known to trigger oxidative stress, and the severity of hepatic steatosis is closely associated with the progression of liver injury and fibrosis. Supporting this, previous studies have shown that CoQ improves MASLD in mice by enhancing fatty acid oxidation and inhibiting fatty acid synthesis via activation of the AMPK pathway [29,30]. However, clinical studies have reported inconsistent results, with CoQ10 intervention showing no significant effects on lipid profiles [31]. Similarly, Se has been reported to regulate lipid metabolism through AMPK activation, but its effects on lipogenesis remain conflicting, with studies showing both increases and decreases in lipid synthesis [12,32]. As demonstrated in this study, the combined use of CoQ and Se may provide a more effective strategy for regulating lipid metabolism and reducing hepatic lipid accumulation.

5. Conclusions

In conclusion, this study demonstrates that co-supplementation with CoQ and Se effectively alleviates MCD diet-induced MASH. The combined treatment significantly reduced hepatic steatosis, inflammation, and fibrosis. Mechanistically, CoQ and Se enhanced antioxidant defenses by increasing CAT and SOD activities, restoring the GSH/GSSG ratio, and reducing lipid peroxidation, as evidenced by lower levels of MDA and 4-HNE in liver tissues. These changes were associated with the downregulation of pro-inflammatory cytokines such as IL-1β and IL-6, as well as fibrosis-related genes, including collagen 1α1, collagen 3α1, and TGF-β. Furthermore, CoQ and Se suppressed proteins involved in ferroptosis, such as ACSL4 and LOX, while upregulating GPX4 expression. These findings suggest the synergistic potential of CoQ and Se co-supplementation as a promising therapeutic strategy for managing MASH and associated liver injury.

Author Contributions: Conceptualization, J.C. (Jayong Chung); methodology, H.C. and J.C. (Jiwon Choi); formal analysis, H.C. and J.C. (Jiwon Choi); data curation, Y.G.; writing—original draft preparation, H.C.; writing—review and editing, H.C., Y.G. and J.C. (Jayong Chung); funding acquisition, J.C. (Jayong Chung). All authors have read and agreed to the published version of the manuscript.

Funding: This research was supported by the National Research Foundation of Korea (NRF) grant supported by the Korean government (MIST): NRF-2020R1F1A1075611.

Institutional Review Board Statement: The animal study protocol was approved by the Institutional Animal Care and Use Committee of Kyung Hee University (#KHSASP-22-116, 2 July 2021).

Data Availability Statement: The original contributions presented in this study are included in the article. Further inquiries can be directed to the corresponding author.

Conflicts of Interest: The authors declare no conflicts of interest.

Abbreviations

The following abbreviations are used in this manuscript:

4-HNE	4-Hydroxynonenal
ACSL4	Acyl-CoA synthetase long-chain family member 4
CAT	Catalase
CoQ	Coenzyme Q
COX2	Cyclooxygenase-2
FSP1	Ferroptosis suppressor protein 1
GPX	Glutathione peroxidase
GSH	Glutathione
GSSG	Oxidized glutathione
LOX	Arachidonate 12-lipoxygenase
MASH	Metabolic dysfunction-associated steatohepatitis
MASLD	Metabolic dysfunction-associated steatotic liver disease
MCD	Methionine choline-deficient
MCS	Methionine choline-sufficient
MDA	Malondialdehyde
NAFLD	Nonalcoholic fatty liver disease
NASH	Nonalcoholic steatohepatitis
NCOA4	Nuclear receptor coactivator 4
Se	Selenium
SOD	Superoxide dismutase

References

1. Powell, E.E.; Wong, V.W.; Rinella, M. Non-alcoholic fatty liver disease. *Lancet* **2021**, *397*, 2212–2224. [CrossRef] [PubMed]
2. Daher, D.; Dahan, K.S.E.; Singal, A.G. Non-alcoholic fatty liver disease-related hepatocellular carcinoma. *J. Liver Cancer* **2023**, *23*, 127–142. [CrossRef]
3. Rinella, M.E.; Lazarus, J.V.; Ratziu, V.; Francque, S.M.; Sanyal, A.J.; Kanwal, F.; Romero, D.; Abdelmalek, M.F.; Anstee, Q.M.; Arab, J.P.; et al. A multisociety Delphi consensus statement on new fatty liver disease nomenclature. *Hepatology* **2023**, *78*, 1966–1986. [CrossRef]
4. Bessone, F.; Razori, M.V.; Roma, M.G. Molecular pathways of nonalcoholic fatty liver disease development and progression. *Cell. Mol. Life Sci.* **2019**, *76*, 99–128. [CrossRef] [PubMed]
5. Marra, F.; Gastaldelli, A.; Svegliati Baroni, G.; Tell, G.; Tiribelli, C. Molecular basis and mechanisms of progression of non-alcoholic steatohepatitis. *Trends Mol. Med.* **2008**, *14*, 72–81. [CrossRef] [PubMed]
6. Qi, J.; Kim, J.W.; Zhou, Z.; Lim, C.W.; Kim, B. Ferroptosis Affects the Progression of Nonalcoholic Steatohepatitis via the Modulation of Lipid Peroxidation-Mediated Cell Death in Mice. *Am. J. Pathol.* **2020**, *190*, 68–81. [CrossRef]
7. Li, X.; Wang, T.X.; Huang, X.; Li, Y.; Sun, T.; Zang, S.; Guan, K.L.; Xiong, Y.; Liu, J.; Yuan, H.X. Targeting ferroptosis alleviates methionine-choline deficient (MCD)-diet induced NASH by suppressing liver lipotoxicity. *Liver Int.* **2020**, *40*, 1378–1394. [CrossRef] [PubMed]
8. Fouad, A.A.; Jresat, I. Hepatoprotective effect of coenzyme Q10 in rats with acetaminophen toxicity. *Environ. Toxicol. Phar.* **2012**, *33*, 158–167. [CrossRef]
9. Ali, S.A.; Faddah, L.; Abdel-Baky, A.; Bayoumi, A. Protective effect of L-carnitine and coenzyme Q10 on CCl4-induced liver injury in rats. *Sci. Pharm.* **2010**, *78*, 881. [CrossRef] [PubMed]
10. Ozardalı, I.l.; Bitiren, M.; Karakılçık, A.Z.; Zerin, M.; Aksoy, N.; Musa, D. Effects of selenium on histopathological and enzymatic changes in experimental liver injury of rats. *Exp. Toxicol. Pathol.* **2004**, *56*, 59–64. [CrossRef]
11. Bioulac-Sage, P.; Dubuisson, L.; Bedin, C.; Gonzalez, P.; de Tinguy-Moreaud, E.; Garcin, H.; Balabaud, C. Nodular regenerative hyperplasia in the rat induced by a selenium-enriched diet: Study of a model. *Hepatology* **1992**, *16*, 418–425. [CrossRef]
12. Zhao, Z.; Barcus, M.; Kim, J.; Lum, K.L.; Mills, C.; Lei, X.G. High Dietary Selenium Intake Alters Lipid Metabolism and Protein Synthesis in Liver and Muscle of Pigs. *J. Nutr.* **2016**, *146*, 1625–1633. [CrossRef]
13. Alim, I.; Caulfield, J.T.; Chen, Y.; Swarup, V.; Geschwind, D.H.; Ivanova, E.; Seravalli, J.; Ai, Y.; Sansing, L.H.; Marie, E.J.S. Selenium drives a transcriptional adaptive program to block ferroptosis and treat stroke. *Cell* **2019**, *177*, 1262–1279.e25. [CrossRef]
14. Bersuker, K.; Hendricks, J.M.; Li, Z.; Magtanong, L.; Ford, B.; Tang, P.H.; Roberts, M.A.; Tong, B.; Maimone, T.J.; Zoncu, R.; et al. The CoQ oxidoreductase FSP1 acts parallel to GPX4 to inhibit ferroptosis. *Nature* **2019**, *575*, 688–692. [CrossRef] [PubMed]

15. Li, Q.W.; Yang, Q.; Liu, H.Y.; Wu, Y.L.; Hao, Y.H.; Zhang, X.Q. Protective Role of Coenzyme Q10 in Acute Sepsis-Induced Liver Injury in BALB/c Mice. *Biomed. Res. Int.* **2020**, *2020*, 7598375. [CrossRef] [PubMed]
16. Choi, J.; Choi, H.; Chung, J. Icariin supplementation suppresses the markers of ferroptosis and attenuates the progression of nonalcoholic steatohepatitis in mice fed a methionine choline-deficient diet. *Int. J. Mol. Sci.* **2023**, *24*, 12510. [CrossRef] [PubMed]
17. Liu, W.; Baker, S.S.; Baker, R.D.; Zhu, L. Antioxidant Mechanisms in Nonalcoholic Fatty Liver Disease. *Curr. Drug Targets* **2015**, *16*, 1301–1314. [CrossRef] [PubMed]
18. Videla, L.A.; Rodrigo, R.; Orellana, M.; Fernandez, V.; Tapia, G.; Quiñones, L.; Varela, N.; Contreras, J.; Lazarte, R.; Csendes, A.; et al. Oxidative stress-related parameters in the liver of non-alcoholic fatty liver disease patients. *Clin. Sci.* **2004**, *106*, 261–268. [CrossRef] [PubMed]
19. Varela-López, A.; Giampieri, F.; Battino, M.; Quiles, J.L. Coenzyme Q and Its Role in the Dietary Therapy against Aging. *Molecules* **2016**, *21*, 373. [CrossRef] [PubMed]
20. Yang, W.S.; SriRamaratnam, R.; Welsch, M.E.; Shimada, K.; Skouta, R.; Viswanathan, V.S.; Cheah, J.H.; Clemons, P.A.; Shamji, A.F.; Clish, C.B.; et al. Regulation of ferroptotic cancer cell death by GPX4. *Cell* **2014**, *156*, 317–331. [CrossRef] [PubMed]
21. Friedmann Angeli, J.P.; Schneider, M.; Proneth, B.; Tyurina, Y.Y.; Tyurin, V.A.; Hammond, V.J.; Herbach, N.; Aichler, M.; Walch, A.; Eggenhofer, E.; et al. Inactivation of the ferroptosis regulator Gpx4 triggers acute renal failure in mice. *Nat. Cell Biol.* **2014**, *16*, 1180–1191. [CrossRef] [PubMed]
22. Doll, S.; Freitas, F.P.; Shah, R.; Aldrovandi, M.; da Silva, M.C.; Ingold, I.; Goya Grocin, A.; Xavier da Silva, T.N.; Panzilius, E.; Scheel, C.H.; et al. FSP1 is a glutathione-independent ferroptosis suppressor. *Nature* **2019**, *575*, 693–698. [CrossRef] [PubMed]
23. Palladini, G.; Di Pasqua, L.G.; Cagna, M.; Croce, A.C.; Perlini, S.; Mannucci, B.; Profumo, A.; Ferrigno, A.; Vairetti, M. MCD Diet Rat Model Induces Alterations in Zinc and Iron during NAFLD Progression from Steatosis to Steatohepatitis. *Int. J. Mol. Sci.* **2022**, *23*, 6817. [CrossRef] [PubMed]
24. Imeryuz, N.; Tahan, V.; Sonsuz, A.; Eren, F.; Uraz, S.; Yuksel, M.; Akpulat, S.; Ozcelik, D.; Haklar, G.; Celikel, C.; et al. Iron preloading aggravates nutritional steatohepatitis in rats by increasing apoptotic cell death. *J. Hepatol.* **2007**, *47*, 851–859. [CrossRef]
25. Kirsch, R.; Sijtsema, H.P.; Tlali, M.; Marais, A.D.; Hall Pde, L. Effects of iron overload in a rat nutritional model of non-alcoholic fatty liver disease. *Liver Int.* **2006**, *26*, 1258–1267. [CrossRef] [PubMed]
26. Yang, W.S.; Kim, K.J.; Gaschler, M.M.; Patel, M.; Shchepinov, M.S.; Stockwell, B.R. Peroxidation of polyunsaturated fatty acids by lipoxygenases drives ferroptosis. *Proc. Natl. Acad. Sci. USA* **2016**, *113*, E4966–E4975. [CrossRef] [PubMed]
27. Huang, Q.; Tian, L.; Zhang, Y.; Qiu, Z.; Lei, S.; Xia, Z.Y. Nobiletin alleviates myocardial ischemia-reperfusion injury via ferroptosis in rats with type-2 diabetes mellitus. *Biomed. Pharmacother.* **2023**, *163*, 114795. [CrossRef]
28. Gao, M.; Monian, P.; Pan, Q.; Zhang, W.; Xiang, J.; Jiang, X. Ferroptosis is an autophagic cell death process. *Cell Res.* **2016**, *26*, 1021–1032. [CrossRef]
29. Chen, K.; Chen, X.; Xue, H.; Zhang, P.; Fang, W.; Chen, X.; Ling, W. Coenzyme Q10 attenuates high-fat diet-induced non-alcoholic fatty liver disease through activation of the AMPK pathway. *Food Funct.* **2019**, *10*, 814–823. [CrossRef] [PubMed]
30. Xu, Z.; Huo, J.; Ding, X.; Yang, M.; Li, L.; Dai, J.; Hosoe, K.; Kubo, H.; Mori, M.; Higuchi, K.; et al. Coenzyme Q10 Improves Lipid Metabolism and Ameliorates Obesity by Regulating CaMKII-Mediated PDE4 Inhibition. *Sci. Rep.* **2017**, *7*, 8253. [CrossRef] [PubMed]
31. Zahedi, H.; Eghtesadi, S.; Seifirad, S.; Rezaee, N.; Shidfar, F.; Heydari, I.; Golestan, B.; Jazayeri, S. Effects of CoQ10 Supplementation on Lipid Profiles and Glycemic Control in Patients with Type 2 Diabetes: A randomized, double blind, placebo-controlled trial. *J. Diabetes Metab. Disord.* **2014**, *13*, 81. [CrossRef] [PubMed]
32. Nido, S.A.; Shituleni, S.A.; Mengistu, B.M.; Liu, Y.; Khan, A.Z.; Gan, F.; Kumbhar, S.; Huang, K. Effects of Selenium-Enriched Probiotics on Lipid Metabolism, Antioxidative Status, Histopathological Lesions, and Related Gene Expression in Mice Fed a High-Fat Diet. *Biol. Trace Elem. Res.* **2016**, *171*, 399–409. [CrossRef] [PubMed]

nutrients

MDPI

Article

Effect of Selol on Tumor Morphology and Biochemical Parameters Associated with Oxidative Stress in a Prostate Tumor-Bearing Mice Model

Małgorzata Sochacka [1,*], Grażyna Hoser [2], Małgorzata Remiszewska [3], Piotr Suchocki [1], Krzysztof Sikora [4] and Joanna Giebułtowicz [1]

1 Department of Drug Chemistry, Pharmaceutical and Biomedical Analysis, Faculty of Pharmacy, Medical University of Warsaw, 1 Banacha Street, PL-02097 Warsaw, Poland; piotr.suchocki@wum.edu.pl (P.S.); joanna.giebultowicz@wum.edu.pl (J.G.)
2 Department of Translational Immunology and Experimental Intensive Care, Centre of Postgraduate Medical Education, Ceglowska 80, PL-01809 Warsaw, Poland
3 Department of Pharmacology, National Medicines Institute, 30/34 Chełmska Street, PL-00725 Warsaw, Poland; malgorzata.remiszewska@nil.gov.pl
4 Pathomorphology Centre, National Medical Institute of the Ministry of the Interior and Administration, 137 Wołoska Street, PL-02507 Warsaw, Poland
* Correspondence: malgorzata.bogucka@wum.edu.pl; Tel.: +48-22-5720630

Abstract: Prostate cancer is the leading cause of cancer death in men. Some studies suggest that selenium Se (+4) may help prevent prostate cancer. Certain forms of Se (+4), such as Selol, have shown anticancer activity with demonstrated pro-oxidative effects, which can lead to cellular damage and cell death, making them potential candidates for cancer therapy. Our recent study in healthy mice found that Selol changes the oxidative–antioxidative status in blood and tissue. However, there are no data on the effect of Selol in mice with tumors, considering that the tumor itself influences this balance. This research investigated the impact of Selol on tumor morphology and oxidative–antioxidative status in blood and tumors, which may be crucial for the formulation's effectiveness. Our study was conducted on healthy and tumor-bearing animal models, which were either administered Selol or not. We determined antioxidant enzyme activities (Se-GPx, GPx, GST, and TrxR) spectrophotometrically in blood and the tumor. Furthermore, we measured plasma prostate-specific antigen (PSA) levels, plasma and tumor malondialdehyde (MDA) concentration as a biomarker of oxidative stress, selenium (Se) concentrations and the tumor ORAC value. Additionally, we assessed the impact of Selol on tumor morphology and the expression of p53, BCL2, and Ki-67. The results indicate that treatment with Selol influences the morphology of tumor cells, indicating a potential role in inducing cell death through necrosis. Long-term supplementation with Selol increased antioxidant enzyme activity in healthy animals and triggered oxidative stress in cancer cells, activating their antioxidant defense mechanisms. This research pathway shows promise in understanding the anticancer effects of Selol. Selol appears to increase the breakdown of cancer cells more effectively in small tumors than in larger ones. In advanced tumors, it may accelerate tumor growth if used as monotherapy. Therefore, further studies are necessary to evaluate its efficacy either in combination therapy or for the prevention of recurrence.

Keywords: cancer; selenium; Selol; antioxidants; tumor

1. Introduction

Prostate cancer (PCa) is the most prevalent cancer in elderly men, characterized by its aggressive nature leading to metastasis and, frequently, fatality [1]. It is currently the second leading cause of death for men in Western societies [2]. Prostate cancer's pathogenesis remains unclear. PCa development and progression involve various factors, including aging, environmental factors, lifestyle choices, physical activity, genetic alterations, and hormonal influences. Oxidative stress (OS) is thought to contribute directly to the development of prostate cancer [3]. Therefore, OS represents a potential therapeutic target for addressing prostate conditions such as prostatic hypertrophy, cancer, or chronic prostatitis. Oxidative stress in cells results from an imbalance between oxidants and antioxidants, leading to damaged lipids, proteins, and DNA structures. Experimental data suggest that cancer cells, as a result of genetic mutations, have reduced activity in certain antioxidant enzymes compared with normal cells [4]. This diminished enzymatic activity can induce oxidative stress, leading to damage to cellular components and structures in cancerous cells. Among the diverse strategies employed in cancer treatment, one approach involves deliberately elevating reactive oxygen species (ROS) levels within cancer cells. Chemotherapeutic agents like cisplatin, arsenic trioxide, and anthracycline antibiotics operate through this mechanism [5].

Selenium (Se), a micronutrient, participates in various physiological processes [6]. Its importance lies in its role in the catalytic centers of antioxidant enzymes, including selenium-dependent glutathione peroxidase (Se-GPx) and thioredoxin reductase (TrxR) [7]. Selenite, in erythrocytes, when interacting with glutathione, forms biologically active selenodiglutathione, with potent anticancer properties that induce cancer cell apoptosis. Inorganic selenium compounds (+4), more than organic ones (+2), have been found to inhibit cancer cell growth and proliferation due to their pro-oxidant properties, particularly at doses exceeding therapeutic levels [8]. This phenomenon presents potential for anticancer therapy; however, the high toxicity of commercially available inorganic Se (+4) compounds limits their applicability. As a result, there is an ongoing search for selenium (+4) compounds that combine high chemoactivity with low toxicity. Consequently, the synthesis of novel chemopreventive compounds is crucial, with a focus on evaluating their efficacy against various cancer types.

Selol is a selenintriglyceride compound derived from sunflower oil. It has lower toxicity compared with sodium selenite (+4) and has no mutagenic effects [9]. In addition, Selol shows strong cytostatic activity against cancer cell lines, with no side effects on normal cells. Selol is a formulation with potential anticancer activity. Previous in vitro studies demonstrated Selol's significant antitumor effects on human HL-60 leukemia cells, including drug-resistant variants (HL-60/Dox and HL-60/Vinc) [10], as well as HeLa [11] and Caco-2 cancer cells [12]. Książek et al. observed that prostate cancer cells, LNCaP, were more susceptible to apoptosis induction caused by the presence of ROS compared with normal prostate cells—PNT1A [13]. The safety of Selol for normal cells was confirmed in PC12 cells. Selol, through the regulation of free radical levels, the enhancement of the antioxidant system, and the inhibition of apoptosis, protects against oxidative damage and death induced by SNP. Selol is believed to induce the production of ROS in cancer cells, leading to excessive oxidative stress. Healthy cells can manage this stress, while in cancer cells, it may result in apoptosis [14].

Under conditions of chronic oxidative stress, cells activate defensive mechanisms, primarily through the activation of phase 2 enzymes via the Nrf2/ARE signaling pathway. In vivo experiments conducted on a healthy animal model have shown that Selol significantly influences changes in non-enzymatic antioxidants (thiols) and the intracellular and extracellular redox status [15].

However, these findings have not been validated in a cancer animal model, where the tumor itself affects the organism's redox status. Considering the physical conditions, our previous study showed that treating mice with Selol resulted in a drop in the rate of body mass reduction and stopped the increase in plasma prostatic specific antigen (PSA) levels. The expression of genes, involved in oxidative stress following treatment with Selol, in LNCaP cells, did not change. However, it is important to remember that gene expression is not directly linked to enzyme activity. Many factors influence the formation of an active protein [16].

Our goal was to investigate the impact of long-term Selol administration on tumor growth and the oxidative–antioxidative status in both blood and the tumor, which could be crucial for the formulation's effectiveness. We assessed the levels of the antioxidant enzymes glutathione S-transferase (GST), glutathione peroxidase (GPx), and thioredoxin reductase (TrxR), regulated by the Nrf2/ARE pathway, in both the blood and tumor of mice with xenografted LNCaP prostate cancer. Additionally, the study considered the marker of oxidative damage malondialdehyde (MDA) and tumor oxygen-radical absorbance capacity (ORAC) and determined the selenium levels. Prostate-specific antigen (PSA) concentrations before and after Selol administration were also determined. Therefore, it was decided to perform a macroscopic examination of the results obtained and analyze the alterations in the tumor at the histopathological level. Histopathological examinations like morphology and p53, BCL2, and Ki-67 expression were conducted.

2. Materials and Methods

2.1. Compound Characterization

The synthesis of Selol was carried out in the Department of Drugs Analysis at Warsaw Medical University (Patent Pol. PL 176,530 (Cl. A61K31/095)). Selol is a mixture of selenitriglicerides obtained by the chemical modification of sunflower oil, in which a minimum of 11 distinct selenium-containing triglycerol derivatives were identified by using mass spectrometry [17]. In the experiments, Selol 5% at a dose of 17 mg Se/kg body mass was used.

2.2. Ethics Statement

All animal experiments were conducted in accordance with the guidelines set forth by European Communities Directive 2010/63/EU. Ethical approval for the study was obtained from the IV Local Ethics Committee for Animal Experimentation in Warsaw, Poland, under protocol number 33/2009 dated 1 April 2009. Every effort was undertaken to minimize animal distress and to limit the number of animals used. The animal experiments adhered to the ARRIVE guidelines.

2.3. Animal Model

Adult, immunodeficient, sexually mature male NSG mice (NOD.Cg-Prkdc/sc dIl2rg), (approximately 27–35 g, 12 weeks old) were purchased from Charles River Laboratories (Germany). Animals were housed in cages (Centre for Postgraduate Medical Training in Warsaw) maintained under controlled environmental conditions at 20 ± 2 °C room temperature, 40 ± 5% relative humidity, and a 12 h light/dark cycle with a dawn/dusk effect. Mice were fed a complete feed mixture for laboratory animals (LSM, Agropol, Lublin, Poland) and had access to water ad libitum. To reduce stress, the animals were handled for 10 minutes each day and acclimated to the oral gavage procedure over a period of one week prior to the start of the experiments.

2.4. Experimental Protocol

The induction of the tumor was performed in accordance with the results of the pilot studies. The procedure involved implanting 5 million LNCaP cells (an epithelial cell line derived from human prostate carcinoma) into the shoulder of mice. Cells were suspended in Matrigel (Corning® Matrigel® Matrix GFR PhenolRF Mouse; Sigma-Aldrich, Sant Louis, MI, USA), a vital protein mixture that promotes optimal cell culture growth, minimizes single-cell dispersion, and contains essential growth factors.

The animal study lasted eight weeks. Tumors were induced in healthy NSG mice (n = 12). At the end of the fifth week after LNCaP cell inoculation, a significant darkening of the skin at the injection site and the development of tumors were observed. Then, the mice were randomly assigned to the following four main groups: (1) Ca—mice with xenografted LNCaP prostate cancer (n = 6); (2) Control—mice without prostatic tumors (n = 5); (3) Control + Se—mice without prostatic tumors treated with Selol (n = 5); (4) Ca + Se—mice with xenografted LNCaP prostate cancer treated with Selol (n = 6). Each of the study groups (Control + Se and Ca + Se) was supplemented daily per os with a single dose of Selol diluted with vegetable oil equivalent to 17 mg Se/kg body weight (which is approx. 20% of LD50—dose based on the in vivo results from the Selol toxicity study; unpublished data). The Control and Ca groups were fed the standard diet with the same rate of pure vegetable oil (placebo) as the study groups. Placebo and Selol were administered to the animals over three weeks. During the treatment period, all mice were weighed and observed for changes in their behavior twice a week. At the end of the experiment, mice were anesthetized with halothane, the blood was collected for the biochemical measurements, and the tumors were isolated from each mouse for further investigation. In the fifth and eighth weeks of the experiment, PSA concentrations were determined to confirm the presence of prostate cancer and/or the effect of Selol supplementation on the marker.

2.5. *Biochemical Analysis*

The animals underwent a 12-h fast before being sacrificed. Blood samples were collected into heparinized tubes and centrifuged at 1000× g for 15 min at 4 °C to obtain plasma. Red blood cells were washed twice with 0.9% NaCl, and the plasma was refrigerated and stored at −80 °C until analysis. On the analysis day, the samples were thawed at room temperature. Red blood cells intended for enzymatic analysis were hemolyzed by using an equal volume of 3 mM phosphate buffer at pH 7.4 containing 1 mM EDTA. The hemolysates were centrifuged at 1000× g for 20 min at 4 °C, and the supernatants were used for further measurements. The tumors were extracted, weighed, and divided into small fragments. The tumor fragments were briefly exposed to liquid nitrogen for preservation before being stored at −80 °C. All tumor samples were processed within a two months. Before measurement, the tumors were homogenized by using a manual glass homogenizer. For enzyme activity measurements, the samples were homogenized in a chilled medium consisting of 5 mM phosphate buffer, 0.25 mM sucrose, and 0.5 mM EDTA at pH 7.2. Meanwhile, for MDA measurements, a cold medium containing 5 mM pyrophosphate buffer at pH 7.4 was used. The cytosolic fraction of the homogenates was separated by centrifugation at 10,000× g for 20 min at 4 °C.

The following parameters were determined in plasma, erythrocytes, and tumor homogenate supernatants: selenium-dependent glutathione peroxidase (Se-GPx) and total glutathione peroxidase (GPx) activities, and thioredoxin reductase (TrxR) and glutathione S-transferase (GST) activities. Furthermore, plasma prostate-specific antigen (PSA) levels, tumor ORAC values (antioxidant capacity), concentrations of malondialdehyde (MDA) in both plasma and tumors (a marker of lipid peroxidation), and selenium concentrations in erythrocytes and tumors were assessed.

2.5.1. Determination of Enzyme Activity

Selenium-dependent glutathione peroxidase (Se-GPx) and glutathione peroxidase (GPx) activities in plasma, red blood cells, and tumor homogenates were determined spectrophotometrically at a wavelength of 340 nm, using a method originally developed by Paglia and Valentine, modified by Wendel [18,19]. The reaction was carried out at 25 °C in 50 mM sodium phosphate buffer containing 0.40 mM EDTA at pH 7.0. A supernatant/plasma volume of 10 µL was utilized for enzyme activity analysis. In the final reaction mixture (total volume of 220 µL), the concentrations were as follows: reduced glutathione (GSH) at 1.0 mM, NADPH at 65 µM, and sodium azide at 0.17 mM. For the Se-GPx activity assay, a substrate tert-butyl hydroperoxide was employed at a concentration of 0.02 mM. Cumene hydroperoxide at 1.05 mM concentration was used for the GPx activity determination.

Glutathione S-transferase (GST) activity in plasma, red blood cells, and tumor homogenates was quantified by using spectrophotometric methods at a wavelength of 340 nm, employing the Habig assay [20]. The enzymatic reaction took place at 25 °C in 50 mM sodium phosphate buffer supplemented with 0.50 mM EDTA at pH 7.5. A 10 µL aliquot of supernatant/plasma was utilized to assess enzyme activity. The final reaction mixture, with a total volume of 200 μL, contained 2 mM reduced glutathione (GSH) and 1 mM 1-chloro-2,4-dinitrobenzene (CDNB) as the substrate.

Thioredoxin reductase (TrxR) activity in plasma, red blood cells, and tumor homogenates was assessed spectrophotometrically at a wavelength of 412 nm, using the modifications outlined by Hill et al. [21]. The enzymatic reaction was conducted at 37 °C in 50 mM sodium phosphate buffer supplemented with 1 mM EDTA at pH 7.0. A 10 μL of the supernatant was used for the enzyme activity analysis. In the final reaction mixture, with a volume of 200 μL, the concentrations were as follows: 4 mM 5,5′-dithiobis(2-nitrobenzoic acid) (DTNB) as the substrate, 2 μM nicotinamide adenine dinucleotide phosphate (NADPH) as the enzymatic reaction cofactor, and 1 mM auranofin (ATM) as a specific inhibitor of the enzyme under study. Thioredoxin reductase activity was determined by measuring the difference in enzymatic activity between samples tested without and with the inhibitor [22,23].

2.5.2. Determination of Malondialdehyde Concentration

The concentration of malondialdehyde (MDA) in both plasma and tumor homogenates was quantified by using an ELISA spectrophotometric assay kit (Wuhan EIAAB Science Co., Ltd., Wuhan, China), following the manufacturer's instructions.

2.5.3. Determination of Oxygen-Radical Absorbance Capacity (ORAC)

The ORAC-FL assay, as described by Ou et al. [24], involved measuring the antioxidant capacity of samples. Hitachi F-7000 (Hitachi, Tokyo, Japan) spectrofluorometer with excitation at 485 nm and emission at 520 nm was used to determine the ORAC value of supernatants of tumor tissues. Black 96-well plates (Greiner Bio-One, Kremsmünster, Austria) were employed in the assay. All solutions (fluorescein and AAPH) were freshly prepared in PBS buffer at pH 7.4 daily. The reaction mixture consisted of 13 mM AAPH and fluorescein at 40 nM.

2.5.4. Determination of Prostate-Specific Antigen (PSA) Concentration

The PSA levels in the mice's plasma were assessed twice, labeled as PSA1 and PSA2. At the end of the fifth week, 150 μL of blood was extracted from the tail of each mouse for the initial PSA measurement (PSA1). After three weeks of administering Selol/placebo, the mice were humanely sacrificed, and their blood was gathered for the subsequent PSA level analysis (PSA2). Following collection, the blood was centrifuged to obtain plasma for the evaluation of PSA levels by using immunodetection (Human PSA-total ELISA Kit; Sigma-Aldrich, Sant Louis, MI, USA; as recommended by the manufacturer).

2.5.5. Determination of Protein and Hemoglobin Concentration

The protein concentration in tumor tissue supernatants was determined by using a spectrophotometric assay with Bradford reagent (Sigma-Aldrich, Sant Louis, MI, USA). The absorbance of the protein-bound Coomassie Brilliant Blue G-250 dye was read at 595 nm. Protein concentrations were calculated based on a standard curve prepared by using bovine serum albumin (BSA) as the reference standard. The hemoglobin concentration of red blood cell (RBC) hemolysates was assessed spectrophotometrically at 546 nm by using a standard immunodetection assay (Human hemoglobin ELISA Kit; Sigma-Aldrich, Sant Louis, MI, USA; as recommended by the manufacturer). Measurements of enzymatic activity, hemoglobin concentration, and protein absorbance were conducted by using a spectrophotometer microplate reader (Synergy MX, BioTek® Instruments, Inc., Winooski, VT, USA).

2.5.6. Determination of Selenium Concentration

To quantify the complete selenium (Se) content in red blood cells and tumor tissues, an inductively coupled plasma mass spectrometer (ICP-MS) (Thermo Fisher Scientific,

Waltham, MA, USA) was used [25,26]. Tissue samples were homogenized in a mixture of 65% HNO_3 and 30% H_2O_2 (in a 3:1 ratio). Subsequently, homogenized samples were transferred to Teflon crucibles and subjected to mineralization by using a microwave mineralizer. For erythrocyte samples, 100 µL aliquots were transferred to Teflon crucibles containing a mineralization mixture as mentioned above, followed by mineralization. The samples were then used for ICPMS analyses, with quality control samples.

2.6. Histopathological Examination

Histopathological evaluation was performed on tissue sections from tumor-bearing animals (n = 5). The lesions assessed were nodules with macroscopic diameters ranging from 3 to 4 mm in control animals and from 3 to 5 mm in animals treated with the active substance. After evaluation, tissues were processed by embedding in 10% buffered formalin, sectioned into 7 µm slices, and stained with hematoxylin and eosin (H&E). Examination of the prepared slides was conducted by using an, Olympus BX41 microscope with an Olympus DP25 camera and cellSens software For immunohistochemical evaluation, slides were cut to a thickness of 4 µm on salinized slides and transferred to a hothouse (50 °C). Staining was performed with DAKO antibodies by using Dako AutostainerLink 48 platform. Slides were transferred to buffer (Target Retrieval Solution EnVision FLEX) at pH 9.0 or 6.0 at PTLink to open antigenic dominance EnVision Detection Kit (Env FLEX, High pH, DAKO) was used. Antibodies against p53, BCL2, and Ki-67 (DAKO Omnis, Agilent Technologies, Santa Clara, CA, USA were used to assess protein expression levels and to evaluate tumor characteristics. Slides were stained with hematoxylin, washed with water, dehydrated with a series of alcohols, overexposed with xylene, and sealed in BDX.

2.7. Statistical Analysis

The data are presented as the means ± standard deviation (SD). Statistical analyses were performed by using one-way ANOVA to compare means among multiple groups, followed by Tukey's and Dunnett's post-hoc tests for pairwise comparisons. The Mann–Whitney U test was used for comparing two independent groups, and the Spearman correlation and multiple regression test was used to assess the strength and direction of the association between two and more than two variables, respectively. A p-value of less than 0.05 was considered significant. Statistical tests were performed by using Statistica software (version 10, StatSoft, TIBCO Software, Warsaw, Poland).

3. Results

3.1. Antioxidant Enzymes

The levels of antioxidant enzymes, such as Se-GPx, GST, and TrxR, in blood plasma were significantly higher in the group of mice with xenografted LNCaP prostate cancer (Ca) compared with the control group (Control) (p = 0.0001, p = 0.0061, and p = 0.02; Table 1). However, no significant differences were observed in the activities of antioxidant enzymes (Se-GPx, GST, TrxR, and GPx) in the erythrocytes of these two groups of mice. In the healthy mice group, the administration of Selol increased Se-GPx activity in blood plasma (Control + Se) (p = 0.0020), as well as Se-GPx, GPx, and GST activities in erythrocytes (p = 0.0003, p = 0.0004, and p = 0.0152, respectively; Table 1).

This effect was not observed in mice with xenografted LNCaP prostate cancer. However, in this group, the activities of Se-GPx, GPx, and GST were higher in the tumor compared with the mice receiving a placebo (Figure 1a,b).

Table 1. Selenoenzyme activities: Se-dependent (Se-GPx), total glutathione peroxidase activity (GPx), and thioredoxin activity (TrxR) in plasma and red blood cells of control mice (Control and Ca) and mice treated with Selol (Control + Se and Ca + Se). Ca + Se—mice with xenografted LNCaP prostate cancer treated with Selol; Ca—mice with xenografted LNCaP prostate cancer treated with placebo; Control—mice without prostatic tumors treated with placebo; Control + Se—mice without prostatic tumors treated with Selol.

Groups	Se-GPx Plasma (U/mL)/ RBC (U/g Hb)	GPx Plasma (U/mL)/ RBC (U/g Hb)	TrxR Plasma (U/mL)/ RBC (U/g Hb)
Ca + Se	$0.83 \pm 0.14^{ab}/1.4 \pm 0.5^{a}$	$0.59 \pm 0.12^{a}/1.68 \pm 1.38^{c}$	$0.053 \pm 0.008^{a}/0.7 \pm 0.5^{b}$
Ca	$0.85 \pm 0.11^{ab}/1.2 \pm 0.3^{a}$	$0.53 \pm 0.07^{a}/1.29 \pm 0.99^{a}$	$0.071 \pm 0.009^{b}/1.6 \pm 0.8^{a}$
Control	$0.49 \pm 0.07^{a}/1.3 \pm 0.2^{a}$	$0.70 \pm 0.13^{b}/1.34 \pm 0.75^{a}$	$0.057 \pm 0.011^{a}/1.5 \pm 0.7^{a}$
Control + Se	$0.63 \pm 0.07^{b}/2.3 \pm 0.4^{b}$	$0.82 \pm 0.19^{b}/2.22 \pm 1.02^{b}$	$0.052 \pm 0.009^{a}/1.4 \pm 0.2^{a}$

Data are presented as means ± standard deviation (SD). For the control groups (Control and Control + Se), $n = 5$, and for the tumor-bearing groups (Ca and Ca + Se), $n = 6$. The mean values in columns with different superscript letter(s) are significantly different at $p < 0.05$, as assessed by Tukey's post hoc test.

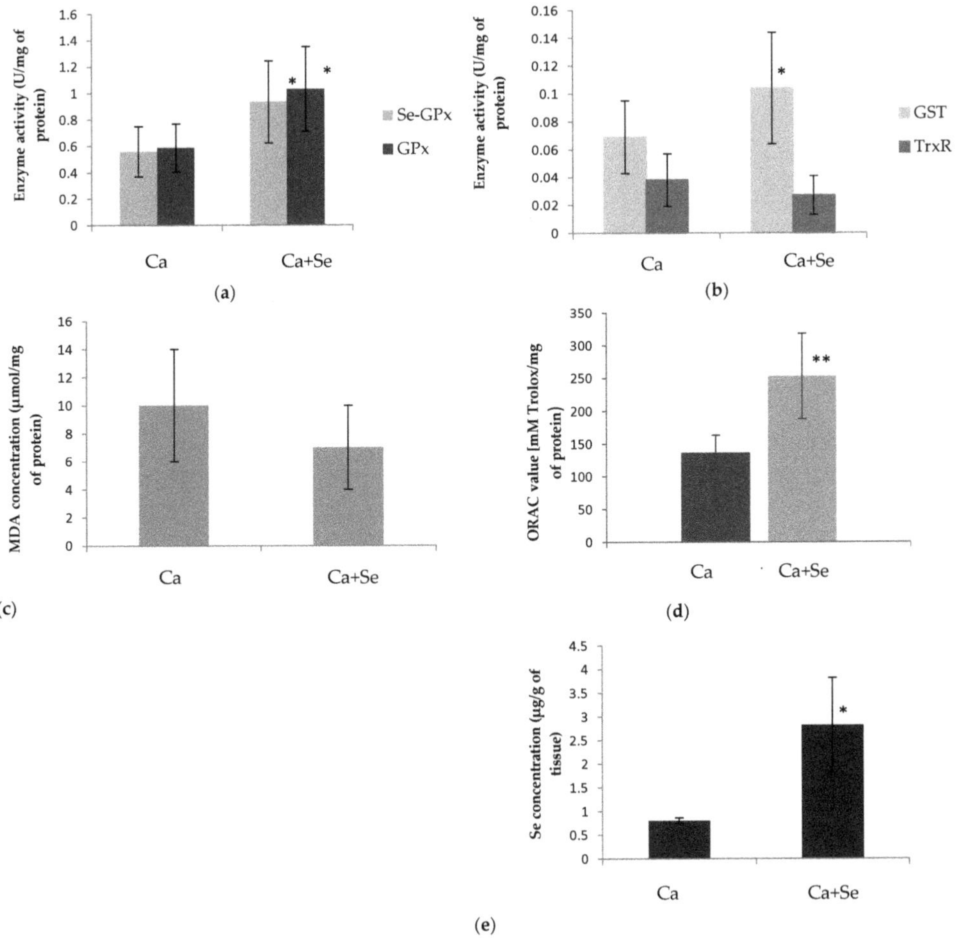

Figure 1. The mean enzyme activities of selenium-dependent glutathione peroxidase (Se-GPx) and total glutathione peroxidase (GPx) (**a**), and glutathione S-transferase (GST) and thioredoxin reductase

(TrxR) (**b**); concentration of malondialdehyde (MDA) (**c**), ORAC value (**d**), and selenium (Se) concentration (**e**) in the tumor tissue of mice with xenografted LNCaP prostate cancer supplemented with Selol (Ca + Se) and control group of mice with xenografted LNCaP prostate supplemented with placebo (Ca). Data are shown as means ± SD (n = 6). The p-values indicate differences between control group (Ca) and study group (Ca + Se) and are indicated by * $p < 0.05$, ** $p < 0.01$.

3.2. Marker of Lipid Peroxidation

The plasma MDA levels were significantly higher in the group with LNCaP prostate cancer compared with the control group ($p = 0.0037$; Table 2). However, Selol administration to the healthy group increased MDA levels ($p = 0.0065$); this effect was not observed in mice with xenografted LNCaP prostate cancer. There were no significant differences observed in the concentration of MDA within the tumor, whether the mice were administered selenium or not (Figure 1c).

Table 2. Glutathione S-transferase activity (GST), malondialdehyde concentration (MDA), and selenium concentration (Se) in plasma and/or red blood cells of control mice (Control and Ca) and mice treated with Selol (Control + Se and Ca + Se). Ca + Se—mice with xenografted LNCaP prostate cancer treated with Selol; Ca—mice with xenografted LNCaP prostate cancer treated with placebo; Control—mice without prostatic tumors treated with placebo; Control + Se—mice without prostatic tumors treated with Selol.

Groups	GST Plasma (U/mL)/ RBC (U/g Hb)	MDA Plasma (nmol/mL)	Se RBC (μg/g Hb)
Ca + Se	0.063 ± 0.004 ^{b}/0.064 ± 0.001 ^{c}	78 ± 19 ^{b}	1.00 ± 0.34 ^{d}
Ca	0.064 ± 0.005 ^{b}/0.062 ± 0.005 ^{c}	87 ± 15 ^{b}	0.54 ± 0.14 ^{c}
Control	0.041 ± 0.001 ^{a}/0.045 ± 0.001 ^{a}	72 ± 12 ^{a}	0.40 ± 0.09 ^{a}
Control + Se	0.046 ± 0.002 ^{a}/0.054 ± 0.001 ^{b}	86 ± 9 ^{b}	0.76 ± 0.08 ^{b}

Data are presented as means ± standard deviation (SD). For the control groups (Control and Control + Se), n = 5, and for the tumor-bearing groups (Ca and Ca + Se), n = 6. The mean values in columns with different superscript letter(s) are significantly different at $p < 0.05$, as assessed by Tukey's post hoc test.

3.3. ORAC Value

The tumor tissue oxygen-radical absorbance capacity (ORAC) was significantly higher in the group of mice treated with Selol (Ca + Se) compared with the placebo group (Ca) (Figure 1d).

3.4. Selenium Concentration

The administration of Selol resulted in an increase in selenium levels in erythrocytes, both in the group of healthy mice and mice with LNCaP prostate cancer ($p = 0.0001$ in both cases). Interestingly, in mice receiving Selol, higher selenium concentrations were observed in LNCaP mice than in healthy mice ($p = 0.0002$; Table 2). As expected, the tumors in mice with xenografted LNCaP prostate cancer that received Selol (Ca + Se) showed significantly higher selenium levels compared with the control group that received the placebo (Ca) (Figure 1e).

3.5. Morphological Study

The tumors of both the study and placebo mice displayed a range of sizes, all characterized by noticeable blood vessel proliferation. Significant differences in tumor appearance were observed between the two experimental groups. Tumors in mice treated with Selol (Ca + Se) appeared darker in color, exhibited swollen interiors, and in some regions, had a "jelly-like" consistency. In contrast, tumors in mice treated with the placebo (Ca) maintained a dense and firm structure. Furthermore, there were no observable alterations in the tissue appearance of other organs in mice that received Selol (Ca + Se and Control + Se).

3.6. PSA Concentration, Tumor Mass, and Body Weight of Mice

Plasma PSA levels were higher in all tumor-bearing mice (n = 12) compared with non-tumor-bearing mice (n = 10), which had PSA levels below 0.003 ng/mL (Table 3). In both the Selol-supplemented (Ca + Se) and placebo (Ca) groups, the plasma PSA levels at the end of the experiment were significantly higher than before treatment ($p = 0.02771$). We noticed the inverse correlation between the tumor mass and the weight of tumor-bearing mice after subtracting tumor mass (M3) at the end of the experiment ($r_s = 0.8936$, $p = 0.0044$) (Table 3), which demonstrates that as the tumor size increases, the mouse mass decreases, and the overall condition worsens.

Table 3. Tumor mass, plasma prostate-specific antigen (PSA) concentration before (PSA1) and after (PSA2) Selol/placebo administration, and weight of mice minus weight of isolated tumor at the end of experiment (M3). Ca + Se—mice with xenografted LNCaP prostate cancer treated with Selol; Ca—mice with xenografted LNCaP prostate cancer treated with placebo; Control—mice without prostatic tumors treated with placebo; Control + Se—mice without prostatic tumors treated with Selol.

Groups	Tumor Mass (g)	PSA1 (ng/mL)	PSA2 (ng/mL)	M3 (g)
Ca + Se	0.75 ± 0.48^{a}	26 ± 19^{a}	117 ± 81^{a}	26.9 ± 3.5^{a}
Ca	0.56 ± 0.17^{a}	20 ± 14^{a}	71 ± 28^{a}	26.57 ± 0.92^{a}
Control	-	<0.003	<0.003	27.1 ± 1.3^{a}
Control + Se	-	<0.003	<0.003	28.4 ± 0.9^{a}

Data are presented as means ± standard deviation (SD). For the control groups (Control and Control + Se), n = 5, and for the tumor-bearing groups (Ca and Ca + Se), n = 6. The mean values in columns with different superscript letter(s) are significantly different at $p < 0.05$, as assessed by Tukey's post hoc test.

Due to the high variability of PSA2 levels and tumor mass in the Ca + Se group, the first step involved plotting the relationship between the PSA values at the beginning (PSA1) and at the end of the study (PSA2), assuming it to be an indicator of cell number. A clear trend was observed for the Ca group, showing a positive correlation between PSA at the beginning and at the end of the experiment ($R^2 = 0.878$, a = 1.846) (Figure 2a). In the Ca + Se group, it was observed that the results for two mice significantly deviated from the trend (marked with red loops) showing higher PSA levels at the end of the study than would be expected based on the initial PSA values. These mice had initial PSA (PSA1) levels greater than 30 ng/mL and were administered Se. If these individuals are excluded from the analysis, it can be noted that for mice with lower initial PSA levels (PSA1), a greater increase in PSA was observed at the end (PSA2) (R^2 =0.626, a= −1.018) (a different trend than in the Ca group, where the relationship was directly proportional). Adding tumor mass to the analysis (Figure 2b), it can be seen that mice with small tumors in the Ca+ Se group exhibited significantly higher PSA2 levels ($R^2 = 0.7252$, a = −0.0158) compared with mice with larger tumors (in the Ca group, this relationship was again directly proportional; $R^2 = 0.8686$, a = 0.0057). Given that high PSA can also be a marker of cell breakdown, it can be inferred that Se is effective in the case of small tumors (PSA < 30 ng/mL at the beginning of the study) but may not be suitable as monotherapy for advanced tumors. In our case, these two individuals (PSA > 30 ng/mL) exhibited significantly larger tumor masses than predicted based on the trend line in the control group. However, the level of secreted PSA was proportional to the tumor size (estimated based on the trend line for the control group), suggesting the lack of Se action in slowing tumor growth.

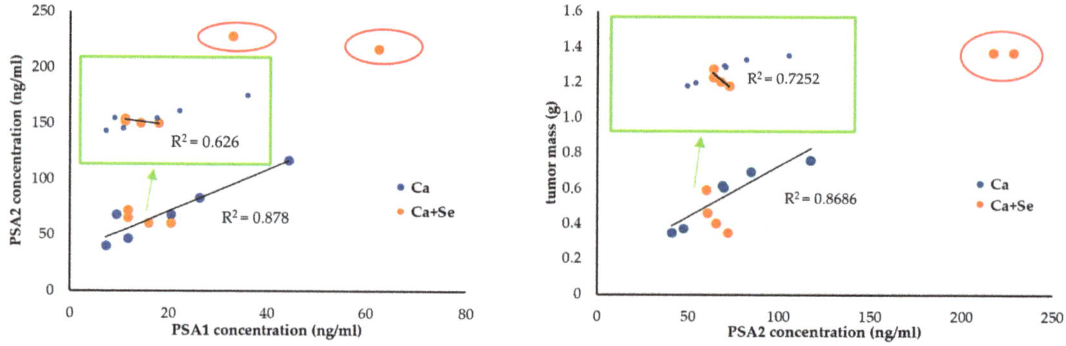

(**a**) (**b**)

Figure 2. Relationship between PSA concentrations at the beginning (PSA1) and end (PSA2) of the experiment in tumor-bearing mice treated with Selol (Ca + Se, *n* = 6) or placebo (Ca, *n* = 6). Notably, two mice in the Ca + Se group significantly deviated from the expected trend (indicated by red loops) (**a**). Relationship between PSA concentration at the end of the experiment (PSA2) and tumor mass in tumor-bearing mice treated with Selol (Ca + Se, *n* = 6) or placebo (Ca, *n* = 6). Two mice in the Ca + Se group showed significant deviations from the overall trend (indicated by red loops) (**b**).

We observed that in the study group (Ca + Se) with small tumors ($n = 4$), an increase in PSA2 levels and the relative increase in PSA positively correlated with higher MDA levels (B = 2.35, $p = 0.016$; B =2.21, $p = 0.020$, respectively) and negatively correlated with ORAC values (B= −2.22, $p = 0.017$; B= −1.65, $p = 0.027$, respectively). Additionally, there was a positive correlation between the animals' weight (M3) and MDA concentration (B = 2.31, $p = 0.0031$) and a negative correlation with ORAC values (B= −2.22, $p = 0.0030$). This indicates that if we use the mice's weight as an indicator of well-being, a higher weight is associated with increased MDA levels in tumors and decreased ORAC values. These findings appear to support the hypothesis that the induction of oxidative stress might be a mechanism through which Selol exerts its effects.

The described relationship was not observed in the placebo group (Ca). In this group, there was only a negative correlation between the relative increase in PSA and the ORAC value (B = −0.89, $p = 0.042$). In contrast, in the study group with small tumors (Ca + Se), cancer cells exhibited greater susceptibility to the pro-oxidant effects of Selol, as evidenced by the increased levels of MDA and high PSA release.

3.7. Histological Study

In the control group (Ca), tumor tissues from animals exhibited intact tumor cells (Figure 3a). In contrast, the Selol-treated group (Ca + Se) displayed focal necrosis ranging from 10% to 30% near blood vessels (Figure 3b). Both groups, control and Selol-treated mice, showed highly proliferative tumor cells with abnormal mitotic figures (Figure 3a–d). Furthermore, tumor tissues in the control group exhibited a compact structure (Figure 3c), whereas after Selol treatment, there was a reduction in tumor foci, with tumor cell nests surrounded by bands of fibrous stroma (Figure 3d). The sparse stroma in both groups (Ca and Ca + Se) exhibited dense vascularization without morphotic elements indicative of an inflammatory reaction.

Additionally, immunohistochemical staining for p53 and BCL2 genes, as well as the Ki-67 protein, revealed no differences in their expression between the groups (Figure 3e–j).

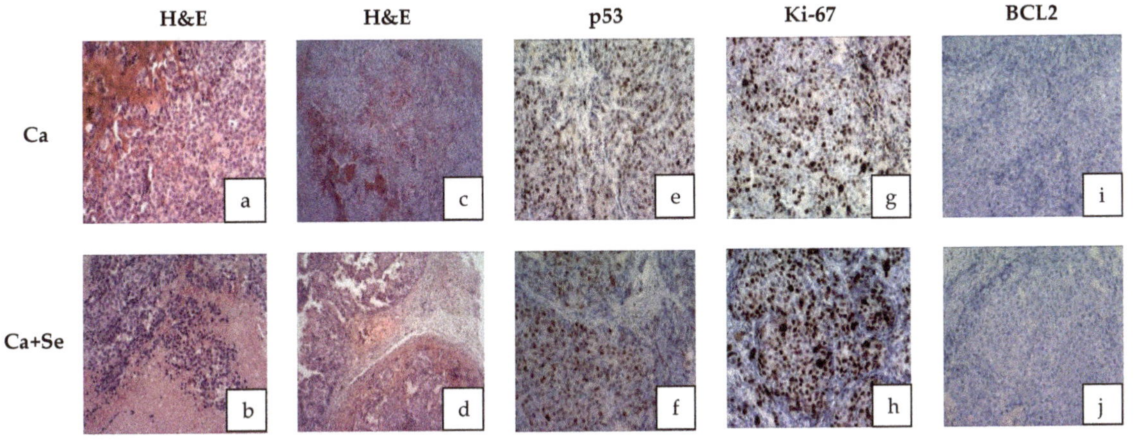

Figure 3. Histological photomicrographs of tumor sections stained with (**a**–**d**) H&E (hematoxylin and eosin): no features of necrosis (**a**); features of necrosis (**b**); lite tumor tissue (**c**) reduction in tumor foci (**d**); (**e**,**f**) stained with p53 (no gene expression in both cases); (**g**,**h**) stained with Ki-67 (features of high proliferation activity in both cases); and (**i**,**j**) stained with BCL2 (no gene expression in both cases). Ca + Se—mice with xenografted LNCaP prostate cancer supplemented with Selol; Ca—control group of mice with xenografted LNCaP prostate supplemented with placebo.

4. Discussion

This study explores the biochemical mechanism of action of Selol, a novel organic selenium compound with promising anticancer and pro-oxidant properties. It investigates how Selol induces oxidative stress, focusing on its impact on cells with heightened metabolic activity and oncogenic signaling. The production of reactive oxygen species (ROS) by pro-oxidant compounds can cause damage to cellular structures, ultimately resulting in the death of cancer cells. This discovery presents a promising opportunity for the development of therapeutic approaches in cancer treatment [27,28].

The presented study shows that Selol administration to animals with prostate cancer increased antioxidant enzyme activity and selenium concentration in tumor tissues. The ORAC value, indicating the antioxidant capacity of tumor tissues, was observed to be higher after Selol treatment. This elevated ORAC value is likely associated with the presence of selenium. It is probable that other tissues or organs in tumor-bearing mice treated with Selol would similarly exhibit enhanced ORAC values. Consistent with this, our recent studies in healthy mice have demonstrated significant increases in ORAC levels in both blood and organs following Selol supplementation [29]. However, there were no significant changes in the concentration of MDA (marker of oxidative stress) in the tumor tissues of the Selol-treated group. It is possible that the levels of oxidative stress in cancer cells may not always correlate with the level of lipid peroxidation products. The concentration of 4-hydroxynonenal, an aldehyde produced during lipid peroxidation, varies depending on the type of cancer and the stage of the tumor [29]. This variation might be due to different levels of activity of aldehyde-metabolizing enzymes that are affected by the progression of cancer, thereby impacting the concentration of aldehyde products from lipid peroxidation [30]. Selol can induce the expression of these enzymes, in the same way as antioxidant enzymes, as they share a common pathway for activation (e.g., through the Nrf2/ARE pathway, which is activated by oxidative stress) [31]. Therefore, the lack of difference in MDA levels despite ongoing oxidative stress may be justified. According to Ksiazek et al., malignant prostate cells (LNCaP) have a weaker antioxidant defense compared with normal cells (PNT1A). Therefore, tumors inducing antioxidant enzymes in response to oxidative stress might not sufficiently counteract its effects, leading to apoptotic changes in cancer cells [13]. In summary, the increase in antioxidant enzyme activity and antioxidant capacity value and the lack of differences in MDA levels in Ca-treated mice may suggest the presence of oxidative stress. This may lead to molecular changes that can result in cell death but also exert anticancer effects. To confirm this hypothesis, further investigation into other markers of oxidation is necessary.

As mentioned previously, after treatment with Selol, we observed an increase in the activity of antioxidant enzymes in tumors, specifically GSH-dependent ones, like Se-GPx, GPx, and GST. The presence of ROS (induced by Selol) causes oxidative stress, leading to the oxidation of sulfhydryl groups and a decrease in the concentration of intracellular GSH. Then, ROS activate the Nrf2-ARE pathway, which leads to the production of antioxidants and an increase in antioxidant enzyme levels in tissues. However, the heightened activity of these antioxidants, including GPx and GST, can deplete further the reduced form of GSH, which serves as a substrate for these enzymes [31]. The enzyme that reduces GSH is TrxR. Here, we observed higher activity of Se-GPx, GPx, and GST as well as antioxidant capacity in the tumor, leading to the consumption of GSH and its conversion into GSSG. However, TrxR activity remained unchanged, indicating no significant effect on the reduction of oxidized proteins that may accumulate in the cell. These findings are supported by previous research, which observed higher GSSG and lower GSH levels in the tumor after Selol treatment [15]. Further decline in glutathione concentration may result from aldehyde products formed during lipid peroxidation, reacting with glutathione (GSH) and forming rapidly eliminated conjugates [32]. All these changes lead to a decrease in the concentration of reduced GSH and an increase in the oxidative form of GSSG. This enhances the oxidoreductive potential in cancer cells, inducing them to undergo apoptosis [33,34]. Interestingly, despite administering Selol, our previous research on the same experimental group showed no significant changes in the expression of oxidative stress-related genes, such as GPx and GST, within the tumor [13]. This finding highlights the importance of phenotypic studies, including the measurement of enzymatic activities, which, although more time-consuming than gene expression screenings, provide crucial insights that might be overlooked in genetic analyses.

In evaluating the effects of Selol administration on tumor size, mouse weight (as a measure of overall well-being), and PSA levels at the end of the experiment, significant variability was observed in the treated group (CV = 62% vs. 31% for tumor weight and 70% vs. 40% for PSA2 levels). This variation suggests the presence of ongoing processes, potentially necrosis, with dynamics that vary among individuals. Based on the notable fluctuations in PSA levels and tumor sizes observed in the study, particularly after excluding individuals with large tumor masses and elevated PSA values (as shown in Section 3.6), our findings indicate that Se may be particularly effective against smaller tumors. This suggests its potential role in preventing metastasis or serving as a complementary treatment alongside therapies like chemotherapy or surgery, especially in advanced cancer stages. The obtained results support the in vitro studies on the Selol interaction with standard chemotherapy drugs, which have shown that it can significantly enhance the antiproliferative effects of doxorubicin, especially in cells resistant to the drug [11]. Additionally, in situations of vincristine-induced hyperalgesia, Selol improved the analgesic effects of fentanyl, buprenorphine, and morphine [10]. However, this hypothesis must be verified.

The elevated PSA levels observed at the end of the experiment in the small-tumor group treated with Selol could be attributed to a temporary rise in PSA, often referred to as a "PSA flare". This phenomenon is likely caused by the breakdown of tumor cells, which releases PSA into the bloodstream as the cancer cells are destroyed [35,36]. This transient increase in PSA is not necessarily indicative of treatment failure. Instead, it reflects the dynamic process of tumor response and should be interpreted in conjunction with other clinical findings and diagnostic tests. Proper evaluation of this PSA fluctuation is essential to distinguishing between actual disease progression and a temporary flare-up due to effective treatment. Furthermore, considering the variations in oxidative stress markers, including MDA and ORAC, as well as PSA levels and animal weights, we can conclude that smaller tumors may be more sensitive to the pro-oxidant effects of Selol.

The tumor morphology in mice treated with Selol differed from that in the placebo group. These differences, supported by histopathological studies, suggest the onset of tumor cell necrosis in the Selol-treated group. Given that the tumors of animals in the Ca + Se group exhibited a different consistency, it may turn out that they are more sensitive to chemotherapy or other types of anticancer therapy. It is worth conducting research in this direction, which suggests promising new therapeutic options for palliative care, especially for patients in the final stages of cancer.

Furthermore, histological study revealed that Selol treatment influences tumors by inducing tumor cell degeneration, focal necrosis, and constriction of tumor cell fields by connective tissue. However, there was no observed effect on the degradation of the mutated p53 gene. The proliferative activity of tumor tissue remained unaffected, and there was no suppression of apoptosis, as evidenced by the absence of BCL2 oncogene expression. The mechanism of Selol's action in this specific type of cancer may differ from its effects in other cell lines, such as A545, where both apoptosis and necrosis contribute to its mechanism [37].

In reassessing the effects of Selol on biochemical parameters, this study found no significant changes in the activities of selenium-dependent glutathione peroxidase (Se-GPx) and glutathione S-transferase (GST) in the plasma and erythrocytes of tumor-bearing mice following Selol supplementation. Additionally, the levels of MDA were comparable in both groups. However, in healthy mice, supplementation with Selol increased the activity of antioxidant enzymes in red blood cells and SeGSHPx activity and MDA concentration in plasma, which supports the previous finding that long-term Selol intake affects antioxidant enzyme activity in the blood of healthy animals [27,38]. The lack of increased antioxidant enzyme activity and the elevation in MDA levels in the plasma of tumor-bearing mice after Selol administration may be attributed to their pre-existing high levels due to the cancerous process. Tumors initiate processes like division, metabolism, and inflammatory cytokine release, leading to increased reactive oxygen species (ROS) production. This aligns with previous studies indicating heightened oxidative stress in tumor cells, impacting antioxidant enzyme activity. In various human tumors, reduced levels of superoxide dismutase and catalase activities have been observed, accompanied by an increase in GSH-dependent enzymes and thioredoxin reductase activity [37].

5. Conclusions

Prolonged supplementation with this novel selenium compound leads to a significant increase in the activity of antioxidant enzymes in the blood of healthy animal models, as shown previously. Selol treatment in tumor-bearing mice influences the morphology of tumor cells, inducing necrotic changes. Additionally, it affects the antioxidant–pro-oxidant potential in the tumor, likely due to oxidative stress. Se appears to increase the breakdown of cancer cells more effectively in small tumors than in larger ones. In advanced tumors, it may accelerate tumor growth if used as monotherapy. Therefore, further studies are necessary to evaluate its efficacy either in combination therapy or for the prevention of recurrence.

Author Contributions: Conceptualization, M.S., J.G. and P.S.; methodology, M.S. and K.S.; software, M.S. and J.G.; validation, M.S. and J.G.; formal analysis, M.S. and J.G.; investigation, M.S., M.R., G.H. and J.G.; resources, M.S. and J.G.; data curation M.S. and J.G.; writing—original draft preparation, M.S. and J.G.; writing—review and editing, M.S. and J.G.; visualization, M.S.; supervision, J.G.; project administration, J.G.; funding acquisition, M.S., P.S. and J.G. All authors have read and agreed to the published version of the manuscript.

Funding: This research was funded by the Polish Ministry of Science and Higher Education based on contract 3606/B/P01/2010/39 as part of research project N N405 360639.

Institutional Review Board Statement: The animal study protocol was approved by the IV Local Ethics Committee for Animal Experimentation in Warsaw, Poland (protocol number 33/2009 on 1 April 2009).

Informed Consent Statement: Not applicable.

Data Availability Statement: The data presented in this study are available upon request form corresponding author.

Conflicts of Interest: The authors declare no conflicts of interest.

References

1. Rawla, P. Epidemiology of Prostate Cancer. *World J. Oncol.* **2019**, *10*, 63–89. [CrossRef] [PubMed]
2. Stangelberger, A.; Waldert, M.; Djavan, B. Prostate cancer in elderly men. *Rev. Urol.* **2008**, *10*, 111–119. [PubMed]
3. Liu, M.; Wang, D.; Luo, Y.; Hu, L.; Bi, Y.; Ji, J.; Huang, H.; Wang, J.; Zhu, L.; Ma, J. Selective killing of cancer cells harboring mutant RAS by concomitant inhibition of NADPH oxidase and glutathione biosynthesis. *Cell Death Dis.* **2021**, *12*, 189. [CrossRef]
4. Yang, H.; Villani, R.M.; Wang, H.; Simpson, M.J.; Roberts, M.S.; Tang, M.; Liang, X. The role of cellular reactive oxygen species in cancer chemotherapy. *J. Exp. Clin. Cancer Res.* **2018**, *37*, 266. [CrossRef]
5. Kieliszek, M.; Bano, I. Selenium as an important factor in various disease states—A review. *Excli J.* **2022**, *21*, 948–966. [CrossRef] [PubMed]
6. Benhar, M. Roles of mammalian glutathione peroxidase and thioredoxin reductase enzymes in the cellular response to nitrosative stress. *Free Radic. Biol. Med.* **2018**, *127*, 160–164. [CrossRef]
7. Gandin, V.; Khalkar, P.; Braude, J.; Fernandes, A.P. Organic selenium compounds as potential chemotherapeutic agents for improved cancer treatment. *Free Radic. Biol. Med.* **2018**, *127*, 80–97. [CrossRef]
8. Radomska, D.; Czarnomysy, R.; Radomski, D.; Bielawski, K. Selenium Compounds as Novel Potential Anticancer Agents. *Int. J. Mol. Sci.* **2021**, *22*, 1009. [CrossRef]
9. Rahden-Staroń, I.; Suchocki, P.; Czeczot, H. Evaluation of mutagenic activity of the organo-selenium compound Selol by use of the Salmonella typhimurium mutagenicity assay. *Mutat. Res.* **2010**, *699*, 44–46. [CrossRef]
10. Suchocki, P.; Misiewicz, I.; Skupinska, K.; Waclawek, K.; Fijalek, Z.; Kasprzycka-Guttman, T. The activity of Selol in multidrug-resistant and sensitive human leukemia cells. *Oncol. Rep.* **2007**, *18*, 893–899. [CrossRef]
11. Dudkiewicz-Wilczyńska, J.; Grabowska, A.; Książek, I.; Sitarz, K.; Suchocki, P.; Anuszewska, E. Comparison of selected gene expression profiles in sensitive and resistant cancer cells treated with doxorubicin and Selol. *Contemp. Oncol.* **2014**, *18*, 90–94. [CrossRef] [PubMed]
12. Suchocki, P.; Misiewicz-Krzemińska, I.; Skupińska, K.; Niedźwiecka, K.; Lubelska, K.; Fijałek, Z.; Kasprzycka-Guttman, T. Selenitetriglicerydes affect CYP1A1 and QR activity by involvement of reactive oxygen species and Nrf2 transcription factor. *Pharmacol. Rep.* **2010**, *62*, 352–361. [CrossRef]
13. Ksiazek, I.; Sitarz, K.; Roslon, M.; Anuszewska, E.; Suchocki, P.; Wilczynska, J.D. The influence of Selol on the expression of oxidative stress genes in normal and malignant prostate cells. *Cancer Genomics. Proteomics.* **2013**, *10*, 225–232.
14. Dominiak, A.; Wilkaniec, A.; Jęśko, H.; Czapski, G.A.; Lenkiewicz, A.M.; Kurek, E.; Wroczyński, P.; Adamczyk, A. Selol, an organic selenium donor, prevents lipopolysaccharide-induced oxidative stress and inflammatory reaction in the rat brain. *Neurochem. Int.* **2017**, *108*, 66–77. [CrossRef]
15. Flis, A.; Suchocki, P.; Królikowska, M.A.; Suchocka, Z.; Remiszewska, M.; Śliwka, L.; Książek, I.; Sitarz, K.; Sochacka, M.; Hoser, G.; et al. Selenitetriglycerides-Redox-active agents. *Pharmacol. Rep.* **2015**, *67*, 1–8. [CrossRef] [PubMed]
16. Ksiazek, I.; Sitarz, K.; Roslon, M.; Anuszewska, E.; Hoser, G.; Wilczyńska, J.D.; Iwanowska, M.; Suchocki, P. The influence of an organic selenium (IV) compound on progression of tumour induced using prostate cancer cells and gene expression connected to the oxidative stress response. *World J. Pharm. Sci.* **2014**, *2*, 1146–1158.
17. Bierla, K.; Flis-Borsuk, A.; Suchocki, P.; Szpunar, J.; Lobinski, R. Speciation of Selenium in Selenium-Enriched Sunflower Oil by High-Performance Liquid Chromatography-Inductively Coupled Plasma Mass Spectrometry/Electrospray-Orbitrap Tandem Mass Spectrometry. *J. Agric. Food Chem.* **2016**, *64*, 4975–4981. [CrossRef]
18. Wendel, A. Glutathione peroxidase. *Methods Enzym.* **1981**, *77*, 325–333. [CrossRef]
19. Paglia, D.E.; Valentine, W.N. Studies on the quantitative and qualitative characterization of erythrocyte glutathione peroxidase. *J. Lab. Clin. Med.* **1967**, *70*, 158–169. [PubMed]
20. Habig, W.H.; Pabst, M.J.; Jakoby, W.B. Glutathione S-Transferases: The First Enzymatic Step in Mercapturic Acid Formation. *J. Biol. Chem.* **1974**, *249*, 7130–7139. [CrossRef]
21. Hill, K.E.; McCollum, G.W.; Burk, R.F. Determination of thioredoxin reductase activity in rat liver supernatant. *Anal. Biochem.* **1997**, *253*, 123–125. [CrossRef]
22. Mustacich, D.; Powis, G. Thioredoxin reductase. *Biochem. J.* **2000**, *346 Pt 1*, 1–8. [CrossRef] [PubMed]
23. Hill, K.E.; McCollum, G.W.; Boeglin, M.E.; Burk, R.F. Thioredoxin reductase activity is decreased by selenium deficiency. *Biochem. Biophys. Res. Commun.* **1997**, *234*, 293–295. [CrossRef]
24. Ou, B.; Hampsch-Woodill, M.; Prior, R.L. Development and validation of an improved oxygen radical absorbance capacity assay using fluorescein as the fluorescent probe. *J. Agric. Food Chem.* **2001**, *49*, 4619–4626. [CrossRef]

25. Nixon, D.E.; Moyer, T.P.; Burritt, M.F. The determination of selenium in serum and urine by inductively coupled plasma mass spectrometry: Comparison with Zeeman graphite furnace atomic absorption spectrometry1This paper is dedicated to the memory of Velmer A. Fassel. This work represents a long standing commitment to the accurate determination of toxic but essential metalloids, such as selenium—My dissertation research under the tutelage of Drs. Fassel and Kniseley.1. *Spectrochim. Acta Part B At. Spectrosc.* **1999**, *54*, 931–942. [CrossRef]
26. Forrer, R.; Gautschi, K.; Stroh, A.; Lutz, H. Direct Determination of Selenium and other Trace Elements in Serum Samples by ICP-MS. *J. Trace Elem. Med. Biol.* **1999**, *12*, 240–247. [CrossRef] [PubMed]
27. Sochacka, M.; Giebułtowicz, J.; Remiszewska, M.; Suchocki, P.; Wroczyński, P. Effects of Selol 5% supplementation on the activity or concentration of antioxidants and malondialdehyde level in the blood of healthy mice. *Pharmacol. Rep.* **2014**, *66*, 301–310. [CrossRef]
28. Raza, M.H.; Siraj, S.; Arshad, A.; Waheed, U.; Aldakheel, F.; Alduraywish, S.; Arshad, M. ROS-modulated therapeutic approaches in cancer treatment. *J. Cancer Res. Clin. Oncol.* **2017**, *143*, 1789–1809. [CrossRef]
29. Hammer, A.; Ferro, M.; Tillian, H.M.; Tatzber, F.; Zollner, H.; Schauenstein, E.; Schaur, R.J. Effect of oxidative stress by iron on 4-hydroxynonenal formation and proliferative activity in hepatomas of different degrees of differentiation. *Free Radic. Biol. Med.* **1997**, *23*, 26–33. [CrossRef]
30. Tjalkens, R.B.; Cook, L.W.; Petersen, D.R. Formation and export of the glutathione conjugate of 4-hydroxy-2,3-E-nonenal (4-HNE) in hepatoma cells. *Arch. Biochem. Biophys.* **1999**, *361*, 113–119. [CrossRef]
31. Vašková, J.; Kočan, L.; Vaško, L.; Perjési, P. Glutathione-Related Enzymes and Proteins: A Review. *Molecules* **2023**, *28*, 1447. [CrossRef] [PubMed]
32. Pizzimenti, S.; Ciamporcero, E.; Daga, M.; Pettazzoni, P.; Arcaro, A.; Cetrangolo, G.; Minelli, R.; Dianzani, C.; Lepore, A.; Gentile, F.; et al. Interaction of aldehydes derived from lipid peroxidation and membrane proteins. *Front. Physiol.* **2013**, *4*, 242. [CrossRef]
33. Lv, H.; Zhen, C.; Liu, J.; Yang, P.; Hu, L.; Shang, P. Unraveling the Potential Role of Glutathione in Multiple Forms of Cell Death in Cancer Therapy. *Oxid. Med. Cell. Longev.* **2019**, *2019*, 3150145. [CrossRef] [PubMed]
34. Averill-Bates, D.A. The antioxidant glutathione. *Vitam Horm* **2023**, *121*, 109–141. [CrossRef] [PubMed]
35. Adhyam, M.; Gupta, A.K. A Review on the Clinical Utility of PSA in Cancer Prostate. *Indian J. Surg. Oncol.* **2012**, *3*, 120–129. [CrossRef]
36. Sidhu, A.; Khan, N.; Phillips, C.; Briones, J.; Kapoor, A.; Zalewski, P.; Fleshner, N.E.; Chow, E.; Emmenegger, U. Prevalence and Prognostic Implications of PSA Flares during Radium-223 Treatment among Men with Metastatic Castration Resistant Prostate Cancer. *J. Clin. Med.* **2023**, *12*, 5604. [CrossRef]
37. Gopčević, K.R.; Rovčanin, B.R.; Tatić, S.B.; Krivokapić, Z.V.; Gajić, M.M.; Dragutinović, V.V. Activity of superoxide dismutase, catalase, glutathione peroxidase, and glutathione reductase in different stages of colorectal carcinoma. *Dig. Dis. Sci.* **2013**, *58*, 2646–2652. [CrossRef]
38. Żarczyńska, K.; Sobiech, P.; Tobolski, D.; Mee, J.F.; Illek, J. Effect of a single, oral administration of selenitetriglycerides, at two dose rates, on blood selenium status and haematological and biochemical parameters in Holstein-Friesian calves. *Ir. Vet. J.* **2021**, *74*, 11. [CrossRef]

nutrients

MDPI

Systematic Review

Does Magnesium Provide a Protective Effect in Crohn's Disease Remission? A Systematic Review of the Literature

Sergiu Costescu [1,2], Felix Bratosin [3], Zoran Laurentiu Popa [2,*], Ingrid Hrubaru [2] and Cosmin Citu [2]

1 Doctoral School Department, "Victor Babes" University of Medicine and Pharmacy Timisoara, 300041 Timisoara, Romania; sergiu.costescu@umft.ro

2 Department of Obstetrics and Gynecology, "Victor Babes" University of Medicine and Pharmacy Timisoara, 300041 Timisoara, Romania; hrubaru.ingrid@umft.ro (I.H.); citu.ioan@umft.ro (C.C.)

3 Department of Infectious Diseases, "Victor Babes" University of Medicine and Pharmacy Timisoara, 300041 Timisoara, Romania; felix.bratosin@umft.ro

* Correspondence: popa.zoran@umft.ro

Abstract: This systematic review evaluates the hypothesis that optimal serum magnesium levels may enhance remission rates in Crohn's disease (CD) and considers whether magnesium supplementation could be beneficial in CD management. This review aims to synthesize available evidence concerning the impact of serum magnesium on disease remission in CD, and to analyze the effectiveness and mechanistic roles of magnesium supplementation. Adhering to the PRISMA guidelines, we searched PubMed, Web of Science, and Scopus up to January 2024 using MeSH terms and free-text queries related to CD and magnesium. The inclusion criteria were studies that investigated serum magnesium levels, effects of supplementation, and the inflammatory mechanisms in CD remission. From the 525 records identified, eight studies met the inclusion criteria after the removal of duplicates and irrelevant records. These studies, conducted between 1998 and 2023, involved a cumulative sample of 453 patients and 292 controls. Key findings include significantly lower serum magnesium levels in CD patients (0.79 ± 0.09 mmol/L) compared to controls (0.82 ± 0.06 mmol/L), with up to 50% prevalence of hypomagnesemia in CD patients observed in one study. Notably, CD patients, particularly men, exhibited lower magnesium intake (men: 276.4 mg/day; women: 198.2 mg/day). Additionally, low magnesium levels correlated with increased sleep latency (95% CI -0.65 to -0.102; $p = 0.011$) and decreased sleep duration (95% CI -0.613 to -0.041; $p = 0.028$). Another key finding was the significant association between low serum magnesium levels and elevated CRP levels as an indicator of CD disease activity. The findings support the hypothesis that serum magnesium levels are significantly lower in CD patients compared to healthy controls and suggest that magnesium supplementation could improve CD management by enhancing remission rates and sleep quality. However, more rigorous, evidence-based research is necessary to define specific supplementation protocols and to fully elucidate the role of magnesium in CD pathophysiology.

Keywords: Crohn's disease; magnesium; micronutrients; nutritional supplementation

1. Introduction

Crohn's disease (CD) represents a significant clinical challenge due to its idiopathic nature and chronic course, characterized by periods of relapse and remission that affect the gastrointestinal tract [1–3]. This inflammatory bowel disease (IBD) is marked by a heterogeneous presentation, which can range from mild to severe intestinal inflammation, leading to symptoms such as abdominal pain, diarrhea, and weight loss [4–6]. These can mimic various gastrointestinal disorders, including malignancies, and require extensive investigations to diagnose and surgical excisions in uncontrolled cases [7–10]. The prevalence of CD varies globally, with recent estimates indicating an increasing incidence in both developed and developing countries, suggesting that environmental and lifestyle factors play critical roles in its pathogenesis alongside genetic susceptibilities [11,12]. Moreover, uncontrolled systemic inflammation and oxidative stress involved in chronic conditions was shown to increase the predisposition of cancers [13–16].

Magnesium, the fourth most abundant mineral in the human body, is crucial for many physiological processes, including energy production, nucleic acid and protein synthesis, ion transport, cell signaling, and the regulation of vascular tone [17–19]. Its role in maintaining immune homeostasis and modulating the inflammatory response is of particular interest in the context of chronic inflammatory diseases like CD [20]. Despite the established importance of magnesium, dietary surveys have consistently shown that a significant portion of the population consumes less than the recommended daily allowance, leading to widespread concern about the health implications of marginal magnesium status [21].

Objective data from epidemiological studies have highlighted an intriguing link between magnesium deficiency and increased risk of chronic inflammatory conditions [22,23]. In the context of Crohn's disease, patients often exhibit disrupted micronutrient homeostasis, attributed to factors such as malabsorption, intestinal loss, and dietary insufficiency, compounded by the disease's impact on the gastrointestinal tract [24]. The exact prevalence of hypomagnesemia in CD patients remains to be clarified, with studies suggesting a range that varies depending on disease location, severity, and the criteria used for magnesium deficiency diagnosis [25].

The potential of magnesium supplementation as a therapeutic strategy in CD is underpinned by its physiological roles and the observation that hypomagnesemia may exacerbate inflammatory pathways relevant to CD pathophysiology and might potentiate the effect of CD treatment and other medications [26–29]. Research indicates that magnesium can influence the immune response by modulating the production of key cytokines such as interleukin-6 (IL-6), tumor necrosis factor-alpha (TNF-α), and interleukin-10 (IL-10). It also affects the leukocyte activity, and the expression of adhesion molecules such as the selectins, integrins LFA-1 and VLA-4, and ICAM-1 (Intercellular Adhesion Molecule 1), VCAM-1 (Vascular Cell Adhesion Molecule 1), and PECAM-1 (Platelet Endothelial Cell Adhesion Molecule), which are pivotal in the inflammatory process [30–32]. Clinical trials and observational studies have begun to explore the effects of magnesium supplementation on various inflammatory diseases, with preliminary findings suggesting potential benefits in reducing disease severity and enhancing quality of life for patients [33–35].

The hypothesis driving this systematic review is that adequate serum magnesium levels are associated with improved remission rates in Crohn's disease, positing that magnesium supplementation could serve as a beneficial adjunctive therapy in managing this condition, and whether it can serve as protective factor for disease remission. Therefore, the primary objective is to consolidate and critically assess the existing evidence regarding the impact of serum magnesium levels on Crohn's disease remission, by evaluating the effectiveness of magnesium supplementation in altering disease outcomes and delineating the mechanistic pathways through which magnesium may exert its anti-inflammatory effects in the context of CD.

2. Materials and Methods

2.1. Protocol and Registration

The protocol for this systematic review was developed in alignment with the Preferred Reporting Items for Systematic Reviews and Meta-Analyses (PRISMA) guidelines [36], ensuring a transparent, reproducible, and methodologically correct approach. For the integrity of our research process, we registered the review protocol with the Open Science Framework (OSF), with the registration code osf.io/754vr.

To conduct the literature search, we employed an extensive search strategy, targeting research published up to January 2024, when the database search was performed. The databases selected comprised PubMed, Web of Science, and Scopus. The search strategy was constructed based on a range of Medical Subject Headings (MeSH) and free-text terms. The following MeSH Terms were used: "Crohn Disease", "Magnesium",

"Micronutrients", "Magnesium Deficiency", "Dietary Magnesium", "Supplementation", "Inflammatory Bowel Diseases", "Remission Induction", "Biomarkers". The free-text terms comprised: "serum magnesium and Crohn's Disease", "magnesium deficiency in IBD", "magnesium supplementation effects", "IBD remission with magnesium", "serum Mg levels in CD", "magnesium therapy for Crohn's", "Crohn's Disease and hypomagnesemia", "nutritional therapy in IBD remission", "inflammatory markers and magnesium".

2.2. Eligibility Criteria and Definitions

The inclusion criteria were set as follows: (1) studies examining the relationship between serum magnesium levels and remission in Crohn's disease; (2) reports on the effects of magnesium supplementation on CD remission rates; (3) investigations into the mechanisms by which magnesium may influence inflammatory processes in CD; and (4) peer-reviewed articles published in English. The exclusion criteria included the following: (1) studies not directly addressing serum magnesium levels or supplementation in the context of Crohn's disease remission; (2) studies where patients with CD were not in remission; (3) articles lacking empirical data or reporting on in vitro or animal studies; (4) reviews, commentaries, and editorials that did not provide original research data; and (5) studies with incomplete information on magnesium assessment methods or outcomes related to CD remission. The decision to exclude studies with active CD patients was based on the existing literature suggesting that micronutrients' levels can be influenced by the systemic inflammatory response [37,38]. Therefore, studies that involved patients with CD before or during treatment were not considered for inclusion.

Crohn's disease in remission was defined as a state where patients experience a significant reduction in or complete absence of the symptoms associated with active Crohn's disease without the need for ongoing acute treatment interventions. Remission was categorized into clinical remission and biochemical remission using the Crohn's Disease Activity Index (CDAI) [39]. Clinical remission refers to the cessation of symptoms such as abdominal pain, diarrhea, and rectal bleeding, allowing patients to return to their normal daily activities without the discomfort and complications associated with active disease phases. Biochemical remission is determined through laboratory markers, including inflammatory markers such as C-reactive protein (CRP) and fecal calprotectin levels, which indicate the absence of underlying inflammation. For the purpose of this systematic review, remission in Crohn's disease will encompass both clinical and biochemical remission, requiring evidence of symptom relief corroborated by relevant laboratory findings. Patients in biochemical remission at baseline were defined as those with albumin >35 g/L, CRP < 10 mg/L (1 mg/dL), and FCP < 250 μg/g [40].

2.3. Data Collection Process

To ensure the relevance of the studies included, we established specific eligibility criteria. The literature search was confined to English-language peer-reviewed journal articles. The initial phase involved the removal of duplicates, followed by a screening of titles and abstracts by two independent reviewers (Z.L.P. and F.B.) to assess relevance to the study objectives. Disagreements were resolved through discussion or, if necessary, consultation with a third reviewer.

For articles advancing to full-text review, the same two reviewers (Z.L.P. and F.B.) conducted an in-depth evaluation to confirm eligibility based on the predefined criteria. Data extraction and management were performed manually, ensuring a systematic approach to synthesizing evidence from selected studies. From a total of 525 records that were screened, 281 were duplicated, 58 did not have available data, and the other 236 articles did not match the inclusion criteria, leaving a total of 8 studies included in the final analysis, as presented in Figure 1.

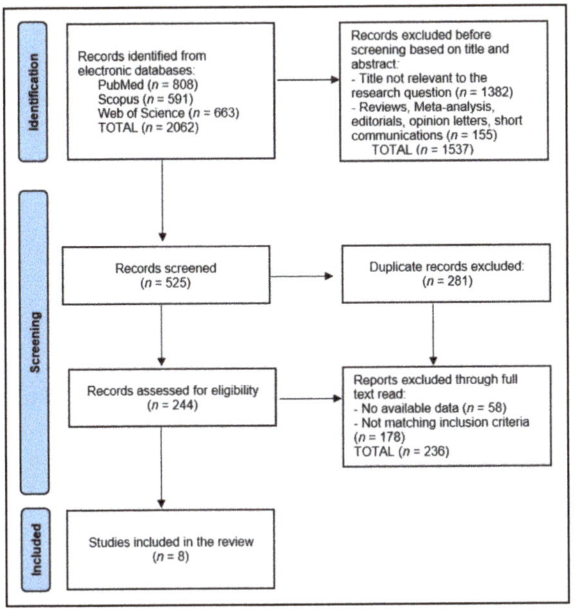

Figure 1. PRISMA flow diagram.

2.4. Risk of Bias and Quality Assessment

For the systematic assessment of study quality and determination of risk of bias within the included studies, our review employed a dual approach, integrating both qualitative and quantitative evaluation methods. Initially, the quality of observational studies was evaluated using the Newcastle–Ottawa Scale, a widely recognized tool that assesses three critical dimensions: the selection of study groups, the comparability of these groups, and the ascertainment of either the exposure or outcome of interest for case–control or cohort studies, respectively. Each study is awarded stars in these categories, cumulating in a score that classifies the study quality as either low, medium, or high. This star system facilitates a nuanced evaluation of study quality, enabling the systematic identification of research that meets high methodological standards. To ensure the objectivity and reproducibility of our quality assessment process, each study was independently evaluated by two researchers. Discrepancies in quality assessment scores were resolved through discussion, or if necessary, consultation with a third researcher.

3. Results

3.1. Study Characteristics

This systematic review included eight distinct studies [40–47] spanning a diverse array of countries, including the Netherlands, Japan, France, Italy, Brazil, and the United Kingdom, signifying a global interest in the subject matter. The timeline of these studies, ranging from 1998 to 2023, underscores a sustained scholarly engagement with the topic over a quarter-century. The inception of this research was marked by a study from Geerling et al. in the Netherlands in 1998 [41], while the most recent investigation by Browson et al. from the United Kingdom was published in 2023 [40].

The studies employed varied methodologies, encompassing both prospective and retrospective cohort studies, as well as cross-sectional designs. Specifically, three studies adopted a prospective cohort approach [41,45,47], four studies were cross-sectional in nature [42–44,46], and one study was characterized as a retrospective cohort [40]. Regarding the quality of these studies, there was a notable variation. Two studies were rated as high in quality [43,46], indicating a robust methodological framework, while the remaining six studies were assessed as medium [40–42,45,47] or low [44] in quality (Table 1).

Table 1. Study characteristics.

Study & Author	Country	Study Year	Study Design	Study Quality
1 [41] Geerling et al.	Netherlands	1998	Prospective Cohort	Medium
2 [42] Geerling et al.	Netherlands	2000	Cross-Sectional	Medium
3 [43] Tajika et al.	Japan	2004	Cross-Sectional	High
4 [44] Filippi et al.	France	2006	Cross-Sectional	Low
5 [45] Valentini al.	Italy	2008	Prospective Cohort	Medium
6 [46] de Castro et al.	Brazil	2019	Cross-Sectional	High
7 [47] MacMaster et al.	United Kingdom	2021	Prospective Cohort	Medium
8 [40] Browson et al.	United Kingdom	2023	Retrospective Cohort	Medium

3.2. Patients' Characteristics

Table 2 elucidates the demographics and clinical attributes of patients across eight studies, offering insight into the characteristics of individuals with Crohn's disease and their comparison groups within the context of serum magnesium levels and disease remission. The collective sample size amounted to 453 patients and 292 controls, revealing a broad spectrum of age, gender distribution, and additional health characteristics.

Table 2. Patient characteristics.

Study Number	Sample Size	Age (Years)	Gender Distribution	Comparison Group	Other Characteristics
1 [41] Geerling et al.	32	40 (median)	18 (56.2%) women; 14 (43.8%) men	32 healthy controls matched for age and gender	Smoking 13 (40.6%); underweight (65–75%); Vitamin D deficiency 18 (56.2%)
2 [42] Geerling et al.	23	30.1 (mean)	15 (65.2%) women; 8 (34.8%) men	23 healthy controls matched for age and gender	Smoking 8 (34.7%)
3 [43] Tajika et al.	33	37 (mean)	8 (24.2%) women; 25 (35.8%) men	15 healthy controls matched for age and gender	Vitamin D deficiency 9 (27.3%)
4 [44] Filippi et al.	54	39.0 (mean)	28 (51.9%) women; 26 (48.1%) men	25 healthy controls	Underweight (30%); low plasma concentration of micronutrients (50%); smoking 17 (31%)
5 [45] Valentini al.	94	37.7 (mean)	61 (64.9%); 33 (35.1%) men	61 healthy controls	Smoking 19 (20.2%); malnutrition 22 (23.7%)
6 [46] de Castro et al.	31	39.7 (mean)	16 (51.6%) women; 15 (48.4%) men	29 patients with active disease	Smoking 1 (3.2%); obesity 5 (16.1%)
7 [47] MacMaster et al.	59	48.0 (median)	22 (37%) women; 37 (63%) men	30 patients with ulcerative colitis	Vitamin D deficiency 16 (32%)
8 [40] Browson et al.	127	43.0 (median)	54 (42.5%) women; 73 (57.5%) men	77 patients with ulcerative colitis	Vitamin D deficiency 12 (9.6%)

The patient ages across these studies showed variability, with median ages reported in two studies by Geerling et al. [41] and Browson et al. [40] at 40 and 43 years, respectively, and mean ages ranging from 30.1 to 39.7 years in the remaining studies. Gender distribution across these studies leaned slightly towards a higher female participation in some studies (e.g., 65.2% women in the study by Geerling et al. [42]), while others had a more balanced or male-dominant ratio (e.g., 63% men in the study by MacMaster et al. [47]).

Notably, all studies included comparison groups, ranging from healthy controls matched for age and gender in studies by Geerling et al. [41,42] to patients with active disease or ulcerative colitis in studies by de Castro et al. [46] and Browson et al. [40]. Other characteristics highlighted include lifestyle factors such as smoking, which varied significantly across studies (from 3.2% in the study by de Castro et al. [46] to 40.6% in the study by Geerling et al. [41]), and nutritional status, with mentions of underweight and malnutrition. Vitamin D deficiency was also a recurrent theme, observed in a significant proportion of participants across several studies, suggesting potential interrelations between vitamin D levels, nutritional status, and Crohn's disease activity or remission status. The heterogeneity among studies reflects the multifaceted nature of Crohn's disease and the myriad factors that can influence disease progression and remission, emphasizing the importance of considering a wide range of demographic and clinical characteristics in understanding the disease's dynamics.

3.3. Disease Characteristics

Disease duration varied significantly across the studies, from as short as 6 months in the study by Geerling et al. [42] to as long as 16 years in the studies by Geerling et al. [41] and Tajika et al. [43], indicating a wide range of disease experiences among the patients. Disease severity, assessed using the Crohn's Disease Activity Index (CDAI) and the Harvey Bradshaw Index (HBI), showed a range of values that indicate different levels of disease activity across the patient cohorts. The CDAI values showed clinical remission of disease, ranging from a median of 139 in the study by Geerling et al. [41], suggesting moderate disease activity, to a mean of 41.4 in the study by de Castro et al. [46], indicating milder disease activity. The use of the Montreal classification in Browson et al.'s work [40] to describe disease behavior further highlights the complexity of assessing Crohn's disease severity.

Surgical history was a common element among the patients, with a significant number undergoing bowel resections, indicative of the severity of their conditions. The percentage of patients with surgical interventions ranged from 17.4% in the study by Geerling et al. [42] to 84.4% in their earlier study [41]. Complications such as colonic and perianal involvement were frequently reported, with percentages indicating a considerable impact on the patients' health and quality of life. For instance, colonic involvement was reported at high rates in several studies, such as 88.3% in the study by Valentini al. [45].

Medication usage varied across the studies, with a wide range of treatments including mesalamine, azathioprine, corticosteroids, immunosuppressants, and biological therapies such as infliximab and vedolizumab. Notably, the use of advanced biological therapies in the study by Browson et al. [40] indicates a shift towards more targeted treatments in recent years compared with the first study from 1998 [41], as presented in Table 3.

Table 3. Disease characteristics.

Study Number	Disease Duration	Disease Severity	Surgical History	Complications	Medication
1 [41] Geerling et al.	16 years (11.0–19.0)	CDAI: 139 (median)	27 (84.4%) small bowel resection	Colonic involvement 18 (56.2%), extent of bowel resection—average of 75.0 cm, ileostomy 2 (6.2%)	Mesalamine (50.0%), azathioprine (34.4%), corticosteroids (40.6%)
2 [42] Geerling et al.	6 months	CDAI: 96.9 (mean)	4 (17.4%) small bowel resection	Small bowel involvement 20 (87.0%)	Mesalamine (100%), azathioprine (4.0%), prednisone 10 mg (26%)
3 [43] Tajika et al.	16.1 years	CDAI: 84.1 (mean)	18 (54.5%) bowel resection	Colonic involvement only 4 (12.1%), small bowel involvement only 7 (21.2%), extent of bowel resection—median of 55.0 cm	Corticosteroids (median dose 1.2 g), mesalamine (48.5%), enteral diets (30.3%)
4 [44] Filippi et al.	NR	CDAI: 89.7 (mean)	23 (42.6%)	NR	Immunosuppressants 28 (52%), corticosteroids 43 (80%)

Table 3. *Cont.*

Study Number	Disease Duration	Disease Severity	Surgical History	Complications	Medication
5 [45] Valentini et al.	7.8 years	CDAI: 71 (median)	38 (40.4%) bowel resection	Colonic involvement 83 (88.3%)	5-Aminosalicylic acid (51%), immunosuppressants (36%), prednisolone (12%)
6 [46] de Castro et al.	12.6 years	CDAI: 41.4 (mean)	17 (54.8%) bowel resection	Colonic involvement only 14 (45.1%), perianal disease 19 (61.3%)	NR
7 [47] MacMaster et al.	55 months in remission	HBI: 1.18 (median)	NR	Colonic involvement only 26 (44%), perianal disease 7 (11.9%)	5-Aminosalicylic acid (27.1%), thiopurine (30.5%), biological (10.2%)
8 [40] Browson et al.	NR	Montreal classification: 33.5% structuring disease, 35.4% penetrating disease	NR	Colonic involvement 36 (28.4%), perianal disease 39 (31.2%)	Infliximab (70.4%), vedolizumab (15.0%), azathioprine (35.4%)

NR—Not Reported; CDAI—Crohn's Disease Activity Index; HBI—Harvey Bradshaw Index.

3.4. Magnesium Measurements

In the studies conducted by Geerling et al. [41,42], Crohn's disease patients exhibited significantly lower magnesium levels (0.79 ± 0.09 mmol/L) compared to controls (0.82 ± 0.06 mmol/L), with a striking 50% prevalence of hypomagnesemia reported in one study. The association with CRP levels in these studies indicates a median CRP level of 2.0 mg/dL in the first study, reflecting a potential link between magnesium levels and inflammation.

Tajika et al. [43] also reported significantly lower magnesium levels in Crohn's disease patients (2.2 ± 0.2 mg/dL) compared to controls, though the study did not report hypomagnesemia rates. The CRP levels in this cohort were comparatively lower (0.9 ± 1.2 mg/dL), suggesting a less pronounced inflammatory state or a different patient population.

Filippi et al. [44] took a unique approach by measuring magnesium intake, reporting significantly lower intake in Crohn's disease patients, with women consuming 198.2 mg/kg/day and men 276.4 mg/kg/day. Valentini al. [45] did not report specific magnesium levels but noted a 28.7% prevalence of hypomagnesemia. The majority of patients in this study (76%) had normal CRP levels, suggesting a lower level of systemic inflammation among the participants.

De Castro et al. [46] found no significant difference in magnesium levels (1.7 ± 0.2 mg/dL) and a relatively low prevalence of hypomagnesemia (15.4%). CRP levels in this study were higher (2.28 ± 0.8 mg/dL), indicating variability in the relationship between magnesium levels and inflammation. MacMaster et al. [47] and Browson et al. [40] also reported no significant findings regarding magnesium levels, with hypomagnesemia prevalence at 1.7% and 2.5%, respectively. CRP levels were notably different, with MacMaster et al. [47] reporting 100% of patients with CRP levels below 1.0 mg/dL, suggesting minimal inflammation, whereas Browson et al. [40] reported 37.8% of patients with CRP levels below 1.0 mg/dL, as presented in Table 4.

Table 4. Magnesium measurements.

Risk Factors	Mg Levels/Intake	Hypomagnesemia *	Magnesium Levels Significantly Associated with CRP	Outcomes/Risk
1 [41] Geerling et al.	0.79 ± 0.09 mmol/L vs. 0.82 ± 0.06 mmol/L in controls	50.0%	2.0 mg/dL	Significantly lower Mg levels than controls
2 [42] Geerling et al.	0.79 ± 0.09 mmol/L vs. 0.82 ± 0.06 mmol/L in controls	NR	1.7 ± 1.9 mg/dL	Significantly lower Mg levels than controls
3 [43] Tajika et al.	2.2 ± 0.2 mg/dL	NR	0.9 ± 1.2 mg/dL	Significantly lower Mg levels than controls

Table 4. *Cont.*

Risk Factors	Mg Levels/Intake	Hypomagnesemia *	Magnesium Levels Significantly Associated with CRP	Outcomes/Risk
4 [44] Filippi et al.	Women: 198.2 mg/kg/day, Men: 276.4 mg/kg/day	NR	0.6 ± 0.8 mg/dL	Significantly lower Mg intake than controls
5 [45] Valentini al.	NR	28.7%	Normal CRP levels in 76% patients	Significantly lower Mg levels than controls
6 [46] de Castro et al.	1.7 ± 0.2 mg/dL	15.4%	2.28 ± 0.8 mg/dL	No significance
7 [47] MacMaster et al.	NR	1.7%	100% < 1.0 mg/dL	No significance
8 [40] Browson et al.	NR	2.5%	37.8% < 1.0 mg/dL	No significance

NR—Not Reported; Mg—Magnesium; CRP—C-reactive protein; *—defined as (<0.75 mmol/L).

4. Discussion

4.1. Summary of Evidence

This systematic review's investigation into the role of serum magnesium levels in Crohn's disease remission offers a comprehensive overview of the varied clinical characteristics and outcomes across multiple studies. The demographic and clinical attributes of 453 patients, as depicted in the patient characteristics data, highlight the heterogeneity inherent in Crohn's disease research. The variability in age, gender distribution, and additional health characteristics such as smoking habits, nutritional status, and vitamin D deficiency underscores the complexity of managing Crohn's disease. This variability necessitates a nuanced understanding of how these factors might influence serum magnesium levels and, by extension, disease remission rates.

The critical examination of disease characteristics further illuminates the diverse nature of Crohn's disease among patients. The wide range of disease durations and severities, as well as the notable differences in surgical histories and complications, points to the multifaceted challenges in treating this condition. The variations in disease severity, assessed using the Crohn's Disease Activity Index (CDAI) and the Harvey Bradshaw Index (HBI), alongside the utilization of different classification systems like the Montreal classification, emphasize the need for a personalized approach to treatment. This personalized approach is further complicated by the broad spectrum of medications used, ranging from mesalamine to advanced biological therapies, reflecting the shift towards more targeted treatments in recent years.

The findings related to magnesium measurements across the studies offer pivotal insights into the potential role of magnesium in Crohn's disease management. The significantly lower magnesium levels observed in Crohn's disease patients compared to controls in several studies suggest a possible link between magnesium deficiency and disease activity or severity. However, the lack of significant findings in other studies, alongside the variability in hypomagnesemia prevalence and its association with CRP levels, indicates that the relationship between serum magnesium levels and Crohn's disease remission is complex and not fully understood. This complexity is further highlighted by the unique approach of measuring magnesium intake in one of the studies, suggesting that dietary factors also play a crucial role in magnesium levels and, potentially, disease outcomes.

For magnesium intake, the recommended replacement dose when a diagnosis of deficiency is considered should be 150 mg, four times a day, and an overall daily requirement from various sources of 400 mg. Of the multiple formulations of magnesium supplements, the best choice for enteral supplementation is the gluconate formulation. Signs and symptoms for deficiency comprise muscle weakness, nausea, palpitations, confusion, and even seizures in severe deficiencies [48].

The study by Zheng et al. [49] provides pivotal objective data on the role of calcium and magnesium concentrations in patients with active Crohn's disease (CD) who had not yet commenced treatment, revealing that serum levels of magnesium and calcium are markedly lower in CD patients compared to healthy controls, with cut-off values set at 0.835 mmol/L for magnesium and 2.315 mmol/L for calcium for CD development. This contrasts with our systematic review, which broadly addresses serum magnesium levels in CD remission without specifically focusing on the treatment-naïve or active phase. Zheng et al.'s findings, highlighting severe deficiencies in magnesium and calcium intake among CD patients, especially those in the active phase of the disease, provide a more nuanced understanding of the nutritional and inflammatory landscape of CD prior to medical intervention. This aspect of temporal specificity and the condition of patients at the onset of their disease journey offer a valuable perspective that complements our study's broader examination of magnesium's importance in CD management, underscoring the potential of these minerals as critical biomarkers for CD diagnosis and monitoring disease activity.

The systematic review by McDonnell et al. [50] provides a comprehensive analysis of micronutrient insufficiencies in adults with CD during clinical remission, identifying prevalent deficiencies in a range of micronutrients, including vitamins D and B12, which are the most consistently reported. This broadens the scope of micronutrient research in CD beyond our study's focus on serum magnesium levels, highlighting a multifaceted nutritional challenge in CD management. Their findings reveal not only the varied micronutrient deficiencies present even during remission but also the inconsistent results when comparing CD patients to healthy controls, particularly with vitamin D being lower in only a quarter of the studies. This juxtaposition underscores the complex nature of micronutrient deficiencies in CD, suggesting that while magnesium plays a crucial role, it is part of a larger spectrum of nutritional insufficiencies that warrant comprehensive assessment and management strategies. McDonnell et al.'s review, by showcasing the significant evidence for vitamins D and B12 deficiencies and the uncertain evidence for others, complements our focused examination of magnesium, illustrating the need for a broader nutritional focus on CD care.

Regarding vitamin D deficiency in CD, the study conducted by Tajika et al. [43] delves into the specific challenges of vitamin D deficiency among CD patients in Japan, revealing that 27.3% of CD patients were vitamin-D-deficient (serum 25-OHD level $\leq$ 10 ng/mL), a stark contrast to only 6.7% of healthy controls exhibiting similar deficiency levels. Objective data from this study further demonstrates the relationship between vitamin D levels and CD severity, with serum 25-OHD levels significantly correlating with disease duration and Crohn's Disease Activity Index (CDAI) score.

Other micronutrients that were reported to be deficient in CD patients, besides magnesium, are folic acid and B12 vitamin. Studies identified a proportion of CD patients with Folate (B9) levels below laboratory reference ranges of 3 ng/mL [51,52]. Particularly notable is the variance in reported deficiencies, with some studies highlighting a higher prevalence of deficiency in patients with mixed clinical activity, whereas others, even among those in remission, found minimal to no deficiency. Comparisons with healthy controls further shape the picture, showing no significant differences in folate levels, suggesting that folate deficiency may not be as distinctive in CD patients as previously thought. However, exploratory analyses hinted at a potential link between dietary intake, disease activity, and folate levels, indicating that while not universally prevalent, certain CD patient subgroups may be more susceptible to folate deficiency.

The investigation into vitamin B12 status among CD patients reveals a significant concern for B12 deficiency, particularly among those who have undergone ileal resections or have terminal ileal inflammation. Existing studies [53,54] reported on the prevalence of low B12 or other biochemical evidence of an impaired B12 status, such as elevated methylmalonic acid levels or reduced holotranscobalamin, highlighting that deficiencies were notably prevalent, with up to 33% in some CD remission groups. The comparison with healthy controls showed that B12 concentrations were lower in the CD group in several studies, suggesting a trend towards B12 insufficiency in CD populations. Objective data underscore ileal resections, especially those exceeding 20 cm, as a significant risk factor for B12 deficiency, emphasizing the critical need for vigilant B12 monitoring and potential supplementation in CD management.

The study by Gilca-Blanaru et al. [29] on hair magnesium concentration in IBD patients offers groundbreaking insights, revealing significantly lower magnesium levels in IBD patients compared to healthy controls, and notably, in CD versus UC. This novel approach not only underscores magnesium's potential role in the pathophysiology of IBD but also its impact on patients' psychological status and sleep quality. The associations between magnesium deficiency and various clinical parameters, such as disease activity, and sleep latency and duration, suggest that magnesium could be pivotal in both the clinical management and the improvement in life quality for IBD patients. The study's implications for future research are vast, hinting at the utility of magnesium in predictive models for disease activity and the potential benefits of supplementation. However, it also calls for evidence-based studies to refine supplementation strategies, emphasizing the need for a deeper understanding of magnesium's role in IBD.

4.2. Limitations

The current study faces some limitations primarily in study variability in terms of patient population and magnesium assessment methods. One significant limitation is the variation in how remission in CD is characterized across the studies included, potentially affecting the uniformity of the data regarding serum magnesium levels' impact on disease activity and remission rates. This variability might obscure the true relationship between magnesium levels and CD remission as the criteria for clinical and biochemical remission differ widely, influencing the interpretation of magnesium's role. Additionally, the exclusion of studies involving patients before or during treatment phases might omit crucial insights into how early or active disease stages could affect, or be affected by, magnesium levels, limiting a comprehensive understanding of magnesium's potential throughout the disease course. Moreover, the reliance on serum magnesium as the primary indicator without considering other factors that influence magnesium status, such as dietary intake or absorption issues, might not fully capture the complex interplay between magnesium and CD pathophysiology.

5. Conclusions

The findings from this systematic review provide compelling evidence that serum magnesium levels are significantly lower in Crohn's disease patients compared to healthy controls, underscoring the potential of magnesium as a critical factor in the management of CD. The observed hypomagnesemia prevalence, particularly pronounced in CD compared to ulcerative colitis, and the established correlation between low magnesium levels and both sleep latency and duration, highlight magnesium's broader impact beyond its direct anti-inflammatory effects. These results suggest that magnesium supplementation could serve as an adjunctive therapy, potentially improving remission rates and ameliorating sleep-related issues in CD patients. This review also suggests that magnesium status may reflect broader nutritional and metabolic challenges faced by individuals with CD, indicating a need for a holistic approach to patient care that includes regular monitoring of micronutrient levels. However, the current body of evidence, while suggestive of these benefits, calls for further research to confirm these hypotheses. Future studies should aim to provide robust, evidence-based recommendations for magnesium supplementation, including optimal dosing, timing, and monitoring strategies, to fully harness magnesium's therapeutic potential in CD management. Moreover, understanding the mechanistic pathways through which magnesium influences CD activity and remission could unveil new avenues for intervention, emphasizing the importance of micronutrients in chronic disease management and patient well-being.

Author Contributions: Conceptualization, S.C.; methodology, S.C.; software, S.C. and I.H.; validation, F.B.; formal analysis, F.B.; investigation, S.C. and F.B.; resources, F.B.; data curation, S.C., I.H. and F.B.; writing—original draft preparation, Z.L.P. and C.C.; writing—review and editing, Z.L.P., I.H. and C.C.; visualization, Z.L.P. and C.C.; supervision, Z.L.P. and C.C.; project administration, Z.L.P. and C.C. All authors have read and agreed to the published version of the manuscript.

Funding: The article processing charge was paid by the "Victor Babes" University of Medicine and Pharmacy Timisoara.

Conflicts of Interest: The authors declare no conflicts of interest.

References

1. Cho, C.W.; You, M.W.; Oh, C.H.; Lee, C.K.; Moon, S.K. Long-term Disease Course of Crohn's Disease: Changes in Disease Location, Phenotype, Activities, and Predictive Factors. *Gut Liver* **2022**, *16*, 157–170. [CrossRef] [PubMed]
2. Woo, V.L. Oral Manifestations of Crohn's Disease: A Case Report and Review of the Literature. *Case Rep. Dent.* **2015**, *2015*, 830472. [CrossRef] [PubMed]
3. Yarur, A.J.; Strobel, S.G.; Deshpande, A.R.; Abreu, M.T. Predictors of Aggressive Inflammatory Bowel Disease. *Gastroenterol. Hepatol.* **2011**, *7*, 652–659.
4. Coates, M.D.; Clarke, K.; Williams, E.; Jeganathan, N.; Yadav, S.; Giampetro, D.; Gordin, V.; Smith, S.; Vrana, K.; Bobb, A.; et al. Abdominal Pain in Inflammatory Bowel Disease: An Evidence-Based, Multidisciplinary Review. *Crohns Colitis 360* **2023**, *5*, otad055. [CrossRef] [PubMed]
5. Sange, A.H.; Srinivas, N.; Sarnaik, M.K.; Modi, S.; Pisipati, Y.; Vaidya, S.; Syed Gaggatur, N.; Sange, I. Extra-Intestinal Manifestations of Inflammatory Bowel Disease. *Cureus* **2021**, *13*, e17187. [CrossRef] [PubMed]
6. Wils, P.; Caron, B.; D'Amico, F.; Danese, S.; Peyrin-Biroulet, L. Abdominal Pain in Inflammatory Bowel Diseases: A Clinical Challenge. *J Clin Med.* **2022**, *11*, 4269. [CrossRef] [PubMed]
7. Fiorillo, C.; Schena, C.A.; Quero, G.; Laterza, V.; Pugliese, D.; Privitera, G.; Rosa, F.; Schepis, T.; Salvatore, L.; Di Stefano, B.; et al. Challenges in Crohn's Disease Management after Gastrointestinal Cancer Diagnosis. *Cancers* **2021**, *13*, 574. [CrossRef] [PubMed]
8. Papadakis, K.A.; Tabibzadeh, S. Diagnosis and Misdiagnosis of Inflammatory Bowel Disease. *Gastrointest. Endosc. Clin. N. Am.* **2002**, *12*, 433–449. [CrossRef]
9. Laredo, V.; García-Mateo, S.; Martínez-Domínguez, S.J.; López de la Cruz, J.; Gargallo-Puyuelo, C.J.; Gomollón, F. Risk of Cancer in Patients with Inflammatory Bowel Diseases and Keys for Patient Management. *Cancers* **2023**, *15*, 871. [CrossRef]
10. M'Koma, A.E. Inflammatory Bowel Disease: Clinical Diagnosis and Surgical Treatment-Overview. *Medicina* **2022**, *58*, 567. [CrossRef]
11. Pasternak, G.; Chrzanowski, G.; Aebisher, D.; Myśliwiec, A.; Dynarowicz, K.; Bartusik-Aebisher, D.; Sosna, B.; Cieślar, G.; Kawczyk-Krupka, A.; Filip, R. Crohn's Disease: Basic Characteristics of the Disease, Diagnostic Methods, the Role of Biomarkers, and Analysis of Metalloproteinases: A Review. *Life* **2023**, *13*, 2062. [CrossRef] [PubMed]
12. M'Koma, A.E. Inflammatory Bowel Disease: An Expanding Global Health Problem. *Clin. Med. Insights Gastroenterol.* **2013**, *6*, 33–47. [CrossRef] [PubMed]
13. Piotrowski, I.; Kulcenty, K.; Suchorska, W. Interplay between Inflammation and Cancer. *Rep. Pract. Oncol. Radiother.* **2020**, *25*, 422–427. [CrossRef]
14. Bînă, A.M.; Sturza, A.; Iancu, I.; Mocanu, A.G.; Bernad, E.; Chiriac, D.V.; Borza, C.; Craina, M.L.; Popa, Z.L.; Muntean, D.M.; et al. Placental Oxidative Stress and Monoamine Oxidase Expression are Increased in Severe Preeclampsia: A Pilot Study. *Mol. Cell. Biochem.* **2022**, *477*, 2851–2861. [CrossRef]
15. Aguilar-Cazares, D.; Chavez-Dominguez, R.; Marroquin-Muciño, M.; Perez-Medina, M.; Benito-Lopez, J.J.; Camarena, A.; Rumbo-Nava, U.; Lopez-Gonzalez, J.S. The Systemic-Level Repercussions of Cancer-Associated Inflammation Mediators Produced in the Tumor Microenvironment. *Front. Endocrinol.* **2022**, *13*, 929572. [CrossRef]
16. Feier, C.V.I.; Muntean, C.; Faur, A.M.; Gaborean, V.; Petrache, I.A.; Cozma, G.V. Exploring Inflammatory Parameters in Lung Cancer Patients: A Retrospective Analysis. *J. Pers. Med.* **2024**, *14*, 552. [CrossRef]
17. Al Alawi, A.M.; Majoni, S.W.; Falhammar, H. Magnesium and Human Health: Perspectives and Research Directions. *Int. J. Endocrinol.* **2018**, *2018*, 9041694. [CrossRef]
18. Razzaque, M.S. Magnesium: Are We Consuming Enough? *Nutrients* **2018**, *10*, 1863. [CrossRef] [PubMed]
19. Barbagallo, M.; Veronese, N.; Dominguez, L.J. Magnesium in Aging, Health and Diseases. *Nutrients* **2021**, *13*, 463. [CrossRef]
20. Ashique, S.; Kumar, S.; Hussain, A.; Mishra, N.; Garg, A.; Gowda, B.H.J.; Farid, A.; Gupta, G.; Dua, K.; Taghizadeh-Hesary, F. A Narrative Review on the Role of Magnesium in Immune Regulation, Inflammation, Infectious Diseases, and Cancer. *J. Health Popul. Nutr.* **2023**, *42*, 74. [CrossRef]
21. Di Nicolantonio, J.J.; O'Keefe, J.H.; Wilson, W. Subclinical Magnesium Deficiency: A Principal Driver of Cardiovascular Disease and a Public Health Crisis. *Open Heart* **2018**, *5*, e000668. [CrossRef] [PubMed]
22. Nielsen, F.H. Effects of Magnesium Depletion on Inflammation in Chronic Disease. *Curr. Opin. Clin. Nutr. Metab. Care* **2014**, *17*, 525–530. [CrossRef] [PubMed]

23. Nielsen, F.H. Magnesium Deficiency and Increased Inflammation: Current Perspectives. *J. Inflamm. Res.* **2018**, *11*, 25–34. [CrossRef] [PubMed]
24. Kilby, K.; Mathias, H.; Boisvenue, L.; Heisler, C.; Jones, J.L. Micronutrient Absorption and Related Outcomes in People with Inflammatory Bowel Disease: A Review. *Nutrients* **2019**, *11*, 1388. [CrossRef] [PubMed]
25. Naser, S.A.; Abdelsalam, A.; Thanigachalam, S.; Naser, A.S.; Alcedo, K. Domino Effect of Hypomagnesemia on the Innate Immunity of Crohn's Disease Patients. *World J. Diabetes* **2014**, *5*, 527–535. [CrossRef] [PubMed]
26. Nakamura, Y.; Kawai, Y.; Nagoshi, S.; Ogawa, T.; Hasegawa, H. Multiple Electrolytes Imbalances in a Patient with Inflammatory Bowel Disease Associated with Vitamin D Deficiency: A Case Report. *J. Med. Case Rep.* **2024**, *18*, 26. [CrossRef] [PubMed]
27. Fernández-Rodríguez, E.; Camarero-González, E. Paciente con enfermedad de Crohn y convulsiones por hipomagnesemia. *Nutr. Hosp.* **2007**, *22*, 720–722.
28. Mukai, A.; Yamamoto, S.; Matsumura, K. Hypocalcemia Secondary to Hypomagnesemia in a Patient with Crohn's Disease. *Clin. J. Gastroenterol.* **2015**, *8*, 22–25. [CrossRef] [PubMed]
29. Gilca-Blanariu, G.E.; Trifan, A.; Ciocoiu, M.; Popa, I.V.; Burlacu, A.; Balan, G.G.; Olteanu, A.V.; Stefanescu, G. Magnesium—A Potential Key Player in Inflammatory Bowel Diseases? *Nutrients* **2022**, *14*, 1914. [CrossRef]
30. Lima, F.D.S.; Fock, R.A. A Review of the Action of Magnesium on Several Processes Involved in the Modulation of Hematopoiesis. *Int. J. Mol. Sci.* **2020**, *21*, 7084. [CrossRef]
31. Yusuf-Makagiansar, H.; Anderson, M.E.; Yakovleva, T.V.; Murray, J.S.; Siahaan, T.J. Inhibition of LFA-1/ICAM-1 and VLA-4/VCAM-1 as a Therapeutic Approach to Inflammation and Autoimmune Diseases. *Med. Res. Rev.* **2002**, *22*, 146–167. [CrossRef] [PubMed]
32. Haydinger, C.D.; Ashander, L.M.; Tan, A.C.R.; Smith, J.R. Intercellular Adhesion Molecule 1: More than a Leukocyte Adhesion Molecule. *Biology* **2023**, *12*, 743. [CrossRef] [PubMed]
33. Veronese, N.; Pizzol, D.; Smith, L.; Dominguez, L.J.; Barbagallo, M. Effect of Magnesium Supplementation on Inflammatory Parameters: A Meta-Analysis of Randomized Controlled Trials. *Nutrients* **2022**, *14*, 679. [CrossRef] [PubMed]
34. Tang, C.F.; Ding, H.; Jiao, R.Q.; Wu, X.X.; Kong, L.D. Possibility of Magnesium Supplementation for Supportive Treatment in Patients with COVID-19. *Eur. J. Pharmacol.* **2020**, *886*, 173546. [CrossRef] [PubMed]
35. Pethő, Á.G.; Fülöp, T.; Orosz, P.; Tapolyai, M. Magnesium Is a Vital Ion in the Body-It Is Time to Consider Its Supplementation on a Routine Basis. *Clin Pract.* **2024**, *14*, 521–535. [CrossRef] [PubMed]
36. Page, M.J.; McKenzie, J.E.; Bossuyt, P.M.; Boutron, I.; Hoffmann, T.C.; Mulrow, C.D.; Shamseer, L.; Tetzlaff, J.M.; Akl, E.A.; Brennan, S.E.; et al. The PRISMA 2020 statement: An updated guideline for reporting systematic reviews. *Syst. Rev.* **2021**, *10*, 89. [CrossRef] [PubMed]
37. Valvano, M.; Capannolo, A.; Cesaro, N.; Stefanelli, G.; Fabiani, S.; Frassino, S.; Monaco, S.; Magistroni, M.; Viscido, A.; Latella, G. Nutrition, Nutritional Status, Micronutrients Deficiency, and Disease Course of Inflammatory Bowel Disease. *Nutrients* **2023**, *15*, 3824. [CrossRef] [PubMed]
38. Balestrieri, P.; Ribolsi, M.; Guarino, M.P.L.; Emerenziani, S.; Altomare, A.; Cicala, M. Nutritional Aspects in Inflammatory Bowel Diseases. *Nutrients* **2020**, *12*, 372. [CrossRef]
39. Freeman, H.J. Use of the Crohn's disease activity index in clinical trials of biological agents. *World J. Gastroenterol.* **2008**, *14*, 4127–4130. [CrossRef]
40. Brownson, E.; Saunders, J.; Jatkowska, A.; White, B.; Gerasimidis, K.; Seenan, J.P.; Macdonald, J. Micronutrient Status and Prediction of Disease Outcome in Adults with Inflammatory Bowel Disease Receiving Biologic Therapy. *Inflamm. Bowel Dis.* **2023**, izad174. [CrossRef] [PubMed]
41. Geerling, B.J.; Badart-Smook, A.; Stockbrügger, R.W.; Brummer, R.J. Comprehensive nutritional status in patients with long-standing Crohn disease currently in remission. *Am. J. Clin. Nutr.* **1998**, *67*, 919–926. [CrossRef] [PubMed]
42. Geerling, B.J.; Badart-Smook, A.; Stockbrügger, R.W.; Brummer, R.J. Comprehensive nutritional status in recently diagnosed patients with inflammatory bowel disease compared with population controls. *Eur. J. Clin. Nutr.* **2000**, *54*, 514–521. [CrossRef] [PubMed]
43. Tajika, M.; Matsuura, A.; Nakamura, T.; Suzuki, T.; Sawaki, A.; Kato, T.; Hara, K.; Ookubo, K.; Yamao, K.; Kato, M.; et al. Risk factors for vitamin D deficiency in patients with Crohn's disease. *J. Gastroenterol.* **2004**, *39*, 527–533. [CrossRef] [PubMed]
44. Filippi, J.; Al-Jaouni, R.; Wiroth, J.B.; Hébuterne, X.; Schneider, S.M. Nutritional deficiencies in patients with Crohn's disease in remission. *Inflamm. Bowel Dis.* **2006**, *12*, 185–191. [CrossRef]
45. Valentini, L.; Schaper, L.; Buning, C.; Hengstermann, S.; Koernicke, T.; Tillinger, W.; Guglielmi, F.W.; Norman, K.; Buhner, S.; Ockenga, J.; et al. Malnutrition and impaired muscle strength in patients with Crohn's disease and ulcerative colitis in remission. *Nutrition* **2008**, *24*, 694–702. [CrossRef] [PubMed]
46. de Castro, M.M.; Corona, L.P.; Pascoal, L.B.; Rodrigues, B.L.; de Lourdes Setsuko Ayrizono, M.; Rodrigues Coy, C.S.; Leal, R.F.; Milanski, M. Impaired nutritional status in outpatients in remission or with active Crohn's disease—Classified by objective endoscopic and imaging assessments. *Clin. Nutr. ESPEN* **2019**, *33*, 60–65. [CrossRef] [PubMed]
47. MacMaster, M.J.; Damianopoulou, S.; Thomson, C.; Talwar, D.; Stefanowicz, F.; Catchpole, A.; Gerasimidis, K.; Gaya, D.R. A prospective analysis of micronutrient status in quiescent inflammatory bowel disease. *Clin. Nutr.* **2021**, *40*, 327–331. [CrossRef] [PubMed]

48. Eiden, K.A. *Nutritional Considerations in Inflammatory Bowel Disease;* Nutrition Issues in Gastroenterology, Series #5; Parrish, C.R., Ed.; Barnes-Jewish Hospita: St. Louis, MO, USA, 2003. Available online: https://med.virginia.edu/ginutrition/wp-content/uploads/sites/199/2015/11/eidenarticle-May-03.pdf (accessed on 12 January 2024).
49. Zheng, Y.; Liao, Y.; Ouyang, Y.; Wu, Z.; Li, Z.; Lin, J.; Zhang, K.; Wang, X.; Cen, Z.; Ma, W.; et al. The effects and predictive value of calcium and magnesium concentrations on nutritional improvement, inflammatory response and diagnosis in patients with Crohn's disease. *J. Hum. Nutr. Diet.* **2023**, *36*, 1649–1660. [CrossRef] [PubMed]
50. McDonnell, M.; Sartain, S.; Westoby, C.; Katarachia, V.; Wootton, S.A.; Cummings, J.R.F. Micronutrient Status in Adult Crohn's Disease during Clinical Remission: A Systematic Review. *Nutrients* **2023**, *15*, 4777. [CrossRef]
51. Roblin, X.; Phelip, J.M.; Genevois, M.; Ducros, V.; Bonaz, B. Hyperhomocysteinaemia is associated with osteoporosis in patients with Crohn's disease. *Aliment. Pharmacol. Ther.* **2007**, *25*, 797–804. [CrossRef]
52. Vagianos, K.; Bector, S.; McConnell, J.; Bernstein, C.N.; Vagianos, K.; Bector, S.; McConnell, J.; Bernstein, C.N. Nutrition assessment of patients with inflammatory bowel disease. *J. Parenter. Enter. Nutr.* **2007**, *31*, 311–319. [CrossRef] [PubMed]
53. Vagianos, K.; Bernstein, C.N. Homocysteinemia and B vitamin status among adult patients with inflammatory bowel disease: A one-year prospective follow-up study. *Inflamm. Bowel Dis.* **2012**, *18*, 718–724. [CrossRef] [PubMed]
54. Bermejo, F.; Algaba, A.; Guerra, I.; Chaparro, M.; De-La-Poza, G.; Valer, P.; Piqueras, B.; Bermejo, A.; Garcia-Alonso, J.; Perez, M.J.; et al. Should we monitor vitamin B12 and folate levels in Crohn's disease patients? *Scand. J. Gastroenterol.* **2013**, *48*, 1272–1277. [CrossRef] [PubMed]

nutrients

MDPI

Article

Exploring the Preventive Potential of Vitamin D against Respiratory Infections in Preschool-Age Children: A Cross-Sectional Study

Oana Silvana Sarau [1,2], Hari Charan Rachabattuni [3], Sai Teja Gadde [4], Sai Praveen Daruvuri [5], Larisa Mihaela Marusca [2,6,*], Florin George Horhat [7], Ariadna Petronela Fildan [8], Elena Tanase [2], Catalin Prodan-Barbulescu [2,9,10] and Delia Ioana Horhat [11]

1 Department V, Internal Medicine, Discipline of Hematology, "Victor Babes" University of Medicine and Pharmacy Timisoara, Eftimie Murgu Square 2, 300041 Timisoara, Romania; oana.sarau@umft.ro
2 Doctoral School, "Victor Babes" University of Medicine and Pharmacy Timisoara, Eftimie Murgu Square 2, 300041 Timisoara, Romania; tanase.elena@umft.ro (E.T.); catalin.prodan-barbulescu@umft.ro (C.P.-B.)
3 Faculty of General Medicine, Dr. Y.S.R. University of Health Sciences, Vijayawada 520008, India; haricharanrachabattuni@gmail.com
4 Faculty of General Medicine, All India Institute of Medical Sciences (AIIMS), Mangalagiri 522503, India; gaddesai0626@gmail.com
5 Faculty of General Medicine, Bukovinian State Medical University, Teatralna Square, 2, 58002 Chernivtsi, Ukraine; praveenzzz39@gmail.com
6 Laboratory Medicine, "Louis Turcanu" Emergency Hospital for Children, Doctor Iosif Nemoianu Street, 300011 Timisoara, Romania
7 Department of Microbiology, Multidisciplinary Research Center on Antimicrobial Resistance (MULTI-REZ), "Victor Babes" University of Medicine and Pharmacy, 300041 Timisoara, Romania; horhat.florin@umft.ro
8 Department of Pulmonology, Faculty of Medicine, "Ovidius" University of Constanta, 900470 Constanta, Romania; petronela.fildan@365.univ-ovidius.ro
9 Department of Anatomy and Embryology, Discipline of Pulmonology, "Victor Babes" University of Medicine and Pharmacy Timisoara, Eftimie Murgu Square 2, 300041 Timisoara, Romania
10 IInd Surgery Clinic, "Victor Babes" University of Medicine and Pharmacy Timisoara, Eftimie Murgu Square 2, 300041 Timisoara, Romania
11 Department of Ear-Nose-Throat, "Victor Babes" University of Medicine and Pharmacy, 300041 Timisoara, Romania; horhat.ioana@umft.ro
* Correspondence: larisa.marusca@umft.ro

Abstract: Recent studies hypothesized that vitamin D supplementation and subsequent higher 25(OH)D serum levels could protect against respiratory infections in children. This cross-sectional study, conducted from May 2022 to December 2023 in Timisoara, Romania, aimed to evaluate the potential influence of vitamin D supplementation on the incidence of respiratory infections among preschool-age children. This study examined 215 children over 18 months who were split into a group of patients with recurrent respiratory infections ($n = 141$) and another group of patients with only one respiratory tract infection in the past 12 months ($n = 74$). Patients were evaluated based on their serum vitamin D levels 25(OH)D, demographic characteristics, and health outcomes. The study identified that preschool-age children with recurrent infections had significantly lower mean vitamin D concentrations (24.5 ng/mL) compared to the control group (29.7 ng/mL, $p < 0.001$). Additionally, a higher proportion of vitamin D deficiency was observed among children with recurrent infections in the past 12 months. Notably, vitamin D supplementation above 600 IU/week significantly reduced the likelihood of respiratory infections, evidenced by an odds ratio of 0.523 ($p < 0.001$), indicating that preschool-age children receiving a dose of vitamin D higher than 600 IU/week were about half as likely to experience respiratory infections compared to those who did not. Furthermore, no significant associations were found between sun exposure, daily sunscreen use, and the incidence of respiratory infections. Conclusively, this study underscores the potential role of vitamin D in helping the immune system against respiratory infections in preschool-age children. The observed protective effect of vitamin D supplementation suggests a potential public health strategy to mitigate the incidence of respiratory infections in preschool children on top of the already known benefits.

Keywords: vitamin D; children; blood tests; respiratory infections

1. Introduction

Vitamin D is synthesized in the skin from 7-dehydrocholesterol when exposed to ultraviolet B (UVB) radiation from sunlight, converting it to cholecalciferol (vitamin D3). Additionally, it can be absorbed through the diet from foods such as fatty fish, egg yolks, and fortified products [1]. Once vitamin D3 is produced or ingested, it undergoes two hydroxylation steps to become biologically active. The first occurs in the liver, where vitamin D3 is converted into 25-hydroxyvitamin D (25(OH)D) by the enzyme 25-hydroxylase. This form of vitamin D is the main circulating form and is what is commonly measured in laboratory analyses to assess vitamin D status. The second hydroxylation takes place in the kidneys, involving the enzyme 1α-hydroxylase, which converts 25(OH)D into the physiologically active form, 1,25-dihydroxyvitamin D (1,25(OH)$_2$D). This active form is crucial for calcium absorption and bone health. The measurement of 25(OH)D is preferred in clinical settings because it has a longer half-life and reflects overall vitamin D reserves more accurately than the highly regulated 1,25(OH)$_2$D [1,2].

Vitamin D, a fat-soluble vitamin, plays an important role in calcium homeostasis and bone metabolism [1–3]. Beyond these traditional roles, emerging evidence suggests a significant impact of vitamin D on the immune system, particularly in the prevention of infections [3–5]. Epidemiological studies have consistently shown a link between vitamin D deficiency and increased susceptibility to infectious diseases, including respiratory infections [6–8]. This association is of particular interest in preschool children who are at a higher risk of developing respiratory infections due to their still-developing immune systems and high exposure rates in communal settings, such as daycare and preschool [9–11].

Respiratory infections, ranging from the common cold to more severe conditions like pneumonia, represent a leading cause of morbidity among preschool-age children worldwide [12–14]. The burden of these infections is not only reflected in the immediate health of the child but also in increased healthcare costs, parental anxiety, and lost days from school and work. Vitamin D's potential to enhance innate and adaptive immune responses suggests a promising adjunctive strategy to reduce the incidence and severity of respiratory infections in this vulnerable population [15–17]. In this context, several large studies and meta-analyses observed the safety and overall protective role of vitamin D supplements and higher 25(OH)D levels against respiratory infections [18,19].

Despite the plausibility of vitamin D's role in modulating immune function, the clinical efficacy of vitamin D supplementation as a preventive measure against respiratory infections in children remains a subject of debate [20,21]. Studies have yielded mixed results, with some showing a significant reduction in the incidence of infections with vitamin D supplementation, while others report no substantial benefits [22,23]. This inconsistency may be attributed to variations in the study design, population, vitamin D dosing, and baseline vitamin D status of participants.

Real-world data underscore the prevalence of vitamin D deficiency in preschool children, which is attributed to factors, such as insufficient dietary intake, limited sun exposure, and the increased use of sunscreen. In the United States, the National Health and Nutrition Examination Survey (NHANES) has documented that approximately 70% of preschool children do not meet the recommended dietary allowance for vitamin D [24,25]. Similar trends are observed globally, emphasizing the need for effective public health strategies to address this deficiency.

Research suggests that vitamin D can influence the production of antimicrobial peptides. such as cathelicidin, which is part of the innate immune system and can annihilate respiratory pathogens [26,27]. In preschool-age children, who are particularly susceptible to respiratory infections due to their developing immune systems and frequent exposure to pathogens in group settings, maintaining optimal levels of vitamin D can be critical. The frequent occurrence of vitamin D insufficiency in this age group further justifies the need for supplementation as a preventative health measure. Therefore, supplementing with vitamin D may not only correct the high prevalence of insufficiency but also enhance the immune responses that are essential in protecting these children from respiratory infections. Therefore, the current study aims to determine the serum vitamin D levels in preschool children and assess their role and supplementation in preventing respiratory infections in this population. By evaluating the efficacy of vitamin D in this context, this study seeks to provide a comprehensive understanding of its potential as a preventive strategy against respiratory infections in preschool children.

2. Materials and Methods

2.1. Study Design and Ethical Considerations

This cross-sectional study was conducted over a period of 1.5 years, spanning from May 2022 to December 2023, and taking place at the County Clinical Hospital from Timisoara, Romania, and private clinics, focusing on the evaluation of preschool children with and without respiratory infections based on their vitamin D status.

This study adhered strictly to the ethical standards set by the institutional research committee and was in alignment with the principles of the 1964 Helsinki Declaration and its subsequent amendments concerning ethical standards in medical research. The research protocol received thorough review and approval from the Ethical Committee for Scientific Research at the "Victor Babes" University of Medicine and Pharmacy Timisoara. The approval, granted in 2022, was documented under approval number 65.

Consent was meticulously obtained by fully informing the parents or legal guardians of the study's scope, potential risks, and benefits. Additionally, age-appropriate explanations were provided to the children to gain their assent. All processes were designed to adhere strictly to ethical standards, ensuring both the protection and comfort of the young participants throughout the study's duration.

2.2. Inclusion and Exclusion Criteria

The inclusion criteria for this study comprised the following: (1) preschool children aged between 2 and 5 years; (2) children whose parents agreed to determine the status of their vitamin D serum levels, allowing for an assessment of their vitamin D status and its potential correlation with respiratory health; (3) the completion of a background check regarding the vitamin D status and influencing factors; (4) children who experienced at least one documented respiratory infection in the past year, providing a direct measure to evaluate the protective role of vitamin D against respiratory infections. Conversely, the exclusion criteria were distinctly defined to maintain the study's focus and integrity as follows: (1) children with chronic respiratory conditions, such as asthma or cystic fibrosis, due to the potential confounding effect on the study's outcomes; (2) children diagnosed with any condition affecting vitamin D metabolism (e.g., renal disease, hyperparathyroidism), which could independently influence the study's findings; (3) cases where medical records were not available or consent for using these records in the study was not obtained; (4) the refusal to measure the vitamin D levels in private clinics at the expense of the participants; (5) and children in the acute phase of respiratory infection.

Children with chronic conditions such as asthma were excluded to avoid complications that could arise from their underlying health issues, which might affect the study's outcomes in relation to respiratory infections and vitamin D's effect on immune function. This exclusion helped when isolating the impact of vitamin D on otherwise healthy children, making the results more interpretable regarding the direct relationship studied. To address potential selection bias, participants were recruited from a wide demographic range using multiple platforms, such as pediatric clinics, community centers, and schools.

2.3. Laboratory Analysis

Within the framework of this study, serum levels of 25-hydroxyvitamin D (25(OH)D) were quantified through the immunoassay method using the COBAS INTEGRA 400 PLUS automated analyzer. According to existing recent guidelines [28], reference values for 25(OH)D levels are defined as follows: (1) the optimal level ranges from 30 to 55.5 ng/mL; (2) the insufficient level ranges from 21 to 29 ng/mL; (3) deficiency is indicated by levels of 20 ng/mL or less; and (4) severe deficiency is marked by levels of 16 ng/mL or less. Each participant's 25-OHD level was measured at physicians' recommendations. A wide range of variables were analyzed to investigate the relationship between vitamin D supplementation and the incidence of respiratory infections among preschool-age children. The collected data encompassed basic demographic details, physiological measurements, vitamin D metabolism markers, inflammatory and infection markers, complete blood count elements, and health outcomes related to infections and hospitalizations.

Demographic and physiological parameters, such as age, gender, body mass index (BMI), height, and weight, were recorded, along with development status (normal, underweight, wasting, stunting) and background (urban or rural). The study also investigated daily calorie intake and nutritional vitamin D supplementation status to determine dietary impacts. Markers critical for understanding vitamin D metabolism, including 25-OHD, PTH (parathyroid hormone), calcitonin, serum calcium, serum phosphate, and creatinine levels, were measured.

Inflammatory and infection markers, such as CRP (C-reactive protein), ferritin, ESR (erythrocyte sedimentation rate), and iron levels, in addition to complete blood count components including WBC (white blood cells), RBC (red blood cells), lymphocytes, hemoglobin, hematocrit, and platelets, were evaluated. Measurements of acid uric and magnesium were also taken. Information regarding vaccinations, the presence of infection, type of infection, site of infection, and the use of antibiotics were used.

2.4. Statistical Analysis

Data management and analysis were conducted utilizing the statistical software SPSS version 26.0 (SPSS Inc., Chicago, IL, USA). Continuous variables were represented as the mean ± standard deviation (SD), while categorical variables were expressed in terms of frequencies and percentages. Student's *t*-test was used to compare two means between the continuous data. The Chi-square test was utilized for the categorical variables. The best cutoff value, sensitivity, specificity, Area Under Curve (AUC), and the Receiver Operating Characteristic were calculated to determine the prediction value of the proposed parameters. A *p*-value threshold of less than 0.05 was set for statistical significance. All results were double-checked through independent re-analysis to ensure accuracy and reliability.

3. Results

Background Characteristics

The study encompassed a sample of 215 children, split into two groups: those with recurrent respiratory infections ($n = 141$) and those without ($n = 74$). Regarding age, the mean age of children with recurrent infections was slightly higher (3.78 years) compared to those without recurrent infections (3.67 years), although the difference was not statistically significant ($p = 0.483$).

A notable finding emerged in the assessment of vitamin D supplementation, where a significant difference was observed. Only 22.70% of children with recurrent infections received vitamin D supplementation above 600 UI/week compared to 59.46% in the non-recurrent group, yielding a highly significant *p*-value (<0.001). Further analysis of the type of respiratory infection (upper versus lower tract) did not yield significant differences ($p = 0.503$). Sun exposure time and daily sunscreen use did not significantly correlate to respiratory infection recurrence, with *p*-values indicating no significant association, as seen in Table 1.

Table 1. Comparison of background characteristics.

Variables	Recurrent Respiratory Infections (n = 141)	No Recurrent Respiratory Infections (n = 74)	p-Value
Age (mean ± SD)	3.78 ± 0.95	3.67 ± 1.03	0.483
Age category, n (%)			0.675
2–3 years	68 (48.23%)	32 (43.24%)	
4–5 years	73 (51.77%)	42 (56.76%)	
BMI (mean ± SD)	16.3 ± 1.6	16.5 ± 1.3	0.389
Development, n (%)			
Normal	108 (76.60%)	56 (75.68%)	0.847
Underweight	16 (11.35%)	12 (16.22%)	0.423
Overweight	11 (7.80%)	5 (6.76%)	0.765
Low weight for height	4 (2.84%)	1 (1.35%)	0.621
Low height for age	2 (1.42%)	0 (0.00%)	0.486
Place of living			0.822
Rural	58 (41.13%)	29 (39.19%)	
Urban	83 (58.87%)	45 (60.81%)	
Daily calorie intake, n (%)			
Low (< 1400 kcal)	29 (20.57%)	16 (21.62%)	0.922
Moderate (1400–1600 kcal)	68 (48.23%)	36 (48.65%)	0.966
High (>1600 kcal)	44 (31.21%)	22 (29.73%)	0.882
Vitamin D supplementation (>600 UI/week), n (%)			4.8×10^{-5}
Yes	32 (22.70%)	44 (59.46%)	
No	109 (77.30%)	30 (40.54%)	
Number of respiratory infections in the past 12 months, n (%)			3.2×10^{-5}
1	0 (0.00%)	74 (100.00%)	
2–3	89 (63.12%)	0 (0.00%)	
>3	52 (36.88%)	0 (0.00%)	
Type of respiratory infection			0.503
Upper tract infection	117 (83.00%)	64 (86.49%)	
Lower tract infection	24 (17.00%)	10 (13.51%)	
Sun exposure per day, n (%)			
5–15 min	52 (36.88%)	25 (33.78%)	0.744
15–30 min	59 (41.84%)	34 (45.95%)	0.679
>30 min	30 (21.28%)	15 (20.27%)	0.888
Daily sunscreen use, n (%)			
Frequently	23 (16.31%)	10 (13.51%)	0.648
Often	44 (31.21%)	28 (37.84%)	0.556
Rarely	58 (41.13%)	26 (35.14%)	0.419
Never	16 (11.35%)	10 (13.51%)	0.764
Antibiotic use in the past 6 months, n (%)			0.257
Yes	81 (57.45%)	37 (50.00%)	
No	60 (42.55%)	37 (50.00%)	

SD—standard deviation; BMI—body mass index; adjusted significance level (p-value threshold) after Bonferroni correction = 0.0041; non-recurrent indicates only 1 respiratory infection.

The concentration of 25-hydroxyvitamin D_3 (25-OHD) showed a significant difference between the groups. Children with recurrent respiratory infections had a lower mean concentration of 24.5 ng/mL, falling below the optimal range and significantly lower than the 29.7 ng/mL observed in children without recurrent infections ($p < 0.001$). Parathyroid hormone (PTH) levels were also higher in the group with recurrent infections, with a mean value of 55.2 ± 15.3 pg/mL compared to 48.7 ± 14.8 pg/mL in the non-recurrent group, which was statistically significant ($p = 0.023$). Other parameters, including calcitonin, calcium, phosphate, and creatinine levels, were within normal ranges and did not show significant differences between the two groups.

However, C-reactive protein levels were significantly higher in children with recurrent respiratory infections (6.8 mg/L) compared to those without (3.1 mg/L), with a p-value of <0.001. ESR showed a moderate but statistically significant difference, with higher rates in the recurrent infection group (18.5 mm/h) compared to the non-recurrent group (14.7 mm/h), indicating a higher level of inflammation ($p = 0.037$). The study also found a significant difference in white blood cell (WBC) counts, with higher counts in children with recurrent respiratory infections (8.3×10^9/L) compared to those without (7.2×10^9/L) ($p = 0.004$). The vitamin D assessment further highlighted the nutritional status, showing a significantly higher percentage of children with optimal vitamin D levels in the non-recurrent group (33.78%) compared to the recurrent group (12.77%) ($p < 0.001$), as presented in Table 2. Conversely, a higher proportion of vitamin D deficiency was noted in children with recurrent infections.

Table 2. Comparison of laboratory parameters between preschool children with and without recurrent respiratory infections.

Variables (Mean ± SD)	Normal Range	Recurrent Respiratory Infections (n = 141)	No Recurrent Respiratory Infections (n = 74)	p-Value
25-OHD (ng/mL)	30–55.5	24.5 ± 5.3	29.7 ± 6.1	3.9×10^{-4}
PTH (pg/mL)	15–65	55.2 ± 15.3	48.7 ± 14.8	0.023
Calcitonin (pg/mL)	<10	7.3 ± 2.5	6.9 ± 2.2	0.311
Calcium (mg/dL)	8.8–10.8	9.4 ± 0.8	9.5 ± 0.7	0.542
Phosphate (mg/dL)	3.4–5.5	4.2 ± 0.5	4.3 ± 0.4	0.376
Creatinine (mg/dL)	0.3–0.7	0.5 ± 0.1	0.5 ± 0.1	0.890
CRP (mg/L)	<5	6.8 ± 2.3	3.1 ± 1.2	6.1×10^{-6}
Ferritin (ng/mL)	15–150	60.3 ± 25.4	55.1 ± 22.3	0.148
ESR (mm/h)	0–20	18.5 ± 8.3	14.7 ± 7.9	0.037
Iron (μg/dL)	50–120	85.2 ± 23.7	91.3 ± 25.1	0.153
WBC ($\times 10^9$/L)	4.0–10.0	8.3 ± 2.1	7.2 ± 1.8	0.004
RBC ($\times 10^{12}$/L)	4.5–5.5	4.8 ± 0.6	4.9 ± 0.5	0.272
Lymphocytes (%)	20–40	35.2 ± 8.4	37.1 ± 7.9	0.154
Neutrophils (%)	40–60	54.6 ± 7.5	52.8 ± 6.9	0.088
Hemoglobin (g/dL)	11.0–14.0	12.3 ± 1.2	12.5 ± 1.1	0.229
Platelets ($\times 10^9$/L)	150–450	310.5 ± 80.2	325.3 ± 75.4	0.197
Vitamin D assessment, n (%)				
Optimal	30–55.5 ng/mL	18 (12.77%)	25 (33.78%)	5.0×10^{-4}
Insufficient	21–29 ng/mL	63 (44.68%)	34 (45.95%)	0.881
Deficient	20–16 ng/mL	52 (36.88%)	12 (16.22%)	6.6×10^{-5}
Severe deficiency	<16 ng/mL	8 (5.67%)	3 (4.05%)	0.717

SD—Standard deviation; optimal level ranges from 30 to 55.5 ng/mL; insufficient level ranges from 21 to 29 ng/mL; deficiency is indicated by levels of 20 ng/mL or less; severe deficiency is marked by levels of 16 ng/mL or less. 25-OHD—25-hydroxyvitamin D_3; PTH—parathyroid hormone; CRP—C-reactive protein; ESR—erythrocyte sedimentation rate; WBC—white blood cells; RBC—red blood cells; adjusted significance level (p-value threshold) after Bonferroni correction = 0.0025; non-recurrent indicates only 1 respiratory infection.

A clear gradient was observed in the levels of 25-hydroxyvitamin D_3 (25-OHD), with children experiencing infections only once after having the highest mean concentration of 29.7 ± 6.1 ng/mL, which decreased to 25.2 ± 5.4 ng/mL in children with two to three infections, and further to 22.8 ± 4.9 ng/mL in those with more than three infections ($p < 0.001$). C-reactive protein levels escalated markedly with the frequency of infections, from 3.1 ± 1.2 mg/L in the group with one infection to 8.7 ± 3.3 mg/L in the group with more than three infections ($p < 0.001$). ESR followed a similar pattern, providing additional evidence of increased inflammatory activity with more frequent infections ($p = 0.002$). White blood cell counts also showed a significant increase, correlating with the frequency of infections ($p < 0.001$).

Children who experienced respiratory infections only once had the highest proportion of optimal vitamin D levels (33.78%), which is within the range of 30 to 55.5 ng/mL. In the groups with multiple respiratory infections, the proportion of optimal vitamin D levels was significantly diminished to 13.48% and 9.62%, respectively. Conversely, the proportion of children classified as vitamin D deficient (levels of 20 ng/mL or less) escalated with the frequency of respiratory infections. This trend is especially notable in children who had more than three infections, where 38.46% were found to be vitamin D deficient, compared to 31.46% in the group with two to three infections and only 16.22% in the once-infected group. Moreover, the analysis extended to children with severe vitamin D deficiency (levels below 16 ng/mL), although the increases in proportions across groups from those infected once (4.05%) to those with more than three infections (9.62%) did not reach the same level of statistical significance, as presented in Table 3.

Table 3. Vitamin D and laboratory assessment based on the prevalence of respiratory infections in preschool children in the past 12 months.

Variables (Mean ± SD)	1 Time (n = 74)	2–3 Times (n = 89)	>3 Times (n = 52)	p-Value
25-OHD (ng/mL)	29.7 ± 6.1	25.2 ± 5.4	22.8 ± 4.9	4.8×10^{-4}
PTH (pg/mL)	48.7 ± 14.8	54.9 ± 15.1	58.3 ± 16.2	0.004
Calcitonin (pg/mL)	6.9 ± 2.2	7.1 ± 2.3	7.5 ± 2.4	0.218
Calcium (mg/dL)	9.5 ± 0.7	9.3 ± 0.8	9.2 ± 0.9	0.076
Phosphate (mg/dL)	4.3 ± 0.4	4.1 ± 0.5	4.0 ± 0.6	0.037
Creatinine (mg/dL)	0.5 ± 0.1	0.5 ± 0.1	0.6 ± 0.1	0.019
CRP (mg/L)	3.1 ± 1.2	6.5 ± 2.1	8.7 ± 3.3	4.2×10^{-5}
Ferritin (ng/mL)	55.1 ± 22.3	61.7 ± 25.1	67.9 ± 27.5	0.031
ESR (mm/hr)	14.7 ± 7.9	18.4 ± 8.2	21.6 ± 9.4	0.002
Iron (μg/dL)	91.3 ± 25.1	86.4 ± 24.8	82.1 ± 23.6	0.053
WBC ($\times 10^9$/L)	7.2 ± 1.8	8.4 ± 2.0	9.1 ± 2.3	3.9×10^{-5}
RBC ($\times 10^{12}$/L)	4.9 ± 0.5	4.8 ± 0.6	4.7 ± 0.7	0.127
Lymphocytes (%)	37.1 ± 7.9	34.5 ± 8.2	32.3 ± 8.5	0.010
Neutrophils (%)	52.8 ± 6.9	55.4 ± 7.2	58.2 ± 7.5	0.003
Hemoglobin (g/dL)	12.5 ± 1.1	12.2 ± 1.2	11.9 ± 1.3	0.017
Platelets ($\times 10^9$/L)	325.3 ± 75.4	308.2 ± 80.1	296.7 ± 82.3	0.044
Vitamin D assessment, n (%)				
Optimal	25 (33.78%)	12 (13.48%)	5 (9.62%)	3.6×10^{-4}
Insufficient	34 (45.95%)	41 (46.07%)	22 (42.31%)	0.912
Deficient	12 (16.22%)	28 (31.46%)	20 (38.46%)	0.001
Severe deficiency	3 (4.05%)	8 (8.99%)	5 (9.62%)	0.258

SD—Standard deviation; optimal level ranges from 30 to 55.5 ng/mL; insufficient level ranges from 21 to 29 ng/mL; deficiency is indicated by levels of 20 ng/mL or less; severe deficiency is marked by levels of 16 ng/mL or less. 25-OHD—25-hydroxyvitamin D_3; PTH—parathyroid hormone; CRP—C-reactive protein; ESR—erythrocyte sedimentation rate; WBC—white blood cells; RBC—red blood cells; adjusted significance level (p-value threshold) after Bonferroni correction = 0.0025; and non-recurrent indicates only 1 respiratory infection.

Figure 1 presents the recurrent versus non-recurrent respiratory infections and compares these based on vitamin D supplementation levels (<600 UI weekly versus >600 UI weekly), illustrating a notable distinction in median vitamin D levels between the groups. Specifically, children receiving more than 600 UI of vitamin D weekly tended to have higher median vitamin D levels regardless of their infection recurrence status. The groups receiving less than 600 UI and more than 600 UI of vitamin D weekly displayed median vitamin D levels of 24.5 ng/mL and 29.7 ng/mL, respectively.

It was observed that groups with more frequent respiratory infections exhibited lower median vitamin D levels, accentuating the potential protective role of vitamin D against such infections. Notably, the subgroup experiencing more than three respiratory infections and receiving less than 600 UI of vitamin D, weekly, showcased a median vitamin D level of 22.8 ng/mL with an IQR of 4.9 ng/mL, compared to their counterparts receiving more than 600 UI, who exhibited a slightly higher median of 26.15 ng/mL and an IQR of 6.31 ng/mL (Figure 2).

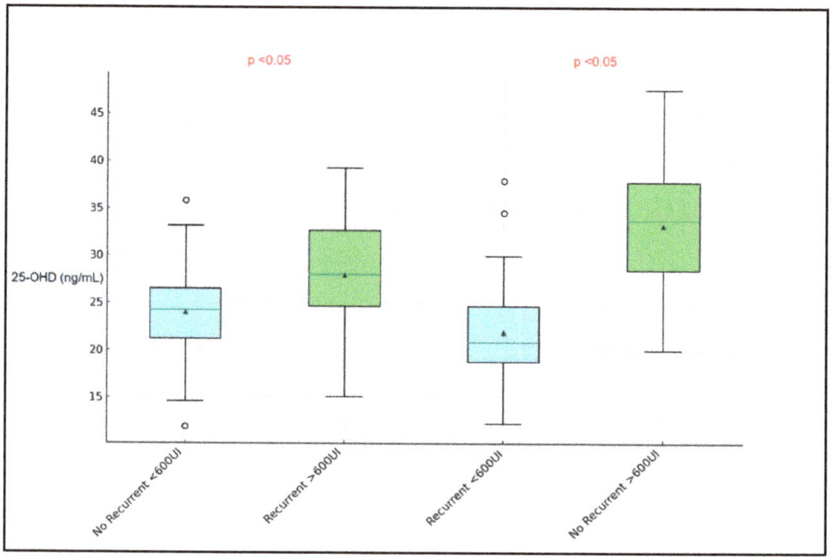

Figure 1. Boxplot analysis of vitamin D levels between preschool children with and without recurrent respiratory infections in the past 12 months (non-recurrent indicates only 1 respiratory infection).

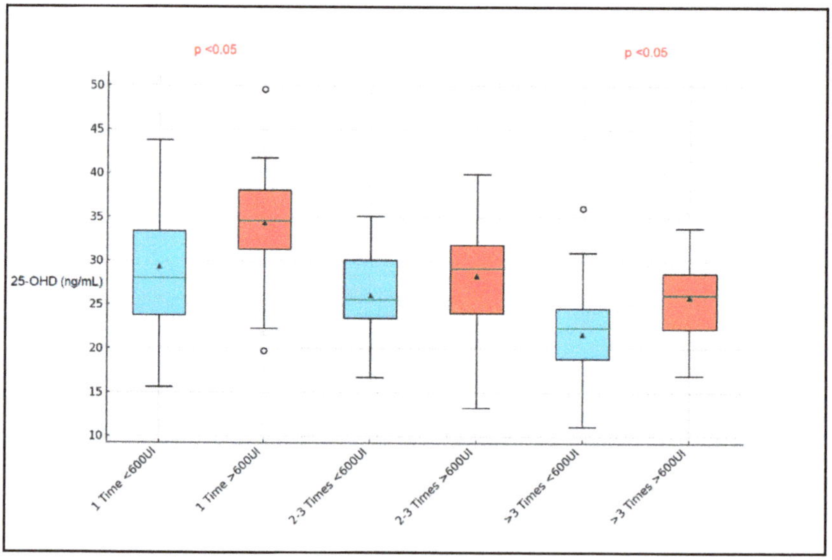

Figure 2. Boxplot analysis by number of respiratory infections in the past 12 months.

Children with severe vitamin D deficiency levels were significantly more likely to suffer from respiratory infections, with an odds ratio (Exp(B)) of 2.967, indicating that they were almost three times as likely to have infections compared to those with optimal vitamin D levels (p-value < 0.001).

Vitamin D supplementation greater than 600 IU/week was associated with a significant decrease in the likelihood of respiratory infections, with an odds ratio of 0.523 (p-value < 0.001), indicating that children receiving this level of supplementation were about half as likely to experience respiratory infections as those who did not receive supplementation, as presented in Table 4.

Table 4. Regression table.

Predictor	B (Coefficients)	Standard Error	Wald	df	*p*-Value	Exp(B) (Odds Ratio)
Vitamin D Status (Reference: Optimal)						
Insufficient	0.143	0.193	0.549	1	0.469	1.154
Deficient	0.289	0.218	1.756	1	0.185	1.335
Severe Deficiency	1.087	0.304	12.785	1	<0.001	2.967
Vitamin D Supplementation (>600 IU/week)	−0.648	0.176	13.519	1	<0.001	0.523
Sun Exposure (Reference: >30 min)						
5–15 min	0.132	0.251	0.276	1	0.599	1.141
15–30 min	0.098	0.205	0.228	1	0.633	1.103
Daily Sunscreen Use (Reference: Never)						
Frequently	0.061	0.265	0.053	1	0.817	1.063
Often	0.034	0.184	0.034	1	0.853	1.035
Rarely	−0.017	0.147	0.013	1	0.909	0.983

df—degrees of freedom.

4. Discussion

4.1. Literature Findings

The findings from our cross-sectional study found a potentially protective role of vitamin D supplementation in reducing the incidence of respiratory infections among preschool-age children. An interesting aspect of this study was the demonstrable effect of vitamin D supplementation above 600 IU/week, which significantly reduced the likelihood of respiratory infections. This correlation supports the hypothesis that vitamin D can have an important role in enhancing immune resilience in this age group.

Critical to our discussion is the contrast in outcomes based on vitamin D status. Children with severe vitamin D deficiency were found to be almost three times more likely to experience respiratory infections compared to those with optimal levels. This significant finding not only highlights the importance of maintaining adequate vitamin D levels for immune health but also indicates the need for targeted interventions in populations at risk of deficiency. Interestingly, our study also found a non-significant relationship between sun exposure, daily sunscreen use, and the incidence of respiratory infections. This finding suggests that the protective effects of vitamin D on respiratory health are not undermined by limited sun exposure or sunscreen use, which are critical factors for skin cancer prevention. It reinforces the importance of dietary supplementation as a reliable method for maintaining adequate vitamin D levels, particularly in regions with limited sunlight or in populations where outdoor activities are minimized.

Moreover, the study's outcomes emphasize the importance of vitamin D supplementation as a public health strategy. The substantial reduction in infection with supplementation greater than 600 IU/week underscores the potential for vitamin D as a preventive measure against respiratory infections. These findings advocate for the incorporation of vitamin D supplementation guidelines into public health policies, especially for children at preschool age, to enhance their overall health status and immune resilience. Further research is warranted to explore the optimal levels of supplementation and to evaluate the long-term benefits of maintaining adequate vitamin D levels in preventing respiratory and other infections in this demographic.

However, in addressing how our findings compare with the existing literature, particularly where they diverge from expected outcomes, it is crucial to consider potential discrepancies. Differences in study design, participant demographics, or methodologies may contribute to these variations. This analysis not only reflects a thorough engagement with the field but also identifies specific areas that warrant further investigation.

The findings from Balan et al. [29] and Esposito et al. [20] converge on the important role of vitamin D in protecting against respiratory tract infections in children, which are a leading cause of morbidity and mortality globally. Balan et al. emphasized the alarming prevalence of vitamin D deficiency among infants and its association with heightened risks of severe respiratory infections, including pneumonia, which is responsible for 19% of all deaths in children under five years old. They advocate for the potential of vitamin D supplementation and improved sun exposure guidelines to significantly reduce these risks; however, no actual threshold values for (25(OH)D) were suggested, reinforcing the novelty that our study brings. On the other hand, Esposito et al. [20]'s review further substantiates the immunomodulatory properties of vitamin D and its link to various RTIs in children, noting the absence of a consensus on the definition of vitamin D deficiency and the adequate levels necessary for immune function. They suggest that maintaining serum 25-hydroxycholecalciferol levels between 20 ng/mL and 50 ng/mL could provide protective immunomodulatory effects against RTIs, including tuberculosis and severe bronchiolitis, similar to our findings where serum levels above a threshold of 26.15 ng/mL were considered protective for RTIs, and with the additional dose-dependent impact of more than 600 UI/week.

Contrary to our findings, Şişmanlar et al.'s case–control study [30] found no significant correlation between vitamin D levels and the incidence or severity of lower respiratory tract infections despite a widespread prevalence of vitamin D deficiency/insufficiency among the children studied. On the contrary, Nicolae et al. [31], through a literature review, highlighted the potential immunomodulatory and antiviral effects of vitamin D, suggesting that its supplementation might lower the risk of acute respiratory tract infections, including COVID-19. While Şişmanlar et al. caution against assuming the direct protective role of vitamin D against such infections due to their findings, Nicolae et al. advocate for the potential benefits of vitamin D in mitigating the severity of RTIs, urging further research to solidify these preliminary observations.

Similarly to our findings, Xiao et al.'s study on children with recurrent respiratory tract infections showed a notable improvement in treatment outcomes with vitamin D supplementation, including a significant total effective treatment rate of 96.67% in the vitamin D group versus 71.19% in the control group [32]. This group also saw improvements in immune function indicators, such as IgA, IgG, IgM, and CD4+ levels, and a reduction in the number of respiratory infection episodes. Abioye et al. [33], examining adults, found that vitamin D supplementation slightly reduced the risk of acute respiratory tract infections with a risk ratio of 0.97 and shortened symptom duration of 6%. Their review also highlights the effectiveness of vitamin C in reducing the risks of RTIs (RR = 0.96) and zinc, significantly shortening symptom duration by 47% and underscoring the potential of micronutrients to enhance immune responses against respiratory infections across different age groups.

Jolliffe et al. [18] and Martineau et al. [34] both underscore the efficacy of vitamin D supplementation in reducing the risk of acute respiratory infections through their meta-analyses, albeit with nuanced differences in their findings. Jolliffe et al., analyzing data from 45 RCTs and involving over 73,000 participants, concluded that vitamin D supplementation offers a modest protective effect against acute respiratory infections (OR 0.91, 95% CI 0.84 to 0.99), with daily doses of 400–1000 IU for up to 12 months being particularly effective. Martineau et al. [34], on the other hand, focusing on 25 RCTs with around 11,000 participants, highlighted that vitamin D supplementation significantly reduced the risk of ARIs (adjusted odds ratio 0.88, 95% CI 0.81 to 0.96), especially in those very deficient in vitamin D (baseline 25[OH]D levels < 25 nmol/L) and in recipients of daily or weekly doses without bolus doses. While both analyses agree on the protective role of vitamin D against ARIs and its safety, Martineau et al. provide a more detailed insight into the effectiveness based on baseline vitamin D levels and dosing strategies.

Other studies, such as those conducted by Jat et al. [35] and Buendia et al. [36], provide complementary insights into the role of vitamin D in pediatric respiratory health, underlining both clinical and economic benefits. Jat et.al's systematic review points to a significant correlation between low vitamin D levels and the increased incidence and severity of lower respiratory tract infections in children, suggesting a potential protective role of vitamin D against such infections. Buendia et al., through a cost-utility analysis, further bolster the argument for vitamin D supplementation by demonstrating its cost-effectiveness in preventing acute respiratory infections in children, showcasing not only a reduction in healthcare costs (USD 1354 with supplementation vs. USD 1948 without) but also a slight improvement in quality-adjusted life years (QALYs) (0.99 with vitamin D supplementation vs. 0.98 without). Regarding the implications for a public health policy, although our study did not include a detailed analysis of the costs of healthcare burden, it should be considered in the context of the universal free healthcare in Romania, where this study took place. Nevertheless, a campaign to supplement preschool-age children's diet with at least 600 UI of vitamin D can be considered according to our findings.

Our study, along with corroborating research, emphasizes vitamin D's significant role in combating respiratory infections in children. We found that children with recurrent infections often had lower vitamin D levels, highlighting the potential protective effect of vitamin D supplementation, particularly at doses over 600 IU/week. This aligns with broader research suggesting vitamin D's efficacy in preventing respiratory ailments across different demographics. Our findings advocate for vitamin D supplementation as a viable public health strategy to enhance immune defense among children. Given the accessible nature and potential benefits of such supplementation, further research should aim to optimize vitamin D intake guidelines for pediatric populations.

The current study findings might not be readily applicable to the general population due to the observed lack of the effect of sun exposure, considering the temperate climate of this country of study and the relatively minor differences in 25-OHD levels between groups, which suggest that precise measurements are essential to discern any significant differences. Moreover, the perceived limited availability of the study suggests that supplementing with vitamin D could be a more feasible solution. To validate these findings in diverse regions, a comparison between groups with and without supplements may offer clearer insights.

4.2. Limitations and Future Perspectives

Despite these insightful findings, our study acknowledges several limitations that merit consideration. First, the cross-sectional design limits the ability to infer causality between vitamin D status or supplementation and the incidence of respiratory infections. Longitudinal studies are necessary to establish a temporal relationship and causality. Additionally, the reliance on parental reports for data on sun exposure and supplementation intake could introduce recall bias, potentially affecting the accuracy of these variables. Another limitation is the study's geographic focus on preschool-age children from specific locations within Romania, which may limit the generalizability of the findings to other climates or populations with different dietary habits and lifestyle factors. Furthermore, this study did not account for all potential confounding variables, such as seasonal variations in vitamin D, indoor air quality, exposure to secondhand smoke, and socioeconomic status, which could influence the risk of respiratory infections.

Based on the findings of this study, future research should explore the optimal dosage and duration of vitamin D supplementation necessary to prevent respiratory infections in preschool-age children effectively. Additionally, longitudinal studies could investigate the long-term effects of maintaining higher 25(OH)D serum levels through regular supplementation, especially in different climatic and geographical settings. Given the observed significant impact of vitamin D on reducing respiratory infections, further studies should also consider the interaction between vitamin D supplementation and other preventive health measures, such as vaccination and hygiene practices, to develop comprehensive public health strategies.

5. Conclusions

The findings from this research highlight the potential benefits of vitamin D in boosting the immune defense against respiratory infections among preschool-age children. Evidenced by the positive impact of vitamin D supplementation, this approach appears to be a promising public health intervention aimed at reducing the frequency of such infections within susceptible pediatric groups. This study supports the idea of integrating vitamin D supplementation recommendations into broader public health policies, especially targeting children in areas with inadequate exposure to sunlight. To fully realize the health benefits for this sensitive population group, additional studies are necessary to refine vitamin D supplementation practices, ensuring they are tailored to effectively enhance the pediatric immune system.

Author Contributions: Conceptualization, O.S.S. and L.M.M.; methodology, O.S.S. and L.M.M.; software, L.M.M., H.C.R. and S.T.G.; validation, F.G.H.; formal analysis, F.G.H. and E.T.; investigation, A.P.F.; resources, S.P.D., A.P.F. and E.T.; data curation, H.C.R., S.T.G. and E.T.; writing—original draft preparation, O.S.S., L.M.M., S.P.D.,and F.G.H.; writing—review and editing, H.C.R., S.T.G., A.P.F. and D.I.H.; visualization, S.P.D., D.I.H. and C.P.-B.; supervision, D.I.H. and C.P.-B.; project administration, F.G.H. and C.P.-B. All authors have read and agreed to the published version of the manuscript.

Funding: The article processing charge was paid by the "Victor Babes", University of Medicine and Pharmacy, Timisoara, Romania.

Institutional Review Board Statement: This study was conducted in accordance with the Declaration of Helsinki and approved by the Scientific Research Ethics Committee of the "Victor Babes" University of Medicine and Pharmacy of Timisoara, (approval number 65 from 2022).

Informed Consent Statement: Informed consent was obtained from all subjects involved in the study.

Data Availability Statement: The original contributions presented in the study are included in the article, further inquiries can be directed to the corresponding author.

Conflicts of Interest: The authors declare no conflicts of interest.

References

1. Sizar, O.; Khare, S.; Goyal, A.; Givler, A. Vitamin D Deficiency. In *StatPearls [Internet]*; StatPearls Publishing: Treasure Island, FL, USA, 2024. [PubMed]
2. Dominguez, L.J.; Farruggia, M.; Veronese, N.; Barbagallo, M. Vitamin D Sources, Metabolism, and Deficiency: Available Compounds and Guidelines for Its Treatment. *Metabolites* **2021**, *11*, 255. [CrossRef] [PubMed] [PubMed Central]
3. Ao, T.; Kikuta, J.; Ishii, M. The Effects of Vitamin D on Immune System and Inflammatory Diseases. *Biomolecules* **2021**, *11*, 1624. [CrossRef] [PubMed]
4. Martens, P.J.; Gysemans, C.; Verstuyf, A.; Mathieu, A.C. Vitamin D's Effect on Immune Function. *Nutrients* **2020**, *12*, 1248. [CrossRef] [PubMed] [PubMed Central]
5. Dahma, G.; Craina, M.; Dumitru, C.; Neamtu, R.; Popa, Z.L.; Gluhovschi, A.; Citu, C.; Bratosin, F.; Bloanca, V.; Alambaram, S.; et al. A Prospective Analysis of Vitamin D Levels in Pregnant Women Diagnosed with Gestational Hypertension after SARS-CoV-2 Infection. *J. Pers. Med.* **2023**, *13*, 317. [CrossRef]
6. Raju, A.; Luthra, G.; Shahbaz, M.; Almatooq, H.; Foucambert, P.; Esbrand, F.D.; Zafar, S.; Panthangi, V.; Cyril Kurupp, A.R.; Khan, S. Role of Vitamin D Deficiency in Increased Susceptibility to Respiratory Infections Among Children: A Systematic Review. *Cureus* **2022**, *14*, e29205. [CrossRef] [PubMed] [PubMed Central]
7. Hughes, D.A.; Norton, R. Vitamin D and respiratory health. *Clin. Exp. Immunol.* **2009**, *158*, 20–25. [CrossRef] [PubMed] [PubMed Central]
8. Taha, R.; Abureesh, S.; Alghamdi, S.; Hassan, R.Y.; Cheikh, M.M.; Bagabir, R.A.; Almoallim, H.; Abdulkhaliq, A. The Relationship Between Vitamin D and Infections Including COVID-19: Any Hopes? *Int. J. Gen. Med.* **2021**, *14*, 3849–3870. [CrossRef] [PubMed] [PubMed Central]
9. de Hoog, M.L.; Venekamp, R.P.; van der Ent, C.K.; Schilder, A.; Sanders, E.A.; Damoiseaux, R.A.; Bogaert, D.; Uiterwaal, C.S.; Smit, H.A.; Bruijning-Verhagen, P. Impact of early daycare on healthcare resource use related to upper respiratory tract infections during childhood: Prospective WHISTLER cohort study. *BMC Med.* **2014**, *12*, 107. [CrossRef] [PubMed]
10. Schuez-Havupalo, L.; Toivonen, L.; Karppinen, S.; Kaljonen, A.; Peltola, V. Daycare attendance and respiratory tract infections: A prospective birth cohort study. *BMJ Open* **2017**, *7*, e014635. [CrossRef] [PubMed] [PubMed Central]

11. Shi, C.; Wang, X.; Ye, S.; Deng, S.; Cong, B.; Lu, B.; Li, Y. Understanding the risk of transmission of respiratory viral infections in childcare centres: Protocol for the DISeases TrANsmission in ChildcarE (DISTANCE) multicentre cohort study. *BMJ Open Respir. Res.* **2023**, *10*, e001617. [CrossRef] [PubMed] [PubMed Central]
12. Al Rajeh, A.M.; Naser, A.Y.; Siraj, R.; Alghamdi, A.; Alqahtani, J.; Aldabayan, Y.; Aldhahir, A.; Al Haykan, A.; Elmosaad, Y.M. Acute upper respiratory infections admissions in England and Wales. *Medicine* **2023**, *102*, e33616. [CrossRef] [PubMed] [PubMed Central]
13. Hon, K.L.; Leung, A.K. Severe childhood respiratory viral infections. *Adv. Pediatr.* **2009**, *56*, 47–73. [CrossRef] [PubMed] [PubMed Central]
14. Grimwood, K.; Chang, A.B. Long-term effects of pneumonia in young children. *Pneumonia* **2015**, *6*, 101–114. [CrossRef] [PubMed] [PubMed Central]
15. Grant, W.B.; Lahore, H.; McDonnell, S.L.; Baggerly, C.A.; French, C.B.; Aliano, J.L.; Bhattoa, H.P. Evidence that Vitamin D Supplementation Could Reduce Risk of Influenza and COVID-19 Infections and Deaths. *Nutrients* **2020**, *12*, 988. [CrossRef] [PubMed] [PubMed Central]
16. Gunville, C.F.; Mourani, P.M.; Ginde, A.A. The role of vitamin D in prevention and treatment of infection. *Inflamm. Allergy Drug Targets* **2013**, *12*, 239–245. [CrossRef] [PubMed] [PubMed Central]
17. Wimalawansa, S.J. Controlling Chronic Diseases and Acute Infections with Vitamin D Sufficiency. *Nutrients* **2023**, *15*, 3623. [CrossRef] [PubMed] [PubMed Central]
18. Jolliffe, D.A.; Camargo, C.A., Jr.; Sluyter, J.D.; Aglipay, M.; Aloia, J.F.; Ganmaa, D.; Bergman, P.; Bischoff-Ferrari, H.A.; Borzutzky, A.; Damsgaard, C.T.; et al. Vitamin D supplementation to prevent acute respiratory infections: A systematic review and meta-analysis of aggregate data from randomised controlled trials. *Lancet Diabetes Endocrinol.* **2021**, *9*, 276–292. [CrossRef] [PubMed]
19. Fang, Q.; Wu, Y.; Lu, J.; Zheng, H. A meta-analysis of the association between vitamin D supplementation and the risk of acute respiratory tract infection in the healthy pediatric group. *Front. Nutr.* **2023**, *10*, 1188958. [CrossRef] [PubMed]
20. Esposito, S.; Lelii, M. Vitamin D and respiratory tract infections in childhood. *BMC Infect. Dis.* **2015**, *15*, 487. [CrossRef] [PubMed]
21. Aranow, C. Vitamin D and the immune system. *J. Investig. Med.* **2011**, *59*, 881–886. [CrossRef] [PubMed] [PubMed Central]
22. Liu, Y.; Clare, S.; D'Erasmo, G.; Heilbronner, A.; Dash, A.; Krez, A.; Zaworski, C.; Haseltine, K.; Serota, A.; Miller, A.; et al. Vitamin D and SARS-CoV-2 Infection: SERVE Study (SARS-CoV-2 Exposure and the Role of Vitamin D among Hospital Employees). *J. Nutr.* **2023**, *153*, 1420–1426. [CrossRef] [PubMed] [PubMed Central]
23. Kearns, M.D.; Alvarez, J.A.; Seidel, N.; Tangpricha, V. Impact of vitamin D on infectious disease. *Am. J. Med. Sci.* **2015**, *349*, 245–262. [CrossRef] [PubMed] [PubMed Central]
24. Calvo, M.S.; Whiting, S.J. Perspective: School Meal Programs Require Higher Vitamin D Fortification Levels in Milk Products and Plant-Based Alternatives-Evidence from the National Health and Nutrition Examination Surveys (NHANES 2001–2018). *Adv. Nutr.* **2022**, *13*, 1440–1449. [CrossRef] [PubMed] [PubMed Central]
25. JaBaay, N.R.; Nel, N.H.; Comstock, S.S. Dietary Intake by Toddlers and Preschool Children: Preliminary Results from a Michigan Cohort. *Children* **2023**, *10*, 190. [CrossRef] [PubMed] [PubMed Central]
26. Vargas Buonfiglio, L.G.; Cano, M.; Pezzulo, A.A.; Vanegas Calderon, O.G.; Zabner, J.; Gerke, A.K.; Comellas, A.P. Effect of vitamin D3 on the antimicrobial activity of human airway surface liquid: Preliminary results of a randomised placebo-controlled double-blind trial. *BMJ Open Respir. Res.* **2017**, *4*, e000211. [CrossRef] [PubMed]
27. Gombart, A.F. The vitamin D-antimicrobial peptide pathway and its role in protection against infection. *Future Microbiol.* **2009**, *4*, 1151–1165. [CrossRef] [PubMed] [PubMed Central]
28. Amrein, K.; Scherkl, M.; Hoffmann, M.; Neuwersch-Sommeregger, S.; Köstenberger, M.; Tmava Berisha, A.; Martucci, G.; Pilz, S.; Malle, O. Vitamin D deficiency 2.0: An update on the current status worldwide. *Eur. J. Clin. Nutr.* **2020**, *74*, 1498–1513. [CrossRef] [PubMed]
29. Balan, K.V.; Babu, U.S.; Godar, D.E.; Calvo, M.S. Vitamin D and respiratory infections in infants and toddlers: A nutri-shine perspective. In *Handbook of Vitamin D in Human Health*; Wageningen Academic: Wageningen, The Netherlands, 2013; Volume 4, pp. 276–297. [PubMed Central]
30. Şişmanlar, T.; Aslan, A.T.; Gülbahar, Ö.; Özkan, S. The effect of vitamin D on lower respiratory tract infections in children. *Türk Pediatri Arşivi* **2016**, *51*, 94–99. [CrossRef] [PubMed] [PubMed Central]
31. Nicolae, M.; Mihai, C.M.; Chisnoiu, T.; Balasa, A.L.; Frecus, C.E.; Mihai, L.; Lupu, V.V.; Ion, I.; Pantazi, A.C.; Nelson Twakor, A.; et al. Immunomodulatory Effects of Vitamin D in Respiratory Tract Infections and COVID-19 in Children. *Nutrients* **2023**, *15*, 3430. [CrossRef] [PubMed] [PubMed Central]
32. Xiao, J.; He, W. The immunomodulatory effects of vitamin D drops in children with recurrent respiratory tract infections. *Am. J. Transl. Res.* **2021**, *13*, 1750–1756. [PubMed] [PubMed Central]
33. Abioye, A.I.; Bromage, S.; Fawzi, W. Effect of micronutrient supplements on influenza and other respiratory tract infections among adults: A systematic review and meta-analysis. *BMJ Glob. Health* **2021**, *6*, e003176. [CrossRef] [PubMed] [PubMed Central]
34. Martineau, A.R.; Jolliffe, D.A.; Hooper, R.L.; Greenberg, L.; Aloia, J.F.; Bergman, P.; Dubnov-Raz, G.; Esposito, S.; Ganmaa, D.; Ginde, A.A.; et al. Vitamin D supplementation to prevent acute respiratory tract infections: Systematic review and meta-analysis of individual participant data. *BMJ* **2017**, *356*, i6583. [CrossRef] [PubMed] [PubMed Central]

35. Jat, K.R. Vitamin D deficiency and lower respiratory tract infections in children: A systematic review and meta-analysis of observational studies. *Trop. Dr.* **2017**, *47*, 77–84. [CrossRef] [PubMed]
36. Buendía, J.A.; Patiño, D.G. Cost-utility of vitamin D supplementation to prevent acute respiratory infections in children. *Cost Eff. Resour. Alloc.* **2023**, *21*, 23. [CrossRef] [PubMed] [PubMed Central]

nutrients

MDPI

Review

Renal Health Through Medicine–Food Homology: A Comprehensive Review of Botanical Micronutrients and Their Mechanisms

Yi Zhao [1], Jian-Ye Song [1], Ru Feng [1], Jia-Chun Hu [1], Hui Xu [1], Meng-Liang Ye [1], Jian-Dong Jiang [1], Li-Meng Chen [2,*] and Yan Wang [1,*]

[1] State Key Laboratory of Bioactive Substance and Function of Natural Medicines, Institute of Materia Medica, Chinese Academy of Medical Sciences and Peking Union Medical College, Beijing 100050, China

[2] Department of Nephrology, State Key Laboratory of Complex Severe and Rare Diseases, Peking Union Medical College Hospital, Chinese Academy of Medical Science and Peking Union Medical College, Beijing 100730, China

* Correspondence: chenlimeng@pumch.cn (L.-M.C.); wangyan@imm.ac.cn (Y.W.)

Abstract: Background: As an ancient concept and practice, "food as medicine" or "medicine–food homology" is receiving more and more attention these days. It is a tradition in many regions to intake medicinal herbal food for potential health benefits to various organs and systems including the kidney. Kidney diseases usually lack targeted therapy and face irreversible loss of function, leading to dialysis dependence. As the most important organ for endogenous metabolite and exogenous nutrient excretion, the status of the kidney could be closely related to daily diet. Therefore, medicinal herbal food rich in antioxidative, anti-inflammation micronutrients are ideal supplements for kidney protection. Recent studies have also discovered its impact on the "gut–kidney" axis. Methods: Here, we review and highlight the kidney-protective effects of botanicals with medicine–food homology including the most frequently used *Astragalus membranaceus* and *Angelica sinensis* (Oliv.) Diels, concerning their micronutrients and mechanism, offering a basis and perspective for utilizing and exploring the key substances in medicinal herbal food to protect the kidney. Results: The index for medicine–food homology in China contains mostly botanicals while many of them are also consumed by people in other regions. Micronutrients including flavonoids, polysaccharides and others present powerful activities towards renal diseases. Conclusions: Botanicals with medicine–food homology are widely speeded over multiple regions and incorporating these natural compounds into dietary habits or as supplements shows promising future for renal health.

Keywords: botanicals; medicine–food homology; kidney protection; gut–kidney axis

1. Introduction

The kidneys are indispensable for human physiological functions, including the excretion of drugs and nutrients. The kidneys maintain the balance of water, electrolytes, and endogenous metabolites throughout the body through the processes of glomerular filtration, tubular reabsorption, and tubular secretion. Additionally, they serve as the predominant organ responsible for the excretion of exogenous substances, including drugs and food nutrients [1]. However, this feature also renders the kidneys highly susceptible to acute or chronic injuries caused by these exogenous substances [2]. For example, drug-induced nephrotoxicity (DIN) accounts for up to 60% of cases of acute kidney injury (AKI) and the correlation increases in elder patients [1,3]. Dietary-resourced substances could also lead to abnormal renal status, for instance, oxalate and oxalate precursors as key determinants of urinary oxalate excretion and stone disease. In addition to certain substances that induce injury, the kidney is also affected by metabolic disorders (e.g., diabetic kidney disease) and immune abnormalities (e.g., membranous glomerulonephritis and immunoglobulin

A nephropathy). The underlying molecular mechanism of kidney disorders is a complex phenomenon involving oxidative stress, inflammation, fibrosis, and mitochondrial dysfunction. Recently, the vital role of the "gut–kidney" axis, which is closely related to daily diet, has been identified and investigated [4]. However, contemporary renal disease therapy is predominantly supportive, comprising diuretics, renin–angiotensin–aldosterone system inhibitors, and immunosuppressants with a paucity of targeted pharmaceutical agents [2]. Meanwhile, these treatments could hardly reverse the continuous decline in renal function and the formation of end-stage renal disease (ESRD) [5]. Compared to drug treatment, certain daily diet patterns may also have an impact on renal function [6,7]. Natural food plants are extremely wealthy in nutrients and biological active compounds worth exploring and utilizing. Therefore, there is a promising future to explore botanicals with medicine–food homology to alleviate or prevent kidney disease.

In fact, the concept of food as medicine, or "Yao Shi Tong Yuan" in Chinese, is a fundamental tenet of Traditional Chinese Medicine (TCM). It underscores the dual function of specific foods in offering both nutritional and therapeutic advantages. The use of herbal food for medical purposes has a long and illustrious history in numerous other regions, including Japan, Korea, South America, and Europe. Despite the complexity of its ingredients, preparation methods, and active components, medicinal herbal food has been shown to have significant effects on a number of disorders, including diabetes mellitus, allergic diseases, pancreatitis, depression, and renal disease [8–11]. In the context of renal disease, a considerable number of botanical foods have been observed to exert a protective effect, as evidenced by a reduction in serum creatinine, blood urea nitrogen, histopathological injury, and fibrosis degree [12–14]. Early in 2002 [15], the National Health Commission (NHC) of the People's Republic of China had published the list of natural medical food including mostly different kinds of herbal ones. Being up to date, the list has expanded to 102 kinds of natural food including *Astragalus membranaceus*, *Codonopsis tangshen* Oliv., and *Poria cocos* (Schw.) Wolf. These herbal foods are frequently consumed by Chinese people either for their flavors or their potential health benefits. Many of them had also demonstrated renal-protective effects through anti-inflammation [16], antioxidation [17,18], and regulating mitochondria [19] and gut microbiota [20] with various micronutrients in them. The Food and Drug Administration (FDA) of the US have also established guidelines for the safety and efficacy of dietary supplements for medical use [21]. The 2020–2030 strategic plan for nutrition research by National Institutes of Health (NIH) had even placed "food as medicine" as one of the strategic goals [22], indicating the potential of medicine–food homology.

Here, we reviewed the frequently used medicinal herbal food in China, the US, and Europe, and summarized the potential renal-protective effects and mechanism of these medicinal herbal foods as shown in Figure 1, providing a better basis for utilizing and exploring the key substances in botanicals with medicine–food homology.

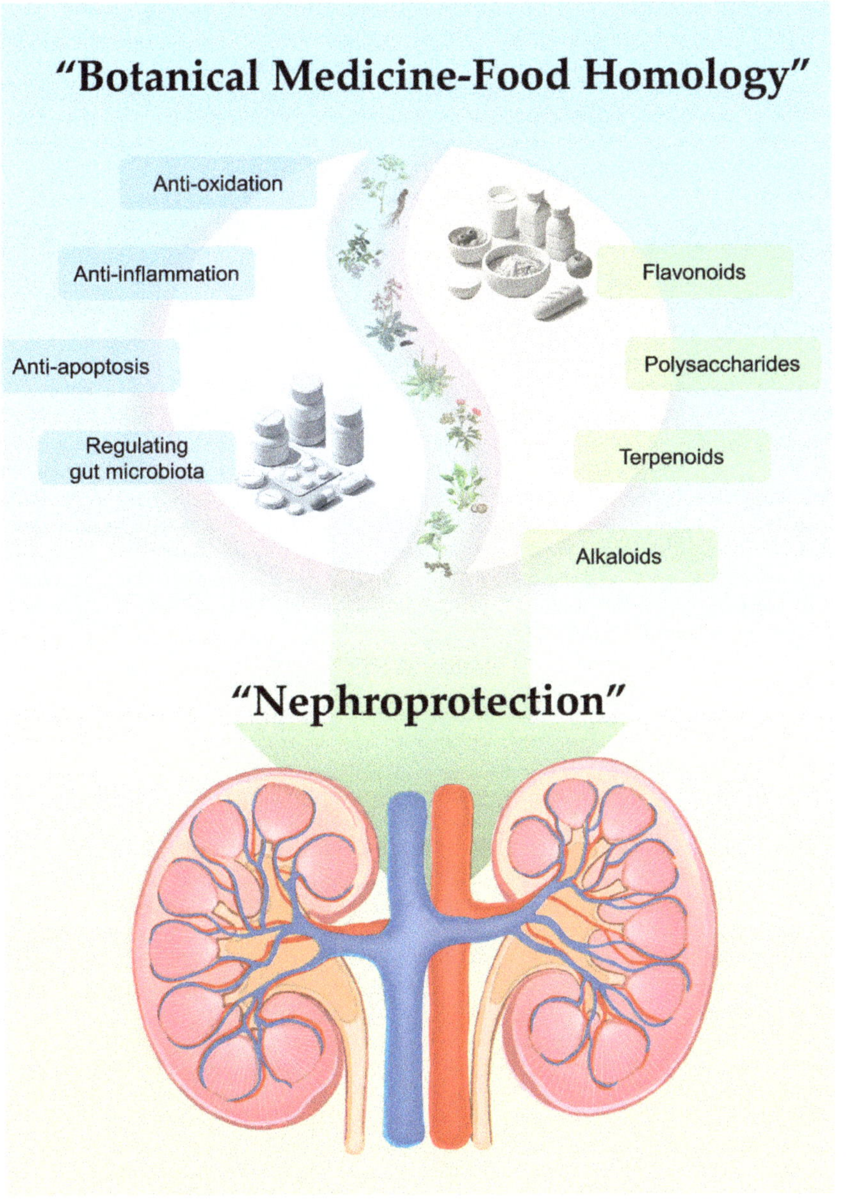

Figure 1. Illustration abstract drawn by authors.

2. Botanical Ingredients with Medicine–Food Homology in China, the US, and Europe

The use of botanical ingredients for dietary supplements or even for food is a widespread tradition around the world. In addition to China, the popularity of botanical dietary supplements is also evident in various European countries. Dietary supplements represent 15–20% of the total botanical market [23]. However, the complex compounds present in botanical ingredients also pose a potential risk. One of the most illustrative examples of a botanical-induced health risk is the aristolochic acid nephropathy (AAN) incident that occurred in the early 1990s [24]. The ingestion of aristolochic acids present in certain herbs had resulted in the development of AAN in numerous patients, leading to chronic renal failure and ESRD in Belgium, China, and Korea [24–26]. Considering the widespread and covert use of herbs, some researchers estimated that the AAN was still underestimated and called for a stronger and systematic supervision system of herbal medicine or ingredients [25]. To ensure the safety and efficiency of botanical ingredients and supplements, many regulations and standards have been published to restrict the addition of botanical ingredients in dietary supplements. In 2002, the NHC of China had published the first index of ingredients that could be both food and medication [15]. The initial version contained 92 unique edible parts including mostly botanical ingredients. Many of them have long been thought to have kidney-protective effects like *Astragalus membranaceus* and *Lycium barbarum* L. [16,27,28]. In recent years, there has been a growing interest in botanical dietary supplements, leading the NHC to edit the index in 2019 [29] and 2023 [30]. This resulted in the addition of 15 new botanical ingredients. In 2021, the NHC had also published related regulations for this index including the criteria for botanical ingredients as both food and medication [31]. The fundamental criteria consist of the following requirements: (i) have been traditionally consumed as food; (ii) have been listed in the *Pharmacopoeia* of the PRC; (iii) no food safety problems have been found in the safety assessment; (iv) comply with relevant laws and regulations on the protection of Chinese herbal medicines, wild animals, plants, and ecological resources. For the first rule, it also requires evidence for the ingredients to have been consumed as food for more than 30 years. Concurrently, all of these ingredients are also included in the *Pharmacopoeia* of the People's Republic of China, which demonstrates their efficacy as medicinal agents. In addition to botanicals that are regarded as both food and medicine, the NHC had also delineated a list of medicinal herbs that may be included in dietary supplements (Table S1) [15]. With regard to the European countries, the regulation of botanical ingredients is also divided into two distinct categories: medicine and food supplements. The European Medicines Agency (EMA) bears the responsibility of assessing the safety and efficacy of herbal preparations when utilized as medicines, while the European Food Safety Authority (EFSA) is tasked with the oversight of herbal preparations employed as food supplements. The evaluation of botanicals used in food products was initiated in 2004, when the EFSA mandated its Scientific Committee to develop a science-based toolkit for the safety assessment of botanicals and botanical preparations [32]. Subsequently, in 2009, the EFSA published the inaugural edition of the Compendium of Botanicals, which provided information regarding the safety risks associated with botanical ingredients in dietary supplements [32]. In the United States, the Dietary Supplement Health and Education Act (DSHEA) of 1994 initially delineated the status of herbs in dietary supplements, alongside that of vitamins, minerals, amino acids, and other substances [33]. While there is no comprehensive list of ingredients used in dietary supplements by the FDA, the NIH has established a Dietary Supplement Label Database (DSLD) [34] that includes as many of these supplements as possible.

Table 1 shows a full list of botanicals in the China index for botanicals with medicine–food homology. It contains a total of 91 botanicals, the majority of which are also included in dietary supplements in the United States and the European Union, as indicated by the EFSA Compendium of Botanicals and the DSLD. However, only a limited number of the listed botanicals are regarded as herbal medicines in accordance with the EMA standard. This is a markedly different situation from that in China, where all the botanicals in Table 1 are also included in the country's *Pharmacopoeia*. Additionally, botanicals such as clove, ginkgo, and ginger are present in all four lists or databases, which suggests their widespread popularity and efficacy as both food and medicine.

Table 1. The full list of botanicals in the China index for medicine–food homology.

Latin Name	English Common Name	EMA Herbal Medicine	EFSA Compendium	NIH DSLD
Eugenia caryophyllata Thunb.	Clove	√	√	√
Illicium verum Hook. f.	Star anise		√	√
Canavalia gladiata (Jacq.) DC.	Sword bean			√
Foeniculum vulgare Mill.	Fennel	√	√	√
Cirsium setosum (Willd.) MB.	Thistle			
Dioscorea opposita Thunb.	Chinese yam			√
Crataegus pinnatifida Bge. var. *major* N.E.Br./*Crataegus pinnatifida* Bge.	Hawthorn	√	√	√
Portulaca oleracea L.	Purslane		√	√
Prunus mume (Sieb.) Sieb. et Zucc.	Japanese apricot		√	√
Chaenomeles speciosa (Sweet) Nakai	Flowering quince		√	
Cannabis sativa L.	Hemp	√		√
Citrus aurantium L. var. *amara* Engl.	Bitter orange			
Polygonatum odoratum (Mill.) Druce	Solomon's seal		√	
Glycyrrhiza uralensis Fisch./*Glycyrrhiza inflata* Bat./*Glycyrrhiza glabra* L.	Licorice	√	√	√
Angelica dahurica (Fisch. ex Hoffm.) Benth. et Hook. f./*Angelica dahurica* (Fisch. ex Hoffm.) Benth. et Hook. f. var. *formosana* (Boiss.) Shan et Yuan	Chinese angelica		√	
Ginkgo biloba L.	Ginkgo	√	√	√
Dolichos lablab L.	Hyacinth bean		√	√
Dimocarpus longan Lour.	Longan		√	√
Cassia obtusifolia L./*Cassia tora* L.	Sicklepod		√	
Lilium lancifolium Thunb./*Lilium pumilum* DC.	Tiger lily		√	√
Myristica fragrans Houtt.	Nutmeg		√	√
Cinnamomum cassia Presl	Cassia	√	√	√
Phyllanthus emblica L.	Amla		√	
Citrus medica L. var. *sarcodactylis* Swingle	Fingered citron			
Prunus armeniaca L. var. *ansu* Maxim/*Prunus sibirica* L./*Prunus mandshurica* (Maxim) Koehne/*Prunus armeniaca* L.	Chinese apricot		√	√
Hippophae rhamnoides L.	Sea buckthorn			
Euryale ferox Salisb.	Euryale ferox		√	
Zanthoxylum schinifolium Sieb. et Zucc./*Zanthoxylum bungeanum* Maxim.	Sichuan pepper			√
Vigna umbeuata Ohwi et Ohashi/*Vigna angularis* Ohwi et Ohashi	Azuki bean			
Hordeum vulgare L.	Barley		√	√
Laminaria japonica Aresch./*Ecklonia kurome* Okam.	Kunbu			
Ziziphus jujuba Mill.	Jujube		√	√

Table 1. *Cont.*

Latin Name	English Common Name	EMA Herbal Medicine	EFSA Compendium	NIH DSLD
Siraitia grosvenorii (Swingle.) C.Jeffrey ex A. M. Lu et Z. Y.Zhang	Luohanguo siraitia fruit		√	
Prunus japonica Thunb.	Pruni semen		√	
Lonicera japonica Thunb.	Japanese honeysuckle		√	
Canarium album Raeusch.	White canarium		√	
Houttuynia cordata Thunb.	Fish mint		√	
Zingiber officinale Rosc.	Ginger	√	√	√
Hovenia dulcis Thunnb./*Hovenia acerba* Lindl./*Hovenia trichocarpa* Chun et Tsiang	Japanese raisin tree		√	
Lycium barbarum L.	Goji berry		√	√
Gardenia jasminoides Ellis	Cape jasmine		√	√
Amomum villosum Lour./*Amomum villosum* Lour. var. *xanthioides* T. L. Wu et Senjen/*Amomum longiligulare* T. L. Wu	Villus amomum		√	√
Sterculia lychnophora Hance	Malva nut tree		√	√
Poria cocos (Schw.) Wolf	Poria, fu ling			
Citrus medica L./*Citrus wilsonii* Tanaka	Citron		√	√
Mosla chinensis Maxim./*Mosla chinensis* Maxim. cv. Jiangxiangru	Chinese mosla		√	
Prunus persica (L.) Batsch/*Prunus davidiana* (Carr.) Franch.	Peach		√	√
Morus alba L.	White mulberry		√	√
Citrus reticulata Blanco	Mandarin orange		√	√
Platycodon grandiflorum (Jacq.) A. DC.	Balloon flower		√	√
Alpinia oxyphylla Miq.	Sharp-leaf galangal		√	√
Nelumbo nucifera Gaertn.	Lotus leaf		√	√
Raphanus sativus L.	Radish seed		√	√
Alpinia officinarum Hance	Lesser galangal		√	√
Lophatherum gracile Brongn.	Lophatherum		√	√
Glycine max (L.) Merr.	Soybean	√	√	√
Chrysanthemum morifolium Ramat.	Chrysanthemum		√	√
Cichorium glandulosum Boiss. et Huet/*Cichorium intybus* L.	Chicory		√	
Polygonatum kingianum Coll.et Hemsl./*Polygonatum sibiricum* Red./*Polygonatum cyrtonema* Hua	Polygonati rhizoma		√	
Sinapis alba L.	White mustard		√	√
Perilla frutescens (L.) Britton	Perilla		√	√
Pueraria lobata (Willd.) Ohwi/*Pueraria thomsonii* Benth.	Kudzu		√	√
Sesamum indicum L.	Sesame		√	√
Piper nigrum L.	Black pepper		√	√

Table 1. *Cont.*

Latin Name	English Common Name	EMA Herbal Medicine	EFSA Compendium	NIH DSLD
Sophora japonica L.	Sophora		√	√
Taraxacum mongolicum Hand. Mazz./*Taraxacum borealisinense* Kitam.	Dandelion	√	√	√
Torreya grandis Fort.	Torreya		√	√
Ziziphus jujuba Mill. var. *spinosa* (Bunge) Hu ex H. F. Chou	Chinese date			
Imperata cylindrical Beauv. var. *major* (nees) C. E. Hubb.	Cogongrass			
Phragmites communis Trin.	Reed		√	√
Mentha haplocalyx Briq.	Chinese mint	√	√	√
Coix lacryma-jobi L. var. *mayuen* (Roman.) Stapf	Job's tears		√	√
Allium macrostemon Bge./*Allium chinense* G. Don	Chinese onion		√	
Rubus chingii Hu	Chinese raspberry	√	√	√
Pogostemon cablin (Blanco) Benth./*Agastache rugosus* (Fisch. et Mey.) O. Ktze.	Patchouli		√	√
Angelica sinensis (Oliv.) Diels	Angelica root	√	√	√
Kaempferia galanga L.	Aromatic ginger		√	√
Crocus sativus L.	Saffron		√	√
Amomum tsao-ko Crevost & Lemarié	Cardamom		√	√
Curcuma longa L.	Turmeric	√	√	√
Piper longum L.	Long pepper		√	√
Codonopsis pilosula (Franch.) Nannf./*Codonopsis pilosula* Nannf. var. *modesta* (Nannf.) L. T. Shen/*Codonopsis tangshen* Oliv.	Dangshen		√	√
Cistanche deserticola Y. C. Ma	Desert cistanche		√	√
Dendrobium officinale Kimura et Migo	Chinese orchid		√	√
Panax quinquefolius L.	American ginseng		√	√
Astragalus membranaceus (Fisch.) Bge.	Mongolian milkvetch (huangqi)		√	√
Ganoderma lucidum (Leyss. ex Fr.) Karst./*Ganoderma sinense* Zhao, Xu et Zhang	Ganoderma			
Cornus officinalis Sieb. et Zucc.	Japanese cornel dogwood		√	
Gastrodia elata Bl.	Gastrodia		√	√
Eucommia ulmoides Oliv.	Hardy rubber tree		√	√

EMA: European Medicines Agency; EFSA: European Food Safety Authority; NIH: National Institutes of Health; DSLD: Dietary Supplement Label Database; √: Indicating this botanical also appears in the index or database of ingredients; var.: Variety; f.: Form; cv.: Cultivar.

3. Nutrients from These Botanical Food Ingredients with Kidney-Protective Effects

3.1. Flavonoids

Flavonoids are polyphenolic compounds that are widely distributed in a variety of botanical foods. The basic chemistry structure of flavonoids consists of two benzene rings with a phenolic hydroxyl group and a heterocyclic ring forming a C6-C3-C6 basic carbon framework [35]. The structure can be further categorized into flavanones, flavones, flavonols, flavanols, dihydroflavonols, and anthocyanins based on different functional groups and their positions [36]. It is one of the most bioactive and common compounds in food resources, especially botanicals. As demonstrated in Table 2, flavonoids that have been validated to have kidney-protective effects include quercetin [37–39], kaempferol [40], myricetin [41,42], isorhamnetin [43,44], fisetin [45,46], icariin [47,48], apigenin [49,50], baicalein [51,52], baicalin [53,54], nobiletin [55], vitexin [56,57], hesperidin [58,59], and hesperetin [60,61]. Quercetin and kaempferol appear in the majority of vegetables and fruits, which accounts for their status as the most prevalent dietary supplement ingredients. A review of the DSLD revealed that dietary supplements containing quercetin constituted 2.3% of the total products [29]. As illustrated in Table 2, citrus botanicals such as *Citrus medica* L. var. *sarcodactylis* Swingle and *Citrus reticulata* Blanco exhibit a notable content of flavonoids, including hesperidin, hesperetin, naringin, quercetin, and kaempferol [62–64]. The flavonoids present in citrus fruits have been demonstrated to possess potent antioxidant properties, making them a promising avenue of research for the development of novel therapeutic agents for the treatment of diabetes, neurodegenerative disorders, and kidney diseases such as AKI and diabetic nephropathy (DN) [65–69]. In addition to citrus, *Glycine max* (L.) Merr. (soybean) in Table 1 contains a unique kind of isoflavones called soy isoflavones, or "phytoestrogens" due to their structural similarity with 17-β-estradiol [70]. Though most of the studies of soy isoflavones fell into their endocrine regulation impacts, one recent study had discovered that the intake of soy isoflavones exhibited favorable effects on renal function and kidney morphology [71]. Puerarin, derived from *Pueraria lobata* (Willd.) Ohwi, is also an isoflavone. Recent studies have demonstrated its influence on the toll-like receptor (TLR) 4/MyD88 pathway and the M1 macrophage differential [72]. Later, flavonoids in *Pueraria thomsonii* Benth. were further found to decrease inflammation in the kidney by regulating the level of Clostridium in the gut [73]. Hesperidin from citrus botanicals could also alter gut microbiota against Zn-induced nephrotoxicity [58], indicating the potential of the gut–kidney axis.

Table 2. Nutrients from these botanical food ingredients with kidney-protective effects.

Botanical Resources	Compounds	Models	Effects	Ref.
		Flavonoids		
Allium macrostemon Bge., *Crocus sativus* L., *Plantago asiatica* L. S	Quercetin	DN rats, ochratoxin A-induced AKI mice	↓ PI3K/AKT signaling ↑ Nrf2/HO-1, fatty acid oxidation	[37–39,74,75]
Glycine max (L.) Merr., *Lonicera japonica* Thunb., *Ginkgo biloba* L., *Lycium barbarum* L., *Plantago asiatica* L. S	Kaempferol	CLP-induced AKI mice, DN mice, DOX-induced AKI mice	↓ ICAM-1, VCAM-1, MCP-1, caspase-3, Bax, MAPK signaling, TGF-β1, and α-SMA ↑ Bcl-2, SOD, and GSH	[40,76–78]
Myricaceae, *Polygonaceae*, *Primulaceae*, *Pinaceae*, and *Anacardiaceae*	Myricetin	DN mice, EG-induced AKI mice	↓ IL-1β, TNF-α, ROCK1/ERK/P38 signaling, and NF-κB signaling ↑ Nrf2, CAT, and SOD	[41,42,79]

Table 2. *Cont.*

Botanical Resources	Compounds	Models	Effects	Ref.
Ginkgo biloba L., *Hippophae rhamnoides* L., *Citrus reticulata* Blanco, *Citrus aurantium* L., *and Citrus medica* L.	Isorhamnetin	LPS-induced AKI mice	↓ IL-1β, IL-6, and TNF-α and M1 macrophage ↑ M2 macrophage	[43,44]
Epimedium brevicornu Maxim. [S]	Icariin	Adenine/UUO-induced CKD rats, DOX-induced AKI mice	↓ TGF-β, α-SMA, and E-cadherin ↑ Nrf2/HO-1, SOD, CAT	[47,48,80–82]
Plantago asiatica L. [S]	Apigenin	DOX/EG/oxonate-induced AKI mice, UAN mice	↓ Oxidative and nitrosative stress, IL-6, TNF-α, NLRP3, caspase-1, IL-1β, TGF-β, Wnt/β-catenin signaling	[49,50,83–87]
Citrus reticulata Blanco, *Citrus aurantium* L., *Citrus medica* L.	Nobiletin	IRI-induced AKI mice	↑ PI3K/AKT signaling	[55]
Crataegus pinnatifida Bge.	Vitexin	UUO-induced CKD mice, oxalate-induced AKI mice	↓ NLRP3, caspase-1, and IL-1β ↑ Nrf2/HO-1, SOD, GSH	[56,57]
Citrus reticulata Blanco, *Citrus aurantium* L., *Citrus medica* L.	Hesperidin, hesperetin	LPS/Zn-induced AKI mice, DDP-induced HK-2 cells	↓ p53, caspase-3 ↑ Nrf2/HO-1, SOD, GSH, and CAT Regulating gut microbiota	[58–61]
Plantago asiatica L. [S]	Luteolin	Cd/$HgCl_2$/$K_2Cr_2O_7$-induced AKI mice, LN mice	↓ HIF-1α, α-SMA, collagen I, and fibronectin ↑ Nrf2/HO-1, GSH, SOD, CAT, and AMPK/mTOR autophagy	[88–92]
Pueraria lobata (Willd.) Ohwi	Puerarin	DN mice, UUO-induced CKD mice	↑ Nrf2, cAMP/PKA/CREB ↓ TLR4/MyD8, and M1 macrophage	[72,93–95]
		Polysaccharides		
Astragalus membranaceus (Fisch.) Bge.	/	DDP-induced AKI mice	↓ ROS generation and mitochondrial vacuolation	[19]
	/	LPS-induced AKI mice	↓ Caspase-3/9 and Bax ↑ Bcl-2	[96]
	/	LPS-induced AKI mice	Regulating gut microbiota ↑ SCFAs	[97]
Bletilla striata [S]	Mw: 260 kDa	Ang II-induced HMCs	↓ ROS generation and NOX4	[18]
	/	TGF-β-induced HMCs	↓ TGF-β, and α-SMA	[98]
Ganoderma lucidum (Leyss. ex Fr.) Karst.	Mw: 72.9 kDa; Ara:Gal:Rha:Glc = 0.08:0.21:0.24:0.47	DN mice	↓ Collagen-1, fibronectin, α-SMA, TGF- β, and MAPK/NF-κB signaling	[99]
	/	IRI-induced AKI mice	↓ p53, caspase-3, Bax, cytochrome c, and ER stress ↑ Bcl-2	[100]
Lycium barbarum L.	Ara:Gal:Glc:GalA:Man:Rha = 12.25: 8.66: 7.66: 2.86: 1.70: 1.00	DN mice	↓ TNF-α, IL-1β, IL-6, and NF-κB signaling	[16]
	/	Lead-induced AKI mice	↓ Bax and caspase-3 ↑ Bcl-2	[101]

Table 2. *Cont.*

Botanical Resources	Compounds	Models	Effects	Ref.
Laminaria japonica Aresch./*Ecklonia kurome* Okam.	Mw: 7 kDa	IRI-induced AKI mice	↓ p53, Bax, MMP, and cytochrome c ↑ Bcl-2	[102]
	Mw: 1960 kDa	DOX-induced AKI mice	↓ TNF-α, IL-1β, MCP-1, and podocyte injury	[103]
	Mw: 8.84 kDa; Fuc:Gal:Man:Glc:Rha:Xyl = 1:0.057:0.041:0.008:0.029:0.019	DN mice	↓ collagen-1, fibronectin, and α-SMA	[104]
	Mw: 7 kDa	DN mice	↓ α-SMA, fibronectin, and TGF-β/Smad ↑ E-cadherin	[105]
	/	DOX-induced CKD mice	↓ α-SMA, fibronectin, and TGF-β/Smad	[106]
	Mw: 7.774 kDa	AGE-induced HRMCs	↓ Fibronectin	[107]
	Mw: 8.84 kDa	TGF-β1- or FGF-2-induced HK-2 cells	↓ α-SMA, MMP9, and EMT	[108]
Polygonatum kingianum Coll.et Hemsl./*Polygonatum sibiricum* Red./*Polygonatum cyrtonema* Hua	Mw: 141 kDa; Gal:GalA:Ara:Glc = 57.67:26.82:4.59:4.54	Uranium-induced HK-2 cells	↓ ROS ↑ GSK-3β/Fyn/Nrf2	[17]
Panax ginseng C. A. Mey. [S]	Glc:Gal:Ara:GalA:Rha:Man = 76.7:6.5:5.1:9.2:1.4:1.1	DDP-induced AKI mice	↓ p53, caspase-3, caspase-6, and ER stress by PERK/eIF2α/ATF4 signaling	[109]
Paeonia × suffruticosa[S]	Mw: 164 kDa; D-Glc:L-Ara = 3.31:2.25;	DN rats	↓ TGF-β, ICAM-1, and VCAM-1	[110]
	Mw: 164 kDa; Ara = 3.31:2.25	DN rats	Regulating gut microbiota ↑ SCFAs	[111]
Plantago asiatica[S]	/	Adenine-induced rats, UAN	↓ IL-6, TNF-α, NLRP3, and caspase-1	[112]
Dendrobium officinale Kimura et Migo	/	HG-induced HK-2 cells, db/db mice	↓ TGF-β, and α-SMA ↑ SIRT1	[113]
Salvia miltiorrhiza Bunge [S]	/	Florfenicol-induced AKI broilers	↓ p53, caspase-3 ↑ Nrf2/HO-1	[114]
Phyllostachys nigra[S]	Mw: 34 kDa	DN mice	Regulating gut microbiota ↑ *Lactobacillales*	[20]
		Terpenoids		
Rehmannia glutinosa[S], *Plantago asiatica*[S], *Scrophularia ningpoensis*[S], *and Crocus sativus* L.	Catalpol	DN mice, DOX/Ang II/Fru/DDP-induced AKI mice, adenine-induced CKD mice	↓ TRPC6, NF-κB, TGF-β1/Smad, TLR4/MyD88 signaling, RAGE/RhoA/ROCK signaling ↑ AMPK signaling	[115–121]
Cornus officinalis Sieb. et Zucc.	Loganin	DN mice, IRI/DOX/CLP-induced AKI mice	↓ NLRP3, AGE/RAGE signaling ↑ Nrf2/HO-1	[122–125]
Gardenia jasminoides Ellis, *Eucommia ulmoides* Oliv., *Rehmannia glutinosa* [S], *and Scrophularia ningpoensis* [S]	Geniposide	DN mice, CLP-induced AKI mice, H_2O_2-induced HK-2 cells	↓ ICAM-1, TNF-α, IL-1, IL-6, NF-κB, and NETs ↑ GSK3β, AMPK-PI3K/AKT, Bcl-2 Regulating gut microbiota	[126–132]

Table 2. *Cont.*

Botanical Resources	Compounds	Models	Effects	Ref.
Cornus officinalis Sieb. et Zucc.	Morroniside	H_2O_2-induced podocytes	↓ NOX4	[133]
Canarium album Raeusch.	Oleuropein	DN mice, acrylamide-induced AKI mice	↓ TNF-α, IFN-γ, IL-2, IL-6, and IL-17α ↑ SOD, GSH-Px, and CAT	[134,135]
Poria cocos (Schw.) Wolf.	Poricoic acid (A, B, C, D, E, F, G, H, AM, AE, BM, DM, and derivatives)	UUO-induced CKD mice	↓ MMP-13, Wnt/β-catenin, TGF-β/Smad3/MAPK ↑ AMPK, Nrf2	[136–142]
Ligustrum lucidum Ait. S	Oleanic acid	UUO-induced CKD mice, DN mice	↓ NF-κB/TNF-α, TGF-β ↑ Nrf2/SIRT1/HO-1 Regulating gut microbiota	[143–147]
Alisma orientatle (Sam.) Juzep. S	Alisol (A, B, and derivatives)	IRI/DDP-induced AKI mice, UUO-induced CKD mice	↓ ICAM-1, MCP-1, COX-2, iNOS, IL-6, TNF-α, FXR activation, TGF-β/Smad3 ↑ SOD and GSH and HO-1	[148–150]
Panax ginseng C. A. Mey.	Ginsenosides	DDP-induced AKI mice, renal carcinoma, DN mice, UUO-induced CKD mice	↓ ER stress, lipid peroxidation, PPARγ, and NOX4-MAPK pathways and TGF-β	[151–158]
Ganoderma lucidum (Leyss. ex Fr.) Karst.	Ganoderic acid, ganodermanontriol, lucidenic acid	ADPKD mice, IRI-induced AKI mice, UUO-induced CKD mice	↓ Ras/MAPK, TGF-β/Smad, IL-6, COX-2, and iNOS ↓ TLR4/MyD88/NF-κB, and caspase-3	[159–161]
Glycyrrhiza uralensis Fisch.	Glycyrrhizinic acid, glycyrrhizic acid	DN mice, TAC/PC-induced AKI mice	↓ ROS, IL-1β, IL-6, TNF-α, CCR2 ↑ AMPK/SIRT1/PGC-1α Regulates autophagy	[162–167]
		Alkaloids		
Ligusticum sinense Chuanxiong S	Tetramethylpyrazine	PC/IRI-induced AKI rats, DN rats	↓ CCL2/CCR2, ROS, NLRP3, TNF-α ↑ AKT, Bcl-2	[168–172]
Leonurus japonicus Houtt. S	Leonurine	DDP/LPS/vancomycin-induced AKI mice, UUO-induced CKD mice	↑ Nrf2 ↓ TLR4/MyD88/NF-κB, TNF-α, IL-1β, TGF-β/Smad3	[173–177]
Coptis chinensis	Berberine	IRI/DOX/DDP/MTX/gentamicin-induced AKI, DN mice, and UUO-induced CKD mice, UAN mice	↓ IL-6, IL-10, TGF-β/Smad3, mitochondrial stress, and ER stress ↑ Nrf2, MDA, SOD, CAT, GSH, and Bcl-2 Regulating gut microbiota	[178–190]
Trigonella foenum-graecum L. S	Trigonelline	ON mice, DN mice	↓ EMT, ROS, α-SMA ↑ AMPK pathway	[191–196]
Piper longum L. S	Piperlonguminine	UUO-induced CKD mice	↓ TRPC6	[197]
Sophora japonica L.	Matrine, oxymatrine	IRI/DDP/gentamicin-induced AKI mice, UUO-induced CKD mice	↓ IL-6, IL-10, TGF-β/Smad3	[198–200]
Nelumbo nucifera Gaertn.	Liensinine, Isoliensinine	IRI-induced AKI rats, LPS-induced AKI mice	↓ TGF-β1/Smad3	[201,202]
Nelumbo nucifera Gaertn.	Neferine, nuciferine	UAN rats, LPS/IRI-induced AKI mice, DN mice	↓ TLR4/MyD88/NF-κB, IL-1β ↑ Bcl-2	[203–210]

Table 2. *Cont.*

Botanical Resources	Compounds	Models	Effects	Ref.
		Others		
Curcuma longa L.	Curcumin	LN mice, patulin-induced AKI mice, CKD patients, UAN rats	↑ Nrf2/FOXO-3a, GSH ↓ PI3K/AKT/NF-κB, TGF-β, ROS Regulating gut microbiota	[211–215]
Rheum palmatum L.	Emodin, aloe emodin, rhein	UUO-induced CKD mice/rats, DN mice	↓ IL-1β, TGF-β, PERK-eIF2α Regulating gut microbiota	[216–220]
Eugenia caryophyllata Thunb.	Eugenol	IRI/patulin-induced AKI mice	↓ TGF-β ↑ Nrf2	[221,222]
Sesamum indicum L.	Sesamin	CKD mice, DDP/LPS-induced AKI mice	↑ GSH, CAT, and SOD Regulating gut microbiota	[223–226]
Ligusticum sinense Chuanxiong [S]	Ferulic acid	UAN mice	↓ TLR4/NF-κB Regulating gut microbiota	[227]
Lonicera japonica Thunb.	Chlorogenic acid	UAN mice	↓ IL-1β, TNF-α, IL-6 Regulating gut microbiota	[228–230]

[S]: These botanicals are medical herbs that could be added to dietary supplements in the index of Table S1; ↑:upregulating or promoting; ↓: downregulating or inhibiting; PI3K: Phosphoinositide 3-kinase; AKT: Protein kinase B; Nrf2: Nuclear factor erythroid 2-related factor 2; HO-1: Heme oxygenase 1; ICAM: Intercellular adhesion molecule; VCAM: Vascular cell adhesion molecule; NLRP3: NOD-, LRR-, and pyrin domain-containing protein 3; Bax: BCL2-associated X; Bcl-2: B-cell lymphoma 2; MAPK: Mitogen-activated protein kinase; AMPK: Adenosine monophosphate-activated protein kinase; NF-κB: Nuclear factor kappa-B; mTOR: Mammalian target of rapamycin; cAMP: Cyclic adenosine monophosphate; PKA: Protein kinase A; CREB: cAMP-response element binding protein; TLR: Toll-like receptor; RAGE: Receptor for AGEs; AGEs: Advanced glycation end products; RhoA: Ras homolog family member A; Ras: Rat sarcoma; ROCK: Rho-associated coiled-coil-containing protein kinase; TGF: Transforming growth factor; iNOS: Inducible nitric oxide synthase; COX: Cyclooxygenase; CCR: Chemokine (C-C motif) receptor; CCL/MCP: Chemokine (C-C motif) ligand; PGC: Peroxisome proliferator-activated receptor-gamma coactivator; FXR: Farnesoid X receptor; α-SMA: α-Smooth muscle actin; ROS: Reactive oxygen species; GSK-3β: Glycogen synthase kinase 3 beta; SOD: Superoxide dismutase; GSH: Glutathione; CAT: Catalase; HIF: Hypoxia-inducible factor; NOX: NADPH oxidase; IL: Interleukin; TNF: Tumor necrosis factor; FOXO: Forkhead box O; ERK: Extracellular regulated protein kinase; MMP: Matrix metalloproteinase; ER: Endoplasmic reticulum; PERK: Protein kinase R-like endoplasmic reticulum kinase; eIF2α: Phosphorylation of eukaryotic initiation factor-2α; ATF4: Activating transcription factor 4; SIRT1: Silent information regulator 1; TRPC: Transient receptor potential canonical; SCFAs: Short-chain fatty acids; CKD: Chronic kidney disease; IRI: Ischemia/reperfusion injury; ADPKD: Autosomal dominant polycystic kidney disease; UUO: Unilateral ureteral obstruction; UAN: Uric acid nephropathy; CLP: Cecum ligation puncture; DOX: Doxorubicin; DDP: Cisplatin; LPS: Lipopolysaccharide; EG: Ethylene glycol; LN: Lupus nephritis; Ang II: Angiotensin II; HMCs: Human mesangial cells; HK-2 cells: Human kidney-2 cells; Fru: Fructose; TAC: Tacrolimus; PC: Post-contrast; MTX: Methotrexate; ON: Oxalate nephropathy.

3.2. Polysaccharides

Natural polysaccharides are a class of complex macromolecules that are formed from a variety of monosaccharide units and diverse glycosidic linkages. The monosaccharide units can be classified into several categories, including hexose, which includes glucose, galactose, and mannose; N-acetyl-hexose (HexNac), which encompasses GalNac and GluNac; pentose (e.g., xylose and arabinose); deoxyhexose (e.g., fucose); and numerous terminal modifications, such as phosphorylation, sulfation, and sialylation. Up to the present date, the identification and isolation still remain a critical challenge. However, the polysaccharides were found to be the principal compounds in some of the botanicals in Table 1 and the pharmacological effects of polysaccharides have also long been confirmed. Table 2 illustrates the representative polysaccharides from botanicals in Tables 1 and S1, along with their impact on kidney diseases.

Laminaria japonica Aresch. is a widespread food ingredient in China with a significant amount of polysaccharides. It contains polysaccharides weighing from 5 kDa to 10^4 kDa [231] with great potential in anti-fibrosis effects, which revealed its capacity to treat CKD [106]. In many kidney diseases including the DN model [104,105], DIN model [103,106], and IRI model [102], polysaccharides from *Laminaria japonica* Aresch. showed strong impact on fibrosis- and apoptosis-related molecules like TGF-β, α-SMA, and Bax/Bcl-2. Polysaccharides are also identified to be the primary compounds in *Polygonatum sibiricum Red* [232]. Polygonat Rhizomai polysaccharides were discovered to be protective against uranium-induced AKI with 141 kDa polysaccharides in them [17]. The polysaccharides from other traditional kidney-protective botanical food like *Lycium barbarum* L. [101] and *Astragalus membranaceus* [19,96,97] showed protective effects against DIN as well.

In consideration of the gut–kidney axis, polysaccharides derived from these botanical ingredients also play a significant role in the intricate interplay of gut–kidney crosstalk. The polysaccharides derived from *Phyllostachys nigra* [20], *Paeonia × suffruticosa* (Moutan Cortex) [111], and *Astragalus membranaceus* (Fisch.) Bge. [97] have been observed to possess the capacity to regulate the gut–kidney axis, thereby conferring benefit to the kidney. The mechanisms involved in remodeling the gut microbiota composition include an increase in the abundance of probiotics, such as *Lactobacillales*, and an upregulation of SCFAs.

3.3. Terpenoids

Terpenoids, which are derived from isoprene, encompass a diverse range of chemical compounds, including monoterpenoids, sesquiterpenoids, diterpenoids, sesterterpenes, triterpenoids, and polyterpenoids [233]. Considering the ingredients in Table 1 and Table S1, *Panax ginseng* C. A. Mey. (ginseng), *Glycyrrhiza uralensis* Fisch. (Liquorice), *Alisma orientatle* (Sam.) Juzep., and *Ganoderma lucidum* (Leyss. ex Fr.) Karst. (Ganoderma) are representative for their great amount and variety of terpenoids.

Ganoderma triterpenoids isolated from Ganoderma are some of the major chemical constituents in Ganoderma and could be further divided into C30 (ganoderic acid, ganodermanontriol, applanoxidic acids, and their derivatives), C27 (lucidenic acid, ganolactone, and their derivatives), and C24 (lucidones and their derivatives), and others according to their skeleton carbons [234]. Among the compounds identified, ganoderic acids had been proven to possess protective properties in the context of ADPKD [159], renal fibrosis [160], and IRI [161]. Licorice is another ingredient that has been demonstrated to possess renal-protective terpenoids, the most prominent of which are glycyrrhizic acid and glycyrrhetinic acid [235]. Glycyrrhizic acid possesses surprising protective effects in DN [162,163] and DIN including tacrolimus [164], contrasts [165], and triptolide [166]-induced kidney injury. Similar effects were also found in glycyrrhetinic acid in DN [162] and IRI [167]. *Alisma orientatle* (Sam.) Juzep. and *Panax ginseng* C. A. Mey. are two botanicals in Table S1, which means that they are not considered daily food but could be added to dietary supplements. However, they have been traditionally used to treat renal disorders in TCM, especially *Alisma orientatle* (Sam.) Juzep. Alisols and their derivatives are tetracyclic triterpene alcohols isolated from *Alisma orientatle* (Sam.) Juzep. and play a significant role in its pharmacological effects [236]. Recent studies had demonstrated the potential of alisols in protecting the kidney from DPP-induced injury and IRI by targeting the farnesoid X receptor and soluble epoxide hydrolase [148,149]. Additionally, alisol B 23-acetate was observed to regulate the gut microbiota, thereby improving renal function in CKD mice [150]. Ginsenosides, the representative compounds in ginseng, are a big family of triterpenoid saponins with a four-ring rigid steroid skeleton [237]. Early in 1998, a study revealed that ginsenoside Rd could protect against IRI by affecting proximal tubule cells [238]. Later, numerous studies had demonstrated that ginsenosides could alleviate AKI [151,152], renal carcinoma [153,154], DN [155,156], and renal fibrosis [157,158].

Iridoids constitute a large and distinctive class of monoterpenoids that are ubiquitous in botanical sources and have been demonstrated to exhibit notable bioactivity [239]. Iridoids are receiving increasing attention for their great pharmacological effects in the liver, kidney, and nervous disorders [240–243]. Catalpol, one of the most common iridoids, for example, showed strong antioxidation and anti-inflammation effects in DN-, CKD-, and DIN-induced AKI models [115–121]. *Cornus officinalis* Sieb. et Zucc. was found to be abundant in iridoids [244], in which loganin and morroniside were shown to be protective for the kidney [122–125,133]. The representative terpenoids including triterpenoids and iridoids from botanicals with medicine–food homology are also shown in Table 2.

3.4. Alkaloids

Isolated from natural herbs, alkaloids are a diverse group of naturally occurring organic compounds that primarily contain basic nitrogen atoms [245]. Structurally, they could be characterized by a heterocyclic ring that incorporates nitrogen, and they often possess complex and varied molecular frameworks, for example, isoquinoline, pyrrolidines, pyridines, indole, and others. Dietary botanicals also contain variable bioactive alkaloids for renal protection. Table 2 provides a list of the principal representative alkaloids with kidney-protective effects derived from the botanicals included in Tables 1 and S1.

Tetramethylpyrazine, the characteristic alkaloid of *Ligusticum sinense* Chuanxiong, has been clinically utilized to inhibit platelet aggregation and reduce blood viscosity [246]. Its renal-protective effects were also validated in multiple models including DIN-induced AKI [168,169], IRI [170], and DN [171,172] with classical mechanisms targeting inflammation and oxidation markers. Leonurine from *Leonurus japonicus* Houtt. also showed protective effects in lipopolysaccharide-, DDP-, and vancomycin-induced AKI [173–177]. Besides AKI, trigonelline, the characteristic alkaloid in *Trigonella foenum-graecum* L. (Fenugreek) and *Coffea arabica* (coffee) was demonstrated to maintain a strong protective effect on oxalate nephropathy (ON) [191,192], which is closely related to diet oxalate. *Nelumbo nucifera* Gaertn. is well known for its abundant alkaloids, especially in its seeds. Liensinine, isoliensinine, neferine, and nuciferine are all alkaloids with kidney-protective effects isolated from *Nelumbo nucifera* Gaertn. Besides AKI and DN, neferine was also revealed to alleviate hyperuricemic nephropathy by targeting the inflammasome pathway [208]. Another alkaloid that has been widely studied for its protective effects on the kidneys is berberine. This isoquinoline alkaloid was initially isolated from *Hydrastis canadensis* and is primarily found in *Coptis chinensis*. Although these botanicals are not typically included in dietary regimens, berberine itself is a frequently utilized compound in dietary supplements. In DSLD, dietary supplements containing berberine reached 865 records. The renal-protective effects and mechanism of berberine have long been studied since 2011 in the DN model [247,248]. Later, the extraordinary effects of berberine were found in multiple nephropathy models including DIN-induced AKI [178–182], IRI-induced AKI [183–185], DN [186–188], and UUO-induced renal fibrosis [189]. The mechanisms involved in the treatment of berberine contained traditional anti-inflammation, oxidation, apoptosis, and also the regulation of gut bacteria. With the increasing interest in the gut microbiota, the interaction between the gut microbiota and berberine in the treatment of renal diseases has shown great promise. Recent studies demonstrated that berberine could improve chronic kidney disease by inhibiting the production of enterogenous toxins such as trimethylamine oxide (TMAO) and p-cresol (pCS), which are metabolites from gut microbiota [190]. Berberine could also increase the abundance of *Coprococcus*, *Bacteroides*, *Akkermansia*, and *Prevotella* to alleviate UAN [249–251]. A growing body of evidence suggests that the mechanisms of renoprotective effects through the gut–renal axis deserve further investigation.

Though many alkaloids possess renal-protective effects, a few studies have yielded contradictory results for the same compounds, for example, matrine from *Sophora japonica* L. Some studies [252,253] found that matrine could lead to kidney injury with mitochondria dysfunction and oxidation while another study demonstrated its protective effect on the DDP-induced AKI model [198]. Its derivate, oxymatrine, was also found to alleviate gentamicin-induced AKI [199], IRI [200], and renal fibrosis [254]. It again reinforces the necessity for the scientific research and regulation of the dietary utilization of botanicals with medicine–food homology.

3.5. Others

In addition to the aforementioned classes of compounds, botanicals with medicine–food homology also contain many other abundant bioactive nutrients including various kinds of polyphenols and anthraquinones, among which some showed great potential in benefiting the kidney as shown in Table 1. Simple phenylpropanoids are a kind of natural polyphenols with a three-carbon side chain linked to a phenyl ring, forming a C6-C3 skeleton. The primary structure also makes them precursors to many other natural compounds, such as flavonoids, lignans, and polyphenols [255]. Simple phenylpropanoids, including the widely distributed ferulic acid and chlorogenic acid, were both found to remodel the composition of the gut microbiota, thereby alleviating UAN [227–229]. Curcumin, the most bioactive and abundant polyphenol [256] in *Curcuma longa* L., has been extensively investigated for its potent antioxidant effects [213]. Together with its derivatives, curcumin displayed potential in treating LN [212], DIN-induced AKI [211], DN [215], and even focal segmental glomerulosclerosis (FSGS) [214]. Additionally, research has indicated that curcumin may mitigate renal impairment by modulating the microbiota in conditions such as CKD and UAN [257,258]. Sesamin, a lignan from dietary sesame, was also demonstrated to decrease uremic toxins by inhibiting the gut microbiota indole pathway [223], indicating importance of the gut–kidney axis. Anthraquinone compounds, for example, emodin and its derivatives, are the most important chemical compounds in *Rheum palmatum* L., which has long been used in TCM and added to dietary supplements [259]. The anthraquinone compounds in *Rheum palmatum* L. also possess renal-protective effects on DN, CKD, and UUO models, mainly targeting TGF-β secretion [216–220]. Interestingly, emodin was found to decrease uremic toxins as well by targeting gut microbiota [260]. An increasing body of evidence is emerging that demonstrates the significance of the gut–kidney axis in relation to dietary nutrients.

4. Mechanisms Involved in the Kidney-Protective Effects of Botanical Ingredients with Medicine–Food Homology

4.1. Antioxidation, Anti-Inflammation, and Anti-Fibrosis

Previous studies had focused on the inflammation/oxidation-oriented mechanisms, which are key pathological changes in kidney diseases. Oxidative stress is characterized by an initial injury in the kidney due to the activities of intra- and extracellular oxygen-derived radicals and the resultant inflammatory response [261]. When the kidney is exposed to harmful stimuli, ROS such as superoxides and hydroxyl radicals are produced in excess and interact with the molecular components and functions of a nephron such as the cell membrane, DNA methylation, histone modifications, and micro-RNAs, which are crucial mechanisms for fetal programming [262]. The production and scavenging of oxygen-derived radicals are in a dynamic balance through enzymatic (SOD, CAT, HO-1) and non-enzymatic (vitamin C, vitamin E, glutathione) antioxidant systems [263]. To deal with increased oxidative stress, several redox signaling response cascades, including Nrf2, could be activated to regulate this antioxidative gene expression [263]. Due to the existence of the oxygen shunt diffusion, the kidney is highly susceptible to oxidative stress and hypoxia [264]. Abnormalities in oxidative stress have been observed in a range of kidney diseases, including CKD, DN, and DIN-induced AKI and CKD [265–268].

The critical role of inflammation in the development of AKI, CKD, and DN was also widely confirmed in animal and clinical studies. The inflammation in the kidney is activated by various mechanisms including endothelial injury, drugs, and infection and causes glomerular, interstitial, and vascular damage [269]. The process of neutrophil infiltration is accompanied by an increase in multiple pro-inflammatory chemotaxes, adhesion factors, and chemokines, including ICAM-1, P- and E-selectin, and IL-1β, IL-6, IL-18, and TNF-α. This process is strongly correlated with fibrosis, autophagy, oxidative stress, and mitochondrial dysfunction [270]. In primary glomerular disease including acute glomerulonephritis, IgA nephropathy, and nephrotic syndrome, complement activation and immune complex deposition, which elicit strong inflammation, were also identified as key pathogenesis [271,272]. Pro-inflammatory signaling pathways include the TLR4/MyD88 signaling pathway, which is also closely related to gut microbiota due to its recognition of pathogen-associated molecular patterns [273]. The activation of TLR4 could lead to the upregulation of another key pro-inflammatory signal, the NF-κB-related pathway [273], which is also the target for most of the anti-inflammation effects in Table 2.

Fibrosis represents another pivotal pathological process following inflammation, especially chronic inflammation. With continuous inflammatory stimulation, various stromal cells in the kidney are transformed to myofibroblasts, which contribute to excessive extracellular matrix production and deposition in the renal parenchyma, eventually leading to loss of renal function [274]. The increase in the secretion of TGF-β and the fibroblast growth factor (EGF) and the secretion of type I collagen, fibronectin, chondroitin sulfate, and other components of the extracellular matrix (ECM) are also directly involved in the epithelial–mesenchymal transition (EMT) and fibrosis [275]. Recent studies had discovered that MMP also contributes to renal fibrosis [276]. There are several severe molecules and pathways involved in the complicated process of renal fibrosis, for instance, the Wnt/β-catenin and TGF-β1/Smad pathways, which are also key targets for botanicals. As the most vital target, Smad3-mediated TGF-β stimulation not only induces collagen production and the inhibition of ECM degradation, but also depresses fatty acid oxidation, leading to a profibrotic phenotype [275].

Botanicals with medicine–food homology happen to be abandoned in natural antioxidant, anti-inflammation, and anti-fibrosis compounds regulating the above pathways and inflammatory cytokines as shown in Table 2. The majority of the mechanisms underlying the protective effects are associated with these mechanisms, underscoring the significant potential and importance of incorporating daily dietary botanicals and supplements into one's routine.

4.2. Regulating the "Gut–Kidney Axis"

In addition to the classical molecular pathological processes centered on inflammation, oxidative stress, and cellular autophagy and apoptosis, a large number of studies have recently revealed a relationship between intestinal disorders and renal disease, a link that has been increasingly emphasized and investigated under the term "gut–kidney axis" [4]. It has been suggested that the gut–renal axis can be subdivided into metabolism-dependent and immunologic pathways [277]. Metabolism-dependent pathways are mainly mediated by metabolites produced by the gut microbiota that have the ability to modulate host physiological functions. For example, alterations in the gut microbiota can lead to intestinal metabolism and dysfunction, thereby increasing uremic toxin production and renal dysfunction [190,278]. On the other hand, kidney disease also affects the composition of gut bacteria and could cause gastrointestinal dysfunction [279,280]. In addition to uremic toxins like pCS, the gut microbiota produces a large number of physiologically active substances such as SCFAs, and bile acids (BAs), which play an important role in the regulation of renal disease and function [4]. Studies have found a reduction in SCFA-producing gut bacteria including *Lactobacillaceae* and *Prevotella* species in ESRD patients compared to healthy individuals [281,282]. However, in some models of kidney disease, a high-fiber diet that promotes the growth of SCFA-producing bacteria and direct supplementation with SCFAs attenuated renal fibrosis [283]. As for the immune pathway, components of the immune system (e.g., lymphocytes, monocytes, and cytokines) play a key role in the communication between the gut and the kidney [284]. A growing number of studies have demonstrated that gut flora play a crucial role in mucosal immunity and systemic inflammation, and that changes in gut flora induce changes in inflammatory cytokine profiles in the bone marrow [285], which are further associated with the development of autoimmune nephropathy [286]. Lymphocytes could even migrate from the gut to the injured kidney via the chemokine pathway [284]. Recent studies have also found that the aberrant galactose-deficient IgA, which is key in the pathogenesis of IgA nephropathy, is associated with aberrant hydrolysis by intestinal bacteria, and is recognized in vivo through the metabolism of the intestinal bacteria exposing aberrant antigenic epitopes, which leads to the formation of immune complexes and renal deposition [286].

As attention is increasingly focused on the gut microbiota, their interaction with botanicals has been discovered and showed a promising future [287–292]. As shown in Table 2, almost all kinds of compounds have the potential in regulating gut microbiota.

Panax notoginseng saponins, the bioactive components of a well-known and widely used botanical, *Panax notoginseng*, in Table S1, could regulate intestinal microorganisms and therefore ameliorate inflammation and fibrosis. Similarly to terpenoids, the renal protection by oleanic acid was also found to be associated with its regulation on gut microbiota [147]. Berberine had also been found to ameliorate chronic kidney disease through inhibiting the production of gut-derived uremic toxins, for example, TMAO and pCS in the gut microbiota [190]. *Astragalus membranaceus*, of which the anti-inflammation and fibrosis effects were confirmed, was also found to influence the gut microbiota, with *Akkermansia muciniphila* and *Lactobacillus* being the main driving bacteria [97]. More and more renal-protective effects of botanicals are found to be associated with the gut–kidney axis. Meanwhile, the gut microbiota exhibit rapid alterations in response to daily diets [293,294], indicating the potential for dietary nutrients to intervene in the gut–kidney axis.

5. Conclusions and Perspective

The concept of "food as medicine" underpins the traditional use of these botanicals, especially within the framework of TCM. This approach, which integrates dietary and medicinal uses, provides a unique and holistic perspective on disease prevention and health maintenance. The review emphasizes that many botanicals have been traditionally used for both food and therapeutic purposes, demonstrating their dual benefits. The diverse bioactive compounds found in these botanicals, such as flavonoids, polysaccharides, saponins, alkaloids, and polyphenols, demonstrate a range of protective effects on renal health. These effects are primarily mediated through antioxidation, anti-inflammation, anti-fibrosis, the modulation of the immune response, and enhancement in mitochondrial function as shown in Figure 2. The integration of these botanicals into modern therapeutic regimes could offer a complementary approach to conventional treatments for kidney diseases, which often focus on symptom management rather than disease reversal. The promising results from experimental studies suggest that incorporating these natural compounds into dietary habits or as supplements could contribute to better renal health outcomes.

A particularly notable aspect highlighted in this review is the interplay between these botanicals and the gut–kidney axis. This emerging area of research emphasizes the complex relationship between gut microbiota and renal function. Botanical compounds can influence the composition and activity of gut microbiota, which in turn affects systemic inflammation, immune responses, and metabolic processes relevant to kidney health. For instance, the modulation of gut microbiota by polysaccharides and polyphenols can lead to the production of beneficial metabolites, such as short-chain fatty acids, which have protective effects on the kidneys. Considering the close relation between daily diets and gut microbiota, the potential for dietary nutrients to intervene in the gut–kidney axis is worth deeper exploration.

In summary, botanical ingredients with medicine–food homology present a valuable resource for developing new strategies in the prevention and management of kidney diseases. By leveraging their effects on the gut–kidney axis and other pathways, these botanicals hold promise for enhancing renal health and improving patient outcomes. Continued research and clinical validation are essential to fully realize their potential in this domain.

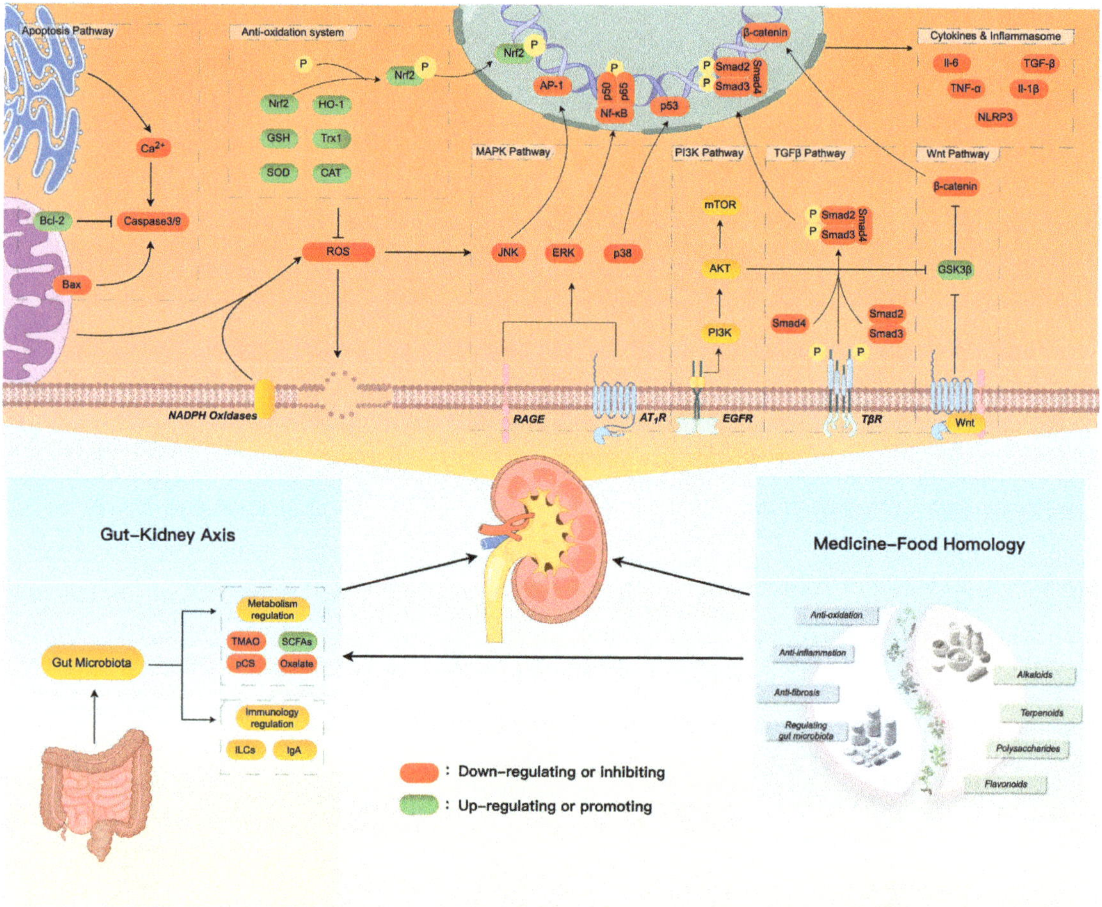

Figure 2. Mechanisms involved in the interplay of dietary medical botanicals and kidney function, drawn by authors using Figdraw (www.figdraw.com).

Supplementary Materials: The following supporting information can be downloaded at: https://www.mdpi.com/article/10.3390/nu16203530/s1, Table S1: Botanicals that are allowed to be added to dietary supplements in China.

Author Contributions: Conceptualization and writing—original draft preparation, Y.Z.; resources, R.F.; methodology, M.-L.Y.; data curation, J.-C.H.; visualization, H.X.; writing—review and editing, J.-Y.S.; funding acquisition, Y.W.; supervision, L.-M.C., J.-D.J., and Y.W. All authors have read and agreed to the published version of the manuscript.

Funding: We acknowledge financial support from the National Key R&D Program of China (Grant No.: 2022YFA0806400), the National Natural Science Foundation of China (Nos. 82173888 and 81973290), the Medical and Health Technology Innovation Project of Chinese Academy of Medical Sciences (2021-I2M-1–007, 2023-12M-2-006, 2021-I2M-1–028), and the Beijing Key Laboratory of Non-Clinical Drug Metabolism and PK/PD study (Z141102004414062).

Institutional Review Board Statement: Not applicable.

Informed Consent Statement: Not applicable.

Data Availability Statement: No new data were created or analyzed in this study. Data sharing is not applicable to this article.

Acknowledgments: We express our gratitude to Bin Zhao (Department of Pharmacy, Peking Union Medical College Hospital) for his help. We would like to thank Shimadzu Co., Ltd. (Shanghai, China) for technological support. Special thanks to Siyu Ou for the help with the illustration.

Conflicts of Interest: The authors declare no conflicts of interest.

References

1. Wu, H.; Huang, J. Drug-Induced Nephrotoxicity: Pathogenic Mechanisms, Biomarkers and Prevention Strategies. *Curr. Drug Metab.* **2018**, *19*, 559–567. [CrossRef] [PubMed]
2. Mody, H.; Ramakrishnan, V.; Chaar, M.; Lezeau, J.; Rump, A.; Taha, K.; Lesko, L.; Ait-Oudhia, S. A Review on Drug-Induced Nephrotoxicity: Pathophysiological Mechanisms, Drug Classes, Clinical Management, and Recent Advances in Mathematical Modeling and Simulation Approaches. *Clin. Pharmacol. Drug Dev.* **2020**, *9*, 896–909. [CrossRef]
3. Schetz, M.; Dasta, J.; Goldstein, S.; Golper, T. Drug-Induced Acute Kidney Injury. *Curr. Opin. Crit. Care* **2005**, *11*, 555–565. [CrossRef]
4. Yang, T.; Richards, E.M.; Pepine, C.J.; Raizada, M.K. The Gut Microbiota and the Brain–Gut–Kidney Axis in Hypertension and Chronic Kidney Disease. *Nat. Rev. Nephrol.* **2018**, *14*, 442–456. [CrossRef]
5. Gaitonde, D.Y.; Cook, D.L.; Rivera, I.M. Chronic Kidney Disease: Detection and Evaluation. *Am. Fam. Physician* **2017**, *96*, 776–783.
6. Tain, Y.L.; Chang, C.I.; Hou, C.Y.; Chang-Chien, G.P.; Lin, S.F.; Hsu, C.N. Resveratrol Propionate Ester Supplement Exerts Antihypertensive Effect in Juvenile Rats Exposed to an Adenine Diet Via Gut Microbiota Modulation. *Nutrients* **2024**, *16*, 2131. [CrossRef] [PubMed]
7. Bellomo, F.; Pugliese, S.; Cairoli, S.; Krohn, P.; De Stefanis, C.; Raso, R.; Rega, L.R.; Taranta, A.; De Leo, E.; Ciolfi, A.; et al. Ketogenic Diet and Progression of Kidney Disease in Animal Models of Nephropathic Cystinosis. *J. Am. Soc. Nephrol.* **2024**, 10-1681. [CrossRef] [PubMed]
8. Yang, C.; Wang, T.; Chen, J.; He, J.; Li, Y.; Chen, C.; Lu, G.; Chen, W. Traditional Chinese Medicine Formulas Alleviate Acute Pancreatitis: Pharmacological Activities and Mechanisms. *Pancreas* **2021**, *50*, 1348–1356. [CrossRef]
9. Wang, Y.; Li, M.; Liang, Y.; Yang, Y.; Liu, Z.; Yao, K.; Chen, Z.; Zhai, S. Chinese Herbal Medicine for the Treatment of Depression: Applications, Efficacies and Mechanisms. *Curr. Pharm. Des.* **2017**, *23*, 5180–5190. [CrossRef]
10. Chan, H.H.L.; Ng, T. Traditional Chinese Medicine (Tcm) and Allergic Diseases. *Curr. Allergy Asthma Rep.* **2020**, *20*, 67. [CrossRef]
11. Wojcikowski, K.; Wohlmuth, H.; Johnson, D.W.; Rolfe, M.; Gobe, G. An In Vitro Investigation of Herbs Traditionally Used for Kidney and Urinary System Disorders: Potential Therapeutic and Toxic Effects. *Nephrology* **2009**, *14*, 70–79. [CrossRef] [PubMed]
12. Li, C.; Huang, H.; Wang, R.; Zhang, C.; Huang, S.; Wu, J.; Mo, P.; Yu, H.; Li, S.; Chen, J.; et al. Formula Restores Iron Metabolism from Dysregulation in Anemic Rats with Adenine-Induced Nephropathy. *J. Ethnopharmacol.* **2023**, *312*, 116526. [CrossRef] [PubMed]
13. Ll, J.; Yu, D.R.; Chen, H.Y.; Zhu, C.F.; Cheng, X.X.; Wang, Y.H.; Ni, J.; Wang, X.J.; Jinag, F. Long-Term Effect of the Treatment of Iga Nephropathy by Tonifying Shen, Activating Blood Stasis, Dispelling Wind-Dampness Combined with Western Medicine. *Zhongguo Zhong Xi Yi Jie He Za Zhi* **2017**, *37*, 28–33. [PubMed]
14. Peng, M.; Cai, P.; Ma, H.; Meng, H.; Xu, Y.; Zhang, X.; Si, G. Chinese Herbal Medicine Shenqi Detoxification Granule Inhibits Fibrosis in Adenine Induced Chronic Renal Failure Rats. *Afr. J. Tradit. Complement. Altern. Med.* **2014**, *11*, 194–204. [PubMed]
15. *Notice of the National Health Commission on Further Regulating the Management of Health Food Raw Materials (No. 51 of 2002)*; National Health Commission of the People's Republic of China: Beijing, China, 2002.
16. Wan, F.; Ma, F.; Wu, J.; Qiao, X.; Chen, M.; Li, W.; Ma, L. Effect of *Lycium barbarum* Polysaccharide on Decreasing Serum Amyloid A3 Expression through Inhibiting Nf-Kb Activation in a Mouse Model of Diabetic Nephropathy. *Anal. Cell. Pathol.* **2022**, *2022*, 7847135. [CrossRef]
17. Li, W.; Yu, L.; Fu, B.; Chu, J.; Chen, C.; Li, X.; Ma, J.; Tang, W. Protective Effects of *Polygonatum kingianum* Polysaccharides and Aqueous Extract on Uranium-Induced Toxicity in Human Kidney (Hk-2) Cells. *Int. J. Biol. Macromol.* **2022**, *202*, 68–79. [CrossRef]
18. Yue, L.; Wang, W.; Wang, Y.; Du, T.; Shen, W.; Tang, H.; Wang, Y.; Yin, H. *Bletilla striata* Polysaccharide Inhibits Angiotensin Ii-Induced Ros and Inflammation Via Nox4 and Tlr2 Pathways. *Int. J. Biol. Macromol.* **2016**, *89*, 376–388. [CrossRef]
19. Ma, Q.; Xu, Y.; Tang, L.; Yang, X.; Chen, Z.; Wei, Y.; Shao, X.; Shao, X.; Xin, Z.; Cai, B.; et al. Astragalus Polysaccharide Attenuates Cisplatin-Induced Acute Kidney Injury by Suppressing Oxidative Damage and Mitochondrial Dysfunction. *BioMed Res. Int.* **2020**, *2020*, 2851349. [CrossRef]
20. Zhao, K.; Wu, X.; Han, G.; Sun, L.; Zheng, C.; Hou, H.; Xu, B.B.; El-Bahy, Z.M.; Qian, C.; Kallel, M.; et al. *Phyllostachys nigra* (Lodd. Ex Lindl.) Derived Polysaccharide with Enhanced Glycolipid Metabolism Regulation and Mice Gut Microbiome. *Int. J. Biol. Macromol.* **2024**, *257 Pt 1*, 128588. [CrossRef]
21. Dwyer, J.T.; Coates, P.M.; Smith, M.J. Dietary Supplements: Regulatory Challenges and Research Resources. *Nutrients* **2018**, *10*, 41. [CrossRef]

22. Nicastro, H.L.; Vorkoper, S.; Sterling, R.; Korn, A.R.; Brown, A.G.M.; Maruvada, P.; Oh, A.Y. Opportunities to Advance Implementation Science and Nutrition Research: A Commentary on the Strategic Plan for Nih Nutrition Research. *Transl. Behav. Med.* **2023**, *13*, 1–6. [CrossRef] [PubMed]
23. Bilia, A.R. Herbal Medicinal Products Versus Botanical-Food Supplements in the European Market: State of Art and Perspectives. *Nat. Prod. Commun.* **2015**, *10*, 125–131. [CrossRef] [PubMed]
24. Luciano, R.L.; Perazella, M.A. Aristolochic Acid Nephropathy: Epidemiology, Clinical Presentation, and Treatment. *Drug Saf.* **2015**, *38*, 55–64. [CrossRef] [PubMed]
25. Ban, T.H.; Min, J.W.; Seo, C.; Kim, D.R.; Lee, Y.H.; Chung, B.H.; Jeong, K.H.; Lee, J.W.; Kim, B.S.; Lee, S.H.; et al. Update of Aristolochic Acid Nephropathy in Korea. *Korean J. Intern. Med.* **2018**, *33*, 961–969. [CrossRef] [PubMed]
26. Dugo, M.; Gatto, R.; Zagatti, R.; Gatti, P.; Cascone, C. Herbal Remedies: Nephrotoxicity and Drug Interactions. *G. Ital. Nefrol.* **2010**, *27* (Suppl. S52), S5–S9.
27. Yang, H.; Zhao, Y.; Ren, B.; Wu, Y.; Qiu, Z.; Cheng, Y.; Qiu, B. Poria Acid Inhibit the Growth and Metastasis of Renal Cell Carcinoma by Inhibiting the Pi3k/Akt/Nf-Kb Signaling Pathway. *Heliyon* **2024**, *10*, e31106. [CrossRef]
28. Lu, M.; Yin, J.; Xu, T.; Dai, X.; Liu, T.; Zhang, Y.; Wang, S.; Liu, Y.; Shi, H.; Zhang, Y.; et al. Fuling-Zexie Formula Attenuates Hyperuricemia-Induced Nephropathy and Inhibits Jak2/Stat3 Signaling and Nlrp3 Inflammasome Activation in Mice. *J. Ethnopharmacol.* **2024**, *319 Pt 2*, 117262. [CrossRef]
29. *Notice on Six New Substances Including Angelica Sinensis and Other Substances Which Are Both Food and Chinese Herbal Medicine According to Tradition (No. 8 of 2019)*; Food Safety Standards and Evaluation Division (Ed.) National Health Commission of the People's Republic of China: Beijing, China, 2019.
30. *Notice on Nine New Substances Including Codonopsis Pilosula and Other Substances Which Are Both Food and Chinese Herbal Medicine According to Tradition (No. 9 of 2023)*; Food Safety Standards and Evaluation Division (Ed.) National Health Commission of the People's Republic of China: Beijing, China, 2023.
31. *Regulations on Catalog of Substances That Are Traditionally Used as Both Food and Herbal Medicine*; Food Safety Standards and Evaluation Division (Ed.) National Health Commission of the People's Republic of China: Beijing, China, 2021.
32. Vettorazzi, A.; de Cerain, A.L.; Sanz-Serrano, J.; Gil, A.G.; Azqueta, A. European Regulatory Framework and Safety Assessment of Food-Related Bioactive Compounds. *Nutrients* **2020**, *12*, 613. [CrossRef]
33. Bailey, R.L. Current Regulatory Guidelines and Resources to Support Research of Dietary Supplements in the United States. *Crit. Rev. Food Sci. Nutr.* **2018**, *60*, 298–309. [CrossRef]
34. US Department of Health and Human Services, National Institutes of Health, Office of Dietary Supplements. *Dietary Supplement Label Database (Dsld)*; US Department of Health and Human Services, National Institutes of Health, Office of Dietary Supplements: Bethesda, MD, USA, 2013.
35. Liu, Y.; Luo, J.; Peng, L.; Zhang, Q.; Rong, X.; Luo, Y.; Li, J. Flavonoids: Potential Therapeutic Agents for Cardiovascular Disease. *Heliyon* **2024**, *10*, e32563. [CrossRef]
36. Frydman, A.; Weisshaus, O.; Bar-Peled, M.; Huhman, D.V.; Sumner, L.W.; Marin, F.R.; Lewinsohn, E.; Fluhr, R.; Gressel, J.; Eyal, Y. Citrus Fruit Bitter Flavors: Isolation and Functional Characterization of the Gene Cm1,2rhat Encoding a 1,2 Rhamnosyltransferase, a Key Enzyme in the Biosynthesis of the Bitter Flavonoids of Citrus. *Plant J.* **2004**, *40*, 88–100. [CrossRef]
37. Zhang, L.; Wang, X.; Chang, L.; Ren, Y.; Sui, M.; Fu, Y.; Zhang, L.; Hao, L. Quercetin Improves Diabetic Kidney Disease by Inhibiting Ferroptosis and Regulating the Nrf2 in Streptozotocin-Induced Diabetic Rats. *Ren. Fail.* **2024**, *46*, 2327495. [CrossRef] [PubMed]
38. Guo, X.; Wen, S.; Wang, J.; Zeng, X.; Yu, H.; Chen, Y.; Zhu, X.; Xu, L. Senolytic Combination of Dasatinib and Quercetin Attenuates Renal Damage in Diabetic Kidney Disease. *Phytomedicine* **2024**, *130*, 155705. [CrossRef] [PubMed]
39. Zeng, Y.F.; Li, J.Y.; Wei, X.Y.; Ma, S.Q.; Wang, Q.G.; Qi, Z.; Duan, Z.C.; Tan, L.; Tang, H. Preclinical Evidence of Reno-Protective Effect of Quercetin on Acute Kidney Injury: A Meta-Analysis of Animal Studies. *Front. Pharmacol.* **2023**, *14*, 1310023. [CrossRef]
40. Xu, Z.; Wang, X.; Kuang, W.; Wang, S.; Zhao, Y. Kaempferol Improves Acute Kidney Injury Via Inhibition of Macrophage Infiltration in Septic Mice. *Biosci. Rep.* **2023**, *43*, BSR20230873. [CrossRef] [PubMed]
41. Yuan, N.; Diao, J.; Dong, J.; Yan, Y.; Chen, Y.; Yan, S.; Liu, C.; He, Z.; He, J.; Zhang, C.; et al. Targeting Rock1 in Diabetic Kidney Disease: Unraveling Mesangial Fibrosis Mechanisms and Introducing Myricetin as a Novel Antagonist. *Biomed. Pharmacother.* **2024**, *171*, 116208. [CrossRef]
42. Yang, Z.J.; Wang, H.R.; Wang, Y.I.; Zhai, Z.H.; Wang, L.W.; Li, L.; Zhang, C.; Tang, L. Myricetin Attenuated Diabetes-Associated Kidney Injuries and Dysfunction Via Regulating Nuclear Factor (Erythroid Derived 2)-Like 2 and Nuclear Factor-Kb Signaling. *Front. Pharmacol.* **2019**, *10*, 647. [CrossRef]
43. Liu, P.; Tang, L.; Li, G.; Wu, X.; Hu, F.; Peng, W. Association between Consumption of Flavonol and Its Subclasses and Chronic Kidney Disease in Us Adults: An Analysis Based on National Health and Nutrition Examination Survey Data from 2007–2008, 2009–2010, and 2017–2018. *Front. Nutr.* **2024**, *11*, 1399251. [CrossRef]
44. Jian, J.; Li, Y.-Q.; Han, R.-Y.; Zhong, X.; Xie, K.-H.; Yan, Y.; Wang, L.; Tan, R.-Z. Isorhamnetin Ameliorates Cisplatin-Induced Acute Kidney Injury in Mice by Activating Slpi-Mediated Anti-Inflammatory Effect in Macrophage. *Immunopharmacol. Immunotoxicol.* **2024**, *46*, 319–329. [CrossRef] [PubMed]
45. Wang, B.; Yang, L.N.; Yang, L.T.; Liang, Y.; Guo, F.; Fu, P.; Ma, L. Fisetin Ameliorates Fibrotic Kidney Disease in Mice Via Inhibiting Acsl4-Mediated Tubular Ferroptosis. *Acta Pharmacol. Sin.* **2024**, *45*, 150–165. [CrossRef]

46. Zou, T.F.; Liu, Z.G.; Cao, P.C.; Zheng, S.H.; Guo, W.T.; Wang, T.X.; Chen, Y.L.; Duan, Y.J.; Li, Q.S.; Liao, C.Z.; et al. Fisetin Treatment Alleviates Kidney Injury in Mice with Diabetes-Exacerbated Atherosclerosis through Inhibiting Cd36/Fibrosis Pathway. *Acta Pharmacol. Sin.* **2023**, *44*, 2065–2074. [CrossRef]
47. Zhang, D.; Liu, S.; Jiang, H.; Liu, S.; Kong, F. Dia Proteomics Analysis Reveals the Mechanism of Folic Acid-Induced Acute Kidney Injury and the Effects of Icariin. *Chem. Biol. Interact.* **2024**, *390*, 110878. [CrossRef] [PubMed]
48. Zhao, Y.; Yang, W.; Zhang, X.; Lv, C.; Lu, J. Icariin, the Main Prenylflavonoid of Epimedii Folium, Ameliorated Chronic Kidney Disease by Modulating Energy Metabolism Via Ampk Activation. *J. Ethnopharmacol.* **2023**, *312*, 116543. [CrossRef] [PubMed]
49. Owumi, S.E.; Kazeem, A.I.; Wu, B.; Ishokare, L.O.; Arunsi, U.O.; Oyelere, A.K. Apigeninidin-Rich *Sorghum bicolor* (L. Moench) Extracts Suppress A549 Cells Proliferation and Ameliorate Toxicity of Aflatoxin B1-Mediated Liver and Kidney Derangement in Rats. *Sci. Rep.* **2022**, *12*, 7438. [CrossRef] [PubMed]
50. Amorim, J.M.; de Souza, L.C.R.; de Souza, R.A.L.; da Silva Filha, R.; de Oliveira Silva, J.; de Almeida Araújo, S.; Tagliti, C.A.; Simões, E.S.A.C.; Castilho, R.O. Costus Spiralis Extract Restores Kidney Function in Cisplatin-Induced Nephrotoxicity Model: Ethnopharmacological Use, Chemical and Toxicological Investigation. *J. Ethnopharmacol.* **2022**, *299*, 115510. [CrossRef] [PubMed]
51. Wang, X.; Kim, C.S.; Adams, B.C.; Wilkinson, R.; Hill, M.M.; Shah, A.K.; Mohamed, A.; Dutt, M.; Ng, M.S.Y.; Ungerer, J.P.J.; et al. Human Proximal Tubular Epithelial Cell-Derived Small Extracellular Vesicles Mediate Synchronized Tubular Ferroptosis in Hypoxic Kidney Injury. *Redox Biol.* **2024**, *70*, 103042. [CrossRef]
52. Guo, S.; Zhou, L.; Liu, X.; Gao, L.; Li, Y.; Wu, Y. Baicalein Alleviates Cisplatin-Induced Acute Kidney Injury by Inhibiting Alox12-Dependent Ferroptosis. *Phytomedicine* **2024**, *130*, 155757. [CrossRef]
53. Hu, H.; Li, W.; Hao, Y.; Peng, Z.; Zou, Z.; Liang, W. Baicalin Ameliorates Renal Fibrosis by Upregulating Cpt1α-Mediated Fatty Acid Oxidation in Diabetic Kidney Disease. *Phytomedicine* **2024**, *122*, 155162. [CrossRef]
54. Miguel, V.; Rey-Serra, C.; Tituaña, J.; Sirera, B.; Alcalde-Estévez, E.; Herrero, J.I.; Ranz, I.; Fernández, L.; Castillo, C.; Sevilla, L.; et al. Enhanced Fatty Acid Oxidation through Metformin and Baicalin as Therapy for COVID-19 and Associated Inflammatory States in Lung and Kidney. *Redox Biol.* **2023**, *68*, 102957. [CrossRef]
55. Liu, B.; Deng, Q.; Zhang, L.; Zhu, W. Nobiletin Alleviates Ischemia/Reperfusion Injury in the Kidney by Activating Pi3k/Akt Pathway. *Mol. Med. Rep.* **2020**, *22*, 4655–4662. [CrossRef]
56. Song, J.; Wang, H.; Sheng, J.; Zhang, W.; Lei, J.; Gan, W.; Cai, F.; Yang, Y. Vitexin Attenuates Chronic Kidney Disease by Inhibiting Renal Tubular Epithelial Cell Ferroptosis Via Nrf2 Activation. *Mol. Med.* **2023**, *29*, 147. [CrossRef]
57. Ding, T.; Zhao, T.; Li, Y.; Liu, Z.; Ding, J.; Ji, B.; Wang, Y.; Guo, Z. Vitexin Exerts Protective Effects against Calcium Oxalate Crystal-Induced Kidney Pyroptosis In Vivo and In Vitro. *Phytomedicine* **2021**, *86*, 153562. [CrossRef] [PubMed]
58. Yang, Q.; Qian, L.; He, S.; Zhang, C. Hesperidin Alleviates Zinc-Induced Nephrotoxicity Via the Gut-Kidney Axis in Swine. *Front. Cell Infect. Microbiol.* **2024**, *14*, 1390104. [CrossRef] [PubMed]
59. Chen, J.; Fan, X.; Chen, J.; Luo, X.; Huang, X.; Zhou, Z.; He, Y.; Feng, S.; Jiao, Y.; Wang, R.; et al. Effects of Hesperidin on the Histological Structure, Oxidative Stress, and Apoptosis in the Liver and Kidney Induced by Nicl(2). *Front. Vet. Sci.* **2024**, *11*, 1424711. [CrossRef] [PubMed]
60. Yang, A.Y.; Choi, H.J.; Kim, K.; Leem, J. Antioxidant, Antiapoptotic, and Anti-Inflammatory Effects of Hesperetin in a Mouse Model of Lipopolysaccharide-Induced Acute Kidney Injury. *Molecules* **2023**, *28*, 2759. [CrossRef]
61. Chen, X.; Wei, W.; Li, Y.; Huang, J.; Ci, X. Hesperetin Relieves Cisplatin-Induced Acute Kidney Injury by Mitigating Oxidative Stress, Inflammation and Apoptosis. *Chem. Biol. Interact.* **2019**, *308*, 269–278. [CrossRef]
62. Chen, C.; Feng, F.; Qi, M.; Chen, Q.; Tang, W.; Diao, H.; Hu, Z.; Qiu, Y.; Li, Z.; Chu, Y.; et al. Dietary Citrus Flavonoids Improved Growth Performance and Intestinal Microbiota of Weaned Piglets Via Immune Function Mediated by Tlr2/Nf-Kb Signaling Pathway. *J. Agric. Food Chem.* **2024**, *72*, 16761–16776. [CrossRef]
63. Chang, Y.W.; Chen, Y.L.; Park, S.H.; Yap, E.E.S.; Sung, W.C. Characterization of Functional Ingredients Extracted with Ethanol Solvents from Ponkan (*Citrus reticulata*) by-Products Using the Microwave Vacuum Drying Method Combined with Ultrasound-Assisted Extraction. *Foods* **2024**, *13*, 2129. [CrossRef]
64. Chen, Y.; Pan, H.; Hao, S.; Pan, D.; Wang, G.; Yu, W. Evaluation of Phenolic Composition and Antioxidant Properties of Different Varieties of Chinese Citrus. *Food Chem.* **2021**, *364*, 130413. [CrossRef]
65. Kamel, K.M.; El-Raouf, O.M.A.; Metwally, S.A.; El-Latif, H.A.A.; El-sayed, M.E. Hesperidin and Rutin, Antioxidant Citrus Flavonoids, Attenuate Cisplatin-Induced Nephrotoxicity in Rats. *J. Biochem. Mol. Toxicol.* **2014**, *28*, 312–319. [CrossRef]
66. Jung, H.A.; Jung, M.J.; Kim, J.Y.; Chung, H.Y.; Choi, J.S. Inhibitory Activity of Flavonoids from Prunus Davidiana and Other Flavonoids on Total Ros and Hydroxyl Radical Generation. *Arch. Pharm. Res.* **2003**, *26*, 809–815. [CrossRef]
67. Mbara, K.C.; Fotsing, M.C.D.; Ndinteh, D.T.; Mbeb, C.N.; Nwagwu, C.S.; Khan, R.; Mokhetho, K.C.; Baijnath, H.; Nlooto, M.; Mokhele, S.; et al. Endoplasmic Reticulum Stress in Pancreatic Β-Cell Dysfunction: The Potential Therapeutic Role of Dietary Flavonoids. *Curr. Res. Pharmacol. Drug Discov.* **2024**, *6*, 100184. [CrossRef] [PubMed]
68. Ramos, F.M.M.; Ribeiro, C.B.; Cesar, T.B.; Milenkovic, D.; Cabral, L.; Noronha, M.F.; Sivieri, K. Lemon Flavonoids Nutraceutical (Eriomin®) Attenuates Prediabetes Intestinal Dysbiosis: A Double-Blind Randomized Controlled Trial. *Food Sci. Nutr.* **2023**, *11*, 7283–7295. [CrossRef] [PubMed]
69. Bellavite, P. Neuroprotective Potentials of Flavonoids: Experimental Studies and Mechanisms of Action. *Antioxidants* **2023**, *12*, 280. [CrossRef] [PubMed]

70. Pabich, M.; Materska, M. Biological Effect of Soy Isoflavones in the Prevention of Civilization Diseases. *Nutrients* **2019**, *11*, 1660. [CrossRef]
71. Misiakiewicz-Has, K.; Maciejewska-Markiewicz, D.; Szypulska-Koziarska, D.; Kolasa, A.; Wiszniewska, B. The Influence of Soy Isoflavones and Soy Isoflavones with Inulin on Kidney Morphology, Fatty Acids, and Associated Parameters in Rats with and without Induced Diabetes Type 2. *Int. J. Mol. Sci.* **2024**, *25*, 5418. [CrossRef]
72. Hu, Z.; Chen, D.; Yan, P.; Zheng, F.; Zhu, H.; Yuan, Z.; Yang, X.; Zuo, Y.; Chen, C.; Lu, H.; et al. Puerarin Suppresses Macrophage M1 Polarization to Alleviate Renal Inflammatory Injury through Antagonizing Tlr4/Myd88-Mediated Nf-Kb P65 and Jnk/Foxo1 Activation. *Phytomedicine* **2024**, *132*, 155813. [CrossRef]
73. Zhang, S.S.; Zhang, N.N.; Guo, S.; Liu, S.J.; Hou, Y.F.; Li, S.; Ho, C.T.; Bai, N.S. Glycosides and Flavonoids from the Extract of Pueraria Thomsonii Benth Leaf Alleviate Type 2 Diabetes in High-Fat Diet Plus Streptozotocin-Induced Mice by Modulating the Gut Microbiota. *Food Funct.* **2022**, *13*, 3931–3945. [CrossRef]
74. Zhou, Y.; Lu, W.; Huang, K.; Gan, F. Ferroptosis Is Involved in Quercetin-Mediated Alleviation of Ochratoxin a-Induced Kidney Damage. *Food Chem. Toxicol.* **2024**, *191*, 114877. [CrossRef] [PubMed]
75. Liu, F.; Feng, Q.; Yang, M.; Yang, Y.; Nie, J.; Wang, S. Quercetin Prevented Diabetic Nephropathy by Inhibiting Renal Tubular Epithelial Cell Apoptosis Via the Pi3k/Akt Pathway. *Phytother. Res.* **2024**, *38*, 3594–3606. [CrossRef]
76. Sheng, H.; Zhang, D.; Zhang, J.; Zhang, Y.; Lu, Z.; Mao, W.; Liu, X.; Zhang, L. Kaempferol Attenuated Diabetic Nephropathy by Reducing Apoptosis and Promoting Autophagy through Ampk/Mtor Pathways. *Front. Med.* **2022**, *9*, 986825. [CrossRef]
77. Wu, Q.; Chen, J.; Zheng, X.; Song, J.; Yin, L.; Guo, H.; Chen, Q.; Liu, Y.; Ma, Q.; Zhang, H.; et al. Kaempferol Attenuates Doxorubicin-Induced Renal Tubular Injury by Inhibiting Ros/Ask1-Mediated Activation of the Mapk Signaling Pathway. *Biomed. Pharmacother.* **2023**, *157*, 114087. [CrossRef] [PubMed]
78. Guan, Y.; Quan, D.; Chen, K.; Kang, L.; Yang, D.; Wu, H.; Yan, M.; Wu, S.; Lv, L.; Zhang, G. Kaempferol Inhibits Renal Fibrosis by Suppression of the Sonic Hedgehog Signaling Pathway. *Phytomedicine* **2023**, *108*, 154246. [CrossRef] [PubMed]
79. Yang, X.; Zhang, P.; Jiang, J.; Almoallim, H.S.; Alharbi, S.A.; Li, Y. Myricetin Attenuates Ethylene Glycol-Induced Nephrolithiasis in Rats Via Mitigating Oxidative Stress and Inflammatory Markers. *Appl. Biochem. Biotechnol.* **2023**, *196*, 5419–5434. [CrossRef] [PubMed]
80. Liu, J.; Xie, L.; Zhai, H.; Wang, D.; Li, X.; Wang, Y.; Song, M.; Xu, C. Exploration of the Protective Mechanisms of Icariin against Cisplatin-Induced Renal Cell Damage in Canines. *Front. Vet. Sci.* **2024**, *11*, 1331409. [CrossRef] [PubMed]
81. Ding, N.; Sun, S.; Zhou, S.; Lv, Z.; Wang, R. Icariin Alleviates Renal Inflammation and Tubulointerstitial Fibrosis Via Nrf2-Mediated Attenuation of Mitochondrial Damage. *Cell Biochem. Funct.* **2024**, *42*, e4005. [CrossRef]
82. Duan, S.; Ding, Z.; Liu, C.; Wang, X.; Dai, E. Icariin Suppresses Nephrotic Syndrome by Inhibiting Pyroptosis and Epithelial-to-Mesenchymal Transition. *PLoS ONE* **2024**, *19*, e0298353. [CrossRef]
83. Wu, Q.; Li, W.; Zhao, J.; Sun, W.; Yang, Q.; Chen, C.; Xia, P.; Zhu, J.; Zhou, Y.; Huang, G.; et al. Apigenin Ameliorates Doxorubicin-Induced Renal Injury Via Inhibition of Oxidative Stress and Inflammation. *Biomed. Pharmacother.* **2021**, *137*, 111308. [CrossRef]
84. Li, Y.; Zhao, Z.; Luo, J.; Jiang, Y.; Li, L.; Chen, Y.; Zhang, L.; Huang, Q.; Cao, Y.; Zhou, P.; et al. Apigenin Ameliorates Hyperuricemic Nephropathy by Inhibiting Urat1 and Glut9 and Relieving Renal Fibrosis Via the Wnt/B-Catenin Pathway. *Phytomedicine* **2021**, *87*, 153585. [CrossRef]
85. Zamani, F.; Samiei, F.; Mousavi, Z.; Azari, M.R.; Seydi, E.; Pourahmad, J. Apigenin Ameliorates Oxidative Stress and Mitochondrial Damage Induced by Multiwall Carbon Nanotubes in Rat Kidney Mitochondria. *J. Biochem. Mol. Toxicol.* **2021**, *35*, 1–7. [CrossRef]
86. Wang, T.; Zhang, Z.; Xie, M.; Li, S.; Zhang, J.; Zhou, J. Apigenin Attenuates Mesoporous Silica Nanoparticles-Induced Nephrotoxicity by Activating Foxo3a. *Biol. Trace Elem. Res.* **2022**, *200*, 2793–2806. [CrossRef]
87. Azimi, A.; Eidi, A.; Mortazavi, P.; Rohani, A.H. Protective Effect of Apigenin on Ethylene Glycol-Induced Urolithiasis Via Attenuating Oxidative Stress and Inflammatory Parameters in Adult Male Wistar Rats. *Life Sci.* **2021**, *279*, 119641. [CrossRef] [PubMed]
88. Zhang, K.; Li, J.; Dong, W.; Huang, Q.; Wang, X.; Deng, K.; Ali, W.; Song, R.; Zou, H.; Ran, D.; et al. Luteolin Alleviates Cadmium-Induced Kidney Injury by Inhibiting Oxidative DNA Damage and Repairing Autophagic Flux Blockade in Chickens. *Antioxidants* **2024**, *13*, 525. [CrossRef]
89. Xu, X.; Yu, Z.; Han, B.; Li, S.; Sun, Y.; Du, Y.; Wang, Z.; Gao, D.; Zhang, Z. Luteolin Alleviates Inorganic Mercury-Induced Kidney Injury Via Activation of the Ampk/Mtor Autophagy Pathway. *J. Inorg. Biochem.* **2021**, *224*, 111583. [CrossRef] [PubMed]
90. Ding, T.; Yi, T.; Li, Y.; Zhang, W.; Wang, X.; Liu, J.; Fan, Y.; Ji, J.; Xu, L. Luteolin Attenuates Lupus Nephritis by Regulating Macrophage Oxidative Stress Via Hif-1α Pathway. *Eur. J. Pharmacol.* **2023**, *953*, 175823. [CrossRef]
91. Li, F.; Wei, R.; Huang, M.; Chen, J.; Li, P.; Ma, Y.; Chen, X. Luteolin Can Ameliorate Renal Interstitial Fibrosis-Induced Renal Anaemia through the Sirt1/Foxo3 Pathway. *Food Funct.* **2022**, *13*, 11896–11914. [CrossRef]
92. Awoyomi, O.V.; Adeoye, Y.D.; Oyagbemi, A.A.; Ajibade, T.O.; Asenuga, E.R.; Gbadamosi, I.T.; Ogunpolu, B.S.; Falayi, O.O.; Hassan, F.O.; Omobowale, T.O.; et al. Luteolin Mitigates Potassium Dichromate-Induced Nephrotoxicity, Cardiotoxicity and Genotoxicity through Modulation of Kim-1/Nrf2 Signaling Pathways. *Environ. Toxicol.* **2021**, *36*, 2146–2160. [CrossRef] [PubMed]
93. Zhu, Q.; Yang, S.; Wei, C.; Lu, G.; Lee, K.; He, J.C.; Liu, R.; Zhong, Y. Puerarin Attenuates Diabetic Kidney Injury through Interaction with Guanidine Nucleotide-Binding Protein Gi Subunit Alpha-1 (Gnai1) Subunit. *J. Cell Mol. Med.* **2022**, *26*, 3816–3827. [CrossRef]

94. Song, Q.; Jian, W.; Zhang, Y.; Li, Q.; Zhao, Y.; Liu, R.; Zeng, Y.; Zhang, F.; Duan, J. Puerarin Attenuates Iron Overload-Induced Ferroptosis in Retina through a Nrf2-Mediated Mechanism. *Mol. Nutr. Food Res.* **2024**, *68*, e2300123. [CrossRef]
95. Jing, G.H.; Liu, Y.D.; Liu, J.N.; Jin, Y.S.; Yu, S.L.; An, R.H. Puerarin Prevents Calcium Oxalate Crystal-Induced Renal Epithelial Cell Autophagy by Activating the Sirt1-Mediated Signaling Pathway. *Urolithiasis* **2022**, *50*, 545–556. [CrossRef]
96. Sun, J.; Wei, S.; Zhang, Y.; Li, J. Protective Effects of Astragalus Polysaccharide on Sepsis-Induced Acute Kidney Injury. *Anal. Cell. Pathol.* **2021**, *2021*, 7178253. [CrossRef]
97. Li, J.; Zhao, J.; Chai, Y.; Li, W.; Liu, X.; Chen, Y. Astragalus Polysaccharide Protects Sepsis Model Rats after Cecum Ligation and Puncture. *Front. Bioeng. Biotechnol.* **2022**, *10*, 1020300. [CrossRef] [PubMed]
98. Wang, Y.; Liu, D.; Chen, S.; Wang, Y.; Jiang, H.; Yin, H. A New Glucomannan from Bletilla Striata: Structural and Anti-Fibrosis Effects. *Fitoterapia* **2014**, *92*, 72–78. [CrossRef] [PubMed]
99. Pan, Y.; Zhang, Y.; Li, J.; Zhang, Z.; He, Y.; Zhao, Q.; Yang, H.; Zhou, P. A Proteoglycan Isolated from Ganoderma Lucidum Attenuates Diabetic Kidney Disease by Inhibiting Oxidative Stress-Induced Renal Fibrosis Both In Vitro and In Vivo. *J. Ethnopharmacol.* **2023**, *310*, 116405. [CrossRef]
100. Zhong, D.; Wang, H.; Liu, M.; Li, X.; Huang, M.; Zhou, H.; Lin, S.; Lin, Z.; Yang, B. Ganoderma Lucidum Polysaccharide Peptide Prevents Renal Ischemia Reperfusion Injury Via Counteracting Oxidative Stress. *Sci. Rep.* **2015**, *5*, 16910. [CrossRef]
101. Xie, W.; Huang, Y.-Y.; Chen, H.-G.; Zhou, X. Study on the Efficacy and Mechanism of Lycium Barbarum Polysaccharide against Lead-Induced Renal Injury in Mice. *Nutrients* **2021**, *13*, 2945. [CrossRef]
102. Chen, J.; Wang, W.; Zhang, Q.; Li, F.; Lei, T.; Luo, D.; Zhou, H.; Yang, B. Low Molecular Weight Fucoidan against Renal Ischemia–Reperfusion Injury Via Inhibition of the Mapk Signaling Pathway. *PLoS ONE* **2013**, *8*, e56224. [CrossRef]
103. Li, X.-Y.; Chen, H.-R.; Zha, X.-Q.; Chen, S.; Pan, L.-H.; Li, Q.-M.; Luo, J.-P. Prevention and Possible Mechanism of a Purified Laminaria Japonica Polysaccharide on Adriamycin-Induced Acute Kidney Injury in Mice. *Int. J. Biol. Macromol.* **2020**, *148*, 591–600. [CrossRef] [PubMed]
104. Wang, Y.; Sun, Y.; Shao, F.; Zhang, B.; Wang, Z.; Li, X. Low Molecular Weight Fucoidan Can Inhibit the Fibrosis of Diabetic Kidneys by Regulating the Kidney Lipid Metabolism. *J. Diabetes Res.* **2021**, *2021*, 7618166. [CrossRef]
105. Chen, J.; Cui, W.; Zhang, Q.; Jia, Y.; Sun, Y.; Weng, L.; Luo, D.; Zhou, H.; Yang, B. Low Molecular Weight Fucoidan Ameliorates Diabetic Nephropathy Via Inhibiting Epithelial-Mesenchymal Transition and Fibrotic Processes. *Am. J. Transl. Res.* **2015**, *7*, 1553–1563.
106. Li, X.-Y.; Chen, H.-R.; Kuang, D.-D.; Pan, L.-H.; Li, Q.-M.; Luo, J.-P.; Zha, X.-Q. Laminaria Japonica Polysaccharide Attenuates Podocyte Epithelial-Mesenchymal Transformation Via Tgf-B1-Mediated Smad3 and P38mapk Pathways. *Int. J. Biol. Macromol.* **2023**, *241*, 124637. [CrossRef]
107. Wang, J.; Zhang, Q.; Li, S.; Chen, Z.; Tan, J.; Yao, J.; Duan, D. Low Molecular Weight Fucoidan Alleviates Diabetic Nephropathy by Binding Fibronectin and Inhibiting Ecm-Receptor Interaction in Human Renal Mesangial Cells. *Int. J. Biol. Macromol.* **2020**, *150*, 304–314. [CrossRef] [PubMed]
108. Li, X.; Li, X.; Zhang, Q.; Zhao, T. Low Molecular Weight Fucoidan and Its Fractions Inhibit Renal Epithelial Mesenchymal Transition Induced by Tgf-B1 or Fgf-2. *Int. J. Biol. Macromol.* **2017**, *105*, 1482–1490. [CrossRef] [PubMed]
109. Wei, X.-M.; Jiang, S.; Li, S.-S.; Sun, Y.-S.; Wang, S.-H.; Liu, W.-C.; Wang, Z.; Wang, Y.-P.; Zhang, R.; Li, W. Endoplasmic Reticulum Stress-Activated Perk-Eif2α-Atf4 Signaling Pathway Is Involved in the Ameliorative Effects of Ginseng Polysaccharides against Cisplatin-Induced Nephrotoxicity in Mice. *ACS Omega* **2021**, *6*, 8958–8966. [CrossRef] [PubMed]
110. Lian, Y.; Zhu, M.; Chen, J.; Yang, B.; Lv, Q.; Wang, L.; Guo, S.; Tan, X.; Li, C.; Bu, W.; et al. Characterization of a Novel Polysaccharide from Moutan Cortex and Its Ameliorative Effect on Ages-Induced Diabetic Nephropathy. *Int. J. Biol. Macromol.* **2021**, *176*, 589–600. [CrossRef]
111. Zhang, M.; Yang, L.; Zhu, M.; Yang, B.; Yang, Y.; Jia, X.; Feng, L. Moutan Cortex Polysaccharide Ameliorates Diabetic Kidney Disease Via Modulating Gut Microbiota Dynamically in Rats. *Int. J. Biol. Macromol.* **2022**, *206*, 849–860. [CrossRef]
112. Zhao, H.; Xu, J.; Wang, R.; Tang, W.; Kong, L.; Wang, W.; Wang, L.; Zhang, Y.; Ma, W. Plantaginis Semen Polysaccharides Ameliorate Renal Damage through Regulating Nlrp3 Inflammasome in Gouty Nephropathy Rats. *Food Funct.* **2021**, *12*, 2543–2553. [CrossRef]
113. Huang, C.; Yu, J.; Da, J.; Dong, R.; Dai, L.; Yang, Y.; Deng, Y.; Yuan, J. Dendrobium Officinale Kimura & Migo Polysaccharide Inhibits Hyperglycaemia-Induced Kidney Fibrosis Via the Mirna-34a-5p/Sirt1 Signalling Pathway. *J. Ethnopharmacol.* **2023**, *313*, 116601.
114. Wang, X.; Liu, W.; Jin, G.; Wu, Z.; Zhang, D.; Bao, Y.; Shi, W. Salvia Miltiorrhiza Polysaccharides Alleviates Florfenicol Induced Kidney Injury in Chicks Via Inhibiting Oxidative Stress and Apoptosis. *Ecotoxicol. Environ. Saf.* **2022**, *233*, 113339. [CrossRef]
115. Zhang, J.; Bi, R.; Meng, Q.; Wang, C.; Huo, X.; Liu, Z.; Wang, C.; Sun, P.; Sun, H.; Ma, X.; et al. Catalpol Alleviates Adriamycin-Induced Nephropathy by Activating the Sirt1 Signalling Pathway In Vivo and In Vitro. *Br. J. Pharmacol.* **2019**, *176*, 4558–4573. [CrossRef]
116. Cong, C.; Yuan, X.; Hu, Y.; Chen, W.; Wang, Y.; Tao, L. Catalpol Alleviates Ang Ii-Induced Renal Injury through Nf-Kb Pathway and Tgf-B1/Smads Pathway. *J. Cardiovasc. Pharmacol.* **2022**, *79*, e116–e121. [CrossRef]
117. Chen, Y.; Liu, Q.; Meng, X.; Zhao, L.; Zheng, X.; Feng, W. Catalpol Ameliorates Fructose-Induced Renal Inflammation by Inhibiting Tlr4/Myd88 Signaling and Uric Acid Reabsorption. *Eur. J. Pharmacol.* **2024**, *967*, 176356. [CrossRef] [PubMed]

118. Zaaba, N.E.; Al-Salam, S.; Beegam, S.; Elzaki, O.; Yasin, J.; Nemmar, A. Catalpol Attenuates Oxidative Stress and Inflammation Via Mechanisms Involving Sirtuin-1 Activation and Nf-Kb Inhibition in Experimentally-Induced Chronic Kidney Disease. *Nutrients* **2023**, *15*, 237. [CrossRef] [PubMed]
119. Zhang, J.; Zhao, T.; Wang, C.; Meng, Q.; Huo, X.; Wang, C.; Sun, P.; Sun, H.; Ma, X.; Wu, J.; et al. Catalpol-Induced Ampk Activation Alleviates Cisplatin-Induced Nephrotoxicity through the Mitochondrial-Dependent Pathway without Compromising Its Anticancer Properties. *Oxid. Med. Cell Longev.* **2021**, *2021*, 7467156. [CrossRef] [PubMed]
120. Chen, J.; Yang, Y.; Lv, Z.; Shu, A.; Du, Q.; Wang, W.; Chen, Y.; Xu, H. Study on the Inhibitive Effect of Catalpol on Diabetic Nephropathy. *Life Sci.* **2020**, *257*, 118120. [CrossRef]
121. Shu, A.; Du, Q.; Chen, J.; Gao, Y.; Zhu, Y.; Lv, G.; Lu, J.; Chen, Y.; Xu, H. Catalpol Ameliorates Endothelial Dysfunction and Inflammation in Diabetic Nephropathy Via Suppression of Rage/Rhoa/Rock Signaling Pathway. *Chem.-Biol. Interact.* **2021**, *348*, 109625. [CrossRef]
122. Zhang, J.; Wang, C.; Kang, K.; Liu, H.; Liu, X.; Jia, X.; Yu, K. Loganin Attenuates Septic Acute Renal Injury with the Participation of Akt and Nrf2/Ho-1 Signaling Pathways. *Drug Des. Devel Ther.* **2021**, *15*, 501–513. [CrossRef]
123. Huang, F.; Wang, X.; Xiao, G.; Xiao, J. Loganin Exerts a Protective Effect on Ischemia-Reperfusion-Induced Acute Kidney Injury by Regulating Jak2/Stat3 and Nrf2/Ho-1 Signaling Pathways. *Drug Dev. Res.* **2022**, *83*, 150–157. [CrossRef]
124. Kong, X.; Zhao, Y.; Wang, X.; Yu, Y.; Meng, Y.; Yan, G.; Yu, M.; Jiang, L.; Song, W.; Wang, B.; et al. Loganin Reduces Diabetic Kidney Injury by Inhibiting the Activation of Nlrp3 Inflammasome-Mediated Pyroptosis. *Chem.-Biol. Interact.* **2023**, *382*, 110640. [CrossRef]
125. Liu, K.; Xu, H.; Lv, G.; Liu, B.; Lee, M.K.K.; Lu, C.; Lv, X.; Wu, Y. Loganin Attenuates Diabetic Nephropathy in C57bl/6j Mice with Diabetes Induced by Streptozotocin and Fed with Diets Containing High Level of Advanced Glycation End Products. *Life Sci.* **2015**, *123*, 78–85. [CrossRef]
126. Li, X.; Ma, A.; Liu, K. Geniposide Alleviates Lipopolysaccharide-Caused Apoptosis of Murine Kidney Podocytes by Activating Ras/Raf/Mek/Erk-Mediated Cell Autophagy. *Artif. Cells Nanomed. Biotechnol.* **2019**, *47*, 1524–1532. [CrossRef]
127. Liu, J.; Zhao, N.; Shi, G.; Wang, H. Geniposide Ameliorated Sepsis-Induced Acute Kidney Injury by Activating Pparγ. *Aging* **2020**, *12*, 22744–22758. [CrossRef] [PubMed]
128. Liu, X.; Qian, N.; Zhu, L.; Fan, L.; Fu, G.; Ma, M.; Bao, J.; Cao, C.; Liang, X. Geniposide Ameliorates Acute Kidney Injury Via Enhancing the Phagocytic Ability of Macrophages Towards Neutrophil Extracellular Traps. *Eur. J. Pharmacol.* **2023**, *957*, 176018. [CrossRef] [PubMed]
129. Cheng, W.; Tan, L.; Yu, S.; Song, J.; Li, Z.; Peng, X.; Wei, Q.; He, Z.; Zhang, W.; Yang, X. Geniposide Reduced Oxidative Stress-Induced Apoptosis in Hk-2 Cell through Pi3k/Akt3/Foxo1 by M6a Modification. *Int. Immunopharmacol.* **2024**, *131*, 111820. [CrossRef]
130. Hu, X.; Zhang, X.; Jin, G.; Shi, Z.; Sun, W.; Chen, F. Geniposide Reduces Development of Streptozotocin-Induced Diabetic Nephropathy Via Regulating Nuclear Factor-Kappa B Signaling Pathways Geniposide Reduces Development of Streptozotocin-Induced Diabetic Nephropathy Via Regulating Nuclear Factor-Kappa B Signaling Pathways. *Fundam. Clin. Pharmacol.* **2017**, *31*, 54–63.
131. Dusabimana, T.; Park, E.J.; Je, J.; Jeong, K.; Yun, S.P.; Kim, H.J.; Kim, H.; Park, S.W. Geniposide Improves Diabetic Nephropathy by Enhancing Ulk1-Mediated Autophagy and Reducing Oxidative Stress through Ampk Activation. *Int. J. Mol. Sci.* **2021**, *22*, 1651. [CrossRef]
132. Peng, J.H.; Leng, J.; Tian, H.J.; Yang, T.; Fang, Y.; Feng, Q.; Zhao, Y.; Hu, Y.Y. Geniposide and Chlorogenic Acid Combination Ameliorates Non-Alcoholic Steatohepatitis Involving the Protection on the Gut Barrier Function in Mouse Induced by High-Fat Diet. *Front. Pharmacol.* **2018**, *9*, 1399. [CrossRef]
133. Gao, X.; Liu, Y.; Wang, L.; Sai, N.; Liu, Y.; Ni, J. Morroniside Inhibits H_2O_2-Induced Podocyte Apoptosis by Down-Regulating Nox4 Expression Controlled by Autophagy in Vitro. *Front. Pharmacol.* **2020**, *11*, 533809. [CrossRef]
134. Liu, Y.; Dai, W.; Ye, S. The Olive Constituent Oleuropein Exerts Nephritic Protective Effects on Diabetic Nephropathy in Db/Db Mice. *Arch. Physiol. Biochem.* **2019**, *128*, 455–462. [CrossRef] [PubMed]
135. Tüfekci, K.K.; Tatar, M. Oleuropein Mitigates Acrylamide-Induced Nephrotoxicity by Affecting Placental Growth Factor Immunoactivity in the Rat Kidney. *Eurasian J. Med.* **2023**, *55*, 228–233.
136. Chen, L.; Cao, G.; Wang, M.; Feng, Y.L.; Chen, D.Q.; Vaziri, N.D.; Zhuang, S.; Zhao, Y.Y. The Matrix Metalloproteinase-13 Inhibitor Poricoic Acid Zi Ameliorates Renal Fibrosis by Mitigating Epithelial-Mesenchymal Transition. *Mol. Nutr. Food Res.* **2019**, *63*, e1900132. [CrossRef]
137. Wang, M.; Chen, D.Q.; Chen, L.; Cao, G.; Zhao, H.; Liu, D.; Vaziri, N.D.; Guo, Y.; Zhao, Y.Y. Novel Inhibitors of the Cellular Renin-Angiotensin System Components, Poricoic Acids, Target Smad3 Phosphorylation and Wnt/B-Catenin Pathway against Renal Fibrosis. *Br. J. Pharmacol.* **2018**, *175*, 2689–2708. [CrossRef] [PubMed]
138. Chen, D.Q.; Wang, Y.N.; Vaziri, N.D.; Chen, L.; Hu, H.H.; Zhao, Y.Y. Poricoic Acid a Activates Ampk to Attenuate Fibroblast Activation and Abnormal Extracellular Matrix Remodelling in Renal Fibrosis. *Phytomedicine* **2020**, *72*, 153232. [CrossRef] [PubMed]
139. Chen, D.Q.; Wu, X.Q.; Chen, L.; Hu, H.H.; Wang, Y.N.; Zhao, Y.Y. Poricoic Acid a as a Modulator of Tph-1 Expression Inhibits Renal Fibrosis Via Modulating Protein Stability of B-Catenin and B-Catenin-Mediated Transcription. *Ther. Adv. Chronic Dis.* **2020**, *11*, 2040622320962648. [CrossRef]

140. Chen, D.Q.; Feng, Y.L.; Chen, L.; Liu, J.R.; Wang, M.; Vaziri, N.D.; Zhao, Y.Y. Poricoic Acid a Enhances Melatonin Inhibition of Aki-to-Ckd Transition by Regulating Gas6/Axlnfκb/Nrf2 Axis. *Free Radic. Biol. Med.* **2019**, *134*, 484–497. [CrossRef] [PubMed]
141. Chen, D.Q.; Chen, L.; Guo, Y.; Wu, X.Q.; Zhao, T.T.; Zhao, H.L.; Zhang, H.J.; Yan, M.H.; Zhang, G.Q.; Li, P. Poricoic Acid a Suppresses Renal Fibroblast Activation and Interstitial Fibrosis in Uuo Rats Via Upregulating Sirt3 and Promoting Β-Catenin K49 Deacetylation. *Acta Pharmacol. Sin.* **2023**, *44*, 1038–1050. [CrossRef]
142. Li, Q.; Ming, Y.; Jia, H.; Wang, G. Poricoic Acid a Suppresses Tgf-Β1-Induced Renal Fibrosis and Proliferation Via the Pdgf-C, Smad3 and Mapk Pathways. *Exp. Ther. Med.* **2021**, *21*, 289. [CrossRef]
143. Chung, S.; Yoon, H.E.; Kim, S.J.; Kim, S.J.; Koh, E.S.; Hong, Y.A.; Park, C.W.; Chang, Y.S.; Shin, S.J. Oleanolic Acid Attenuates Renal Fibrosis in Mice with Unilateral Ureteral Obstruction Via Facilitating Nuclear Translocation of Nrf2. *Nutr. Metab.* **2014**, *11*, 2. [CrossRef] [PubMed]
144. Nataraju, A.; Saini, D.; Ramachandran, S.; Benshoff, N.; Liu, W.; Chapman, W.; Mohanakuma, T.r. Oleanolic Acid, a Plant Triterpenoid, Significantly Improves Survival and Function of Islet Allograft. *Transplantation* **2009**, *88*, 987–994. [CrossRef]
145. Alqrad, M.A.I.; El-Agamy, D.S.; Ibrahim, S.R.M.; Sirwi, A.; Abdallah, H.M.; Abdel-Sattar, E.; El-Halawany, A.M.; Elsaed, W.M.; Mohamed, G.A. Sirt1/Nrf2/Nf-Kb Signaling Mediates Anti-Inflammatory and Anti-Apoptotic Activities of Oleanolic Acid in a Mouse Model of Acute Hepatorenal Damage. *Medicina* **2023**, *59*, 1351. [CrossRef]
146. Liu, Y.; Zheng, J.Y.; Wei, Z.T.; Liu, S.K.; Sun, J.L.; Mao, Y.H.; Xu, Y.D.; Yang, Y. Therapeutic Effect and Mechanism of Combination Therapy with Ursolic Acid and Insulin on Diabetic Nephropathy in a Type I Diabetic Rat Model. *Front. Pharmacol.* **2022**, *13*, 969207. [CrossRef]
147. Wang, K.; Xu, X.; Shan, Q.; Ding, R.; Lyu, Q.; Huang, L.; Chen, X.; Han, X.; Yang, Q.; Sang, X.; et al. Integrated Gut Microbiota and Serum Metabolomics Reveal the Protective Effect of Oleanolic Acid on Liver and Kidney-Injured Rats Induced by Euphorbia Pekinensis. *Phytother. Res.* **2022**. [CrossRef] [PubMed]
148. Zhang, J.; Luan, Z.L.; Huo, X.K.; Zhang, M.; Morisseau, C.; Sun, C.P.; Hammock, B.D.; Ma, X.C. Direct Targeting of Seh with Alisol B Alleviated the Apoptosis, Inflammation, and Oxidative Stress in Cisplatin-Induced Acute Kidney Injury. *Int. J. Biol. Sci.* **2023**, *19*, 294–310. [CrossRef] [PubMed]
149. Luan, Z.L.; Ming, W.H.; Sun, X.W.; Zhang, C.; Zhou, Y.; Zheng, F.; Yang, Y.L.; Guan, Y.F.; Zhang, X.Y. A Naturally Occurring Fxr Agonist, Alisol B 23-Acetate, Protects against Renal Ischemia-Reperfusion Injury. *Am. J. Physiol. Renal Physiol.* **2021**, *321*, F617–F628. [CrossRef] [PubMed]
150. Chen, H.; Wang, M.C.; Chen, Y.Y.; Chen, L.; Wang, Y.N.; Vaziri, N.D.; Miao, H.; Zhao, Y.Y. Alisol B 23-Acetate Attenuates Ckd Progression by Regulating the Renin-Angiotensin System and Gut-Kidney Axis. *Ther. Adv. Chronic Dis.* **2020**, *11*, 2040622320920025. [CrossRef] [PubMed]
151. Wang, L.; Hao, X.; Li, X.; Li, Q.; Fang, X. Effects of Ginsenoside Rh2 on Cisplatin-Induced Nephrotoxicity in Renal Tubular Epithelial Cells by Inhibiting Endoplasmic Reticulum Stress. *J. Biochem. Mol. Toxicol.* **2024**, *38*, e23768. [CrossRef]
152. Guo, J.; Chen, L.; Ma, M. Ginsenoside Rg1 Suppresses Ferroptosis of Renal Tubular Epithelial Cells in Sepsis-Induced Acute Kidney Injury Via the Fsp1-Coq(10)-Nad(P)H Pathway. *Curr. Med. Chem.* **2024**, *31*, 2119–2132. [CrossRef]
153. Zhao, H.; Ding, R.; Han, J. Ginsenoside Rh4 Facilitates the Sensitivity of Renal Cell Carcinoma to Ferroptosis Via the Nrf2 Pathway. *Arch. Esp. Urol.* **2024**, *77*, 119–128. [CrossRef]
154. Hwang, H.J.; Hong, S.H.; Moon, H.S.; Yoon, Y.E.; Park, S.Y. Ginsenoside Rh2 Sensitizes the Anti-Cancer Effects of Sunitinib by Inducing Cell Cycle Arrest in Renal Cell Carcinoma. *Sci. Rep.* **2022**, *12*, 19752. [CrossRef]
155. Chen, Y.; Peng, Y.; Li, P.; Jiang, Y.; Song, D. Ginsenoside Rg3 Induces Mesangial Cells Proliferation and Attenuates Apoptosis by Mir-216a-5p/Mapk Pathway in Diabetic Kidney Disease. *Aging* **2024**, *16*, 9933–9943. [CrossRef]
156. Sui, Z.; Sui, D.; Li, M.; Yu, Q.; Li, H.; Jiang, Y. Ginsenoside Rg3 Has Effects Comparable to Those of Ginsenoside Re on Diabetic Kidney Disease Prevention in Db/Db Mice by Regulating Inflammation, Fibrosis and Pparγ. *Mol. Med. Rep.* **2023**, *27*, 84. [CrossRef]
157. Liu, Y.; Mou, L.; Yi, Z.; Lin, Q.; Banu, K.; Wei, C.; Yu, X. Integrative Informatics Analysis Identifies That Ginsenoside Re Improves Renal Fibrosis through Regulation of Autophagy. *J. Nat. Med.* **2024**, *78*, 722–731. [CrossRef] [PubMed]
158. Ji, P.; Shi, Q.; Liu, Y.; Han, M.; Su, Y.; Sun, R.; Zhou, H.; Li, W.; Li, W. Ginsenoside Rg1 Treatment Alleviates Renal Fibrosis by Inhibiting the Nox4-Mapk Pathway in T2dm Mice. *Ren. Fail.* **2023**, *45*, 2197075. [CrossRef] [PubMed]
159. Su, L.; Liu, L.; Jia, Y.; Lei, L.; Liu, J.; Zhu, S.; Zhou, H.; Chen, R.; Lu, H.A.J.; Yang, B. Ganoderma Triterpenes Retard Renal Cyst Development by Downregulating Ras/Mapk Signaling and Promoting Cell Differentiation. *Kidney Int.* **2017**, *92*, 1404–1418. [CrossRef]
160. Geng, X.Q.; Ma, A.; He, J.Z.; Wang, L.; Jia, Y.L.; Shao, G.Y.; Li, M.; Zhou, H.; Lin, S.Q.; Ran, J.H.; et al. Ganoderic Acid Hinders Renal Fibrosis Via Suppressing the Tgf-Β/Smad and Mapk Signaling Pathways. *Acta Pharmacol. Sin.* **2020**, *41*, 670–677. [CrossRef]
161. Shao, G.; He, J.; Meng, J.; Ma, A.; Geng, X.; Zhang, S.; Qiu, Z.; Lin, D.; Li, M.; Zhou, H.; et al. Ganoderic Acids Prevent Renal Ischemia Reperfusion Injury by Inhibiting Inflammation and Apoptosis. *Int. J. Mol. Sci.* **2021**, *22*, 10229. [CrossRef]
162. Cai, L.; Horowitz, M.; Islam, M.S. Potential Therapeutic Targets for the Prevention of Diabetic Nephropathy: Glycyrrhetinic Acid. *World J. Diabetes* **2023**, *14*, 1717–1720. [CrossRef]
163. Hou, S.; Zhang, T.; Li, Y.; Guo, F.; Jin, X. Glycyrrhizic Acid Prevents Diabetic Nephropathy by Activating Ampk/Sirt1/Pgc-1α Signaling in Db/Db Mice. *J. Diabetes Res.* **2017**, *2017*, 2865912. [CrossRef] [PubMed]

164. Cao, R.; Li, Y.; Hu, X.; Qiu, Y.; Li, S.; Xie, Y.; Xu, C.; Lu, C.; Chen, G.; Yang, J. Glycyrrhizic Acid Improves Tacrolimus-Induced Renal Injury by Regulating Autophagy. *Faseb J.* **2023**, *37*, e22749. [CrossRef] [PubMed]
165. Oh, H.; Choi, A.; Seo, N.; Lim, J.S.; You, J.S.; Chung, Y.E. Protective Effect of Glycyrrhizin, a Direct Hmgb1 Inhibitor, on Post-Contrast Acute Kidney Injury. *Sci. Rep.* **2021**, *11*, 15625. [CrossRef]
166. Li, Z.; Yan, M.; Cao, L.; Fang, P.; Guo, Z.; Hou, Z.; Zhang, B. Glycyrrhetinic Acid Accelerates the Clearance of Triptolide through P-Gp in Vitro. *Phytother. Res.* **2017**, *31*, 1090–1096. [CrossRef]
167. Jiang, Y.; Cai, C.; Zhang, P.; Luo, Y.; Guo, J.; Li, J.; Rong, R.; Zhang, Y.; Zhu, T. Transcriptional Profile Changes after Treatment of Ischemia Reperfusion Injury-Induced Kidney Fibrosis with 18β-Glycyrrhetinic Acid. *Ren. Fail.* **2022**, *44*, 660–671. [CrossRef] [PubMed]
168. Zhu, Z.; Li, J.; Song, Z.; Li, T.; Li, Z.; Gong, X. Tetramethylpyrazine Attenuates Renal Tubular Epithelial Cell Ferroptosis in Contrast-Induced Nephropathy by Inhibiting Transferrin Receptor and Intracellular Reactive Oxygen Species. *Clin. Sci.* **2024**, *138*, 235–249. [CrossRef] [PubMed]
169. Gong, X.; Duan, Y.; Zheng, J.; Ye, Z.; Hei, T.K. Tetramethylpyrazine Prevents Contrast-Induced Nephropathy Via Modulating Tubular Cell Mitophagy and Suppressing Mitochondrial Fragmentation, Ccl2/Ccr2-Mediated Inflammation, and Intestinal Injury. *Oxid. Med. Cell Longev.* **2019**, *2019*, 7096912. [CrossRef] [PubMed]
170. Sun, W.; Li, A.; Wang, Z.; Sun, X.; Dong, M.; Qi, F.; Wang, L.; Zhang, Y.; Du, P. Tetramethylpyrazine Alleviates Acute Kidney Injury by Inhibiting Nlrp3/Hif-1α and Apoptosis. *Mol. Med. Rep.* **2020**, *22*, 2655–2664. [CrossRef]
171. Rai, U.; Kosuru, R.; Prakash, S.; Tiwari, V.; Singh, S. Tetramethylpyrazine Alleviates Diabetic Nephropathy through the Activation of Akt Signalling Pathway in Rats. *Eur. J. Pharmacol.* **2019**, *865*, 172763. [CrossRef]
172. Jing, M.; Cen, Y.; Gao, F.; Wang, T.; Jiang, J.; Jian, Q.; Wu, L.; Guo, B.; Luo, F.; Zhang, G.; et al. Nephroprotective Effects of Tetramethylpyrazine Nitrone Tbn in Diabetic Kidney Disease. *Front. Pharmacol.* **2021**, *12*, 680336. [CrossRef]
173. Hu, J.; Gu, W.; Ma, N.; Fan, X.; Ci, X. Leonurine Alleviates Ferroptosis in Cisplatin-Induced Acute Kidney Injury by Activating the Nrf2 Signalling Pathway. *Br. J. Pharmacol.* **2022**, *179*, 3991–4009. [CrossRef]
174. Yin, X.; Gao, Q.; Li, C.; Yang, Q.; Dong, H.; Li, Z. Leonurine Alleviates Vancomycin Nephrotoxicity Via Activating Pparγ and Inhibiting the Tlr4/Nf-Kb/Tnf-A Pathway. *Int. Immunopharmacol.* **2024**, *131*, 111898. [CrossRef]
175. Cheng, H.; Bo, Y.; Shen, W.; Tan, J.; Jia, Z.; Xu, C.; Li, F. Leonurine Ameliorates Kidney Fibrosis Via Suppressing Tgf-B and Nf-Kb Signaling Pathway in Uuo Mice. *Int. Immunopharmacol.* **2015**, *25*, 406–415. [CrossRef]
176. Xu, D.; Chen, M.; Ren, X.; Ren, X.; Wu, Y. Leonurine Ameliorates Lps-Induced Acute Kidney Injury Via Suppressing Ros-Mediated Nf-Kb Signaling Pathway. *Fitoterapia* **2014**, *97*, 148–155. [CrossRef]
177. Cheng, R.; Wang, X.; Huang, L.; Lu, Z.; Wu, A.; Guo, S.; Li, C.; Mao, W.; Xie, Y.; Xu, P.; et al. Novel Insights into the Protective Effects of Leonurine against Acute Kidney Injury: Inhibition of Er Stress-Associated Ferroptosis Via Regulating Atf4/Chop/Acsl4 Pathway. *Chem. Biol. Interact.* **2024**, *395*, 111016. [CrossRef] [PubMed]
178. Hassanein, E.H.M.; Shalkami, A.-G.S.; Khalaf, M.M.; Mohamed, W.R.; Hemeida, R.A.M. The Impact of Keap1/Nrf2, P_{38}Mapk/Nf-Kb and Bax/Bcl2/Caspase-3 Signaling Pathways in the Protective Effects of Berberine against Methotrexate-Induced Nephrotoxicity. *Biomed. Pharmacother.* **2019**, *109*, 47–56. [CrossRef]
179. Fouad, G.I.; Ahmed, K.A. The Protective Impact of Berberine against Doxorubicin-Induced Nephrotoxicity in Rats. *Tissue Cell* **2021**, *73*, 101612. [CrossRef]
180. Malaviya, A.N. Landmark Papers on the Discovery of Methotrexate for the Treatment of Rheumatoid Arthritis and Other Systemic Inflammatory Rheumatic Diseases: A Fascinating Story. *Int. J. Rheum. Dis.* **2016**, *19*, 844–851. [CrossRef] [PubMed]
181. Domitrovic, R.; Cvijanovic, O.; Pernjak-Pugel, E.; Skoda, M.; Mikelic, L.; Crncevic-Orlic, Z. Berberine Exerts Nephroprotective Effect against Cisplatin-Induced Kidney Damage through Inhibition of Oxidative/Nitrosative Stress, Inflammation, Autophagy and Apoptosis. *Food Chem. Toxicol.* **2013**, *62*, 397–406. [CrossRef]
182. Adil, M.; Kandhare, A.D.; Dalvi, G.; Ghosh, P.; Venkata, S.; Raygude, K.S.; Bodhankar, S.L. Ameliorative Effect of Berberine against Gentamicin-Induced Nephrotoxicity in Rats Via Attenuation of Oxidative Stress, Inflammation, Apoptosis and Mitochondrial Dysfunction. *Ren. Fail.* **2016**, *38*, 996–1006. [CrossRef] [PubMed]
183. Kumas, M.; Esrefoglu, M.; Karatas, E.; Duymac, N.; Kanbay, S.; Ergun, I.S.; Uyuklu, M.; Kocyigit, A. Investigation of Dose-Dependent Effects of Berberine against Renal Ischemia/Reperfusion Injury in Experimental Diabetic Rats. *Nefrologia* **2019**, *39*, 411–423. [CrossRef]
184. Lu, J.; Yi, Y.; Pan, R.; Zhang, C.; Han, H.; Chen, J.; Liu, W. Berberine Protects Hk-2 Cells from Hypoxia/Reoxygenation Induced Apoptosis Via Inhibiting Sphk1 Expression. *J. Nat. Med.* **2018**, *72*, 390–398. [CrossRef]
185. Visnagri, A.; Kandhare, A.D.; Bodhankar, S.L. Renoprotective Effect of Berberine Via Intonation on Apoptosis and Mitochondrial-Dependent Pathway in Renal Ischemia Reperfusion-Induced Mutilation. *Ren. Fail.* **2015**, *37*, 482–493. [CrossRef]
186. Zhang, X.; He, H.; Liang, D.; Jiang, Y.; Liang, W.; Chi, Z.-H.; Ma, J. Protective Effects of Berberine on Renal Injury in Streptozotocin (Stz)-Induced Diabetic Mice. *Int. J. Mol. Sci.* **2016**, *17*, 1327. [CrossRef]
187. Yang, G.; Zhao, Z.; Zhang, X.; Wu, A.; Huang, Y.; Miao, Y.; Yang, M. Effect of Berberine on the Renal Tubular Epithelial-to-Mesenchymal Transition by Inhibition of the Notch/Snail Pathway in Diabetic Nephropathy Model Kkay Mice. *Drug Des. Dev. Ther.* **2017**, *11*, 1065–1079. [CrossRef] [PubMed]
188. Zhang, X.; Guan, T.; Yang, B.; Chi, Z.; Wan, Q.; Gu, H.F. Protective Effect of Berberine on High Glucose and Hypoxia-Induced Apoptosis Via the Modulation of Hif-1α in Renal Tubular Epithelial Cells. *Am. J. Transl. Res.* **2019**, *11*, 669–682. [PubMed]

189. Wang, F.-M.; Yang, Y.-J.; Ma, L.-L.; Tian, X.-J.; He, Y.-Q. Berberine Ameliorates Renal Interstitial Fibrosis Induced by Unilateral Ureteral Obstruction in Rats. *Nephrology* **2014**, *19*, 542–551. [CrossRef] [PubMed]
190. Pan, L.; Yu, H.; Fu, J.; Hu, J.; Xu, H.; Zhang, Z.; Bu, M.; Yang, X.; Zhang, H.; Lu, J.; et al. Berberine Ameliorates Chronic Kidney Disease through Inhibiting the Production of Gut-Derived Uremic Toxins in the Gut Microbiota. *Acta Pharm. Sin. B* **2023**, *13*, 1537–1553. [CrossRef]
191. Peerapen, P.; Thongboonkerd, V. Protective Roles of Trigonelline against Oxalate-Induced Epithelial-to-Mesenchymal Transition in Renal Tubular Epithelial Cells: An in Vitro Study. *Food Chem. Toxicol.* **2020**, *135*, 110915. [CrossRef]
192. Peerapen, P.; Boonmark, W.; Putpeerawit, P.; Sassanarakkit, S.; Thongboonkerd, V. Proteomic and Computational Analyses Followed by Functional Validation of Protective Effects of Trigonelline against Calcium Oxalate-Induced Renal Cell Deteriorations. *Comput. Struct. Biotechnol. J.* **2023**, *21*, 5851–5867. [CrossRef]
193. Sheweita, S.A.; ElHady, S.A.; Hammoda, H.M. Trigonella Stellata Reduced the Deleterious Effects of Diabetes Mellitus through Alleviation of Oxidative Stress, Antioxidant- and Drug-Metabolizing Enzymes Activities. *J. Ethnopharmacol.* **2020**, *256*, 112821. [CrossRef]
194. Chen, C.; Ma, J.; Miao, C.S.; Zhang, H.; Zhang, M.; Cao, X.; Shi, Y. Trigonelline Induces Autophagy to Protect Mesangial Cells in Response to High. Glucose Via Activating the Mir-5189-5p-Ampk Pathway. *Phytomedicine* **2021**, *92*, 153614. [CrossRef]
195. Gong, M.; Guo, Y.; Dong, H.; Wu, W.; Wu, F.; Lu, F. Trigonelline Inhibits Tubular Epithelial-Mesenchymal Transformation in Diabetic Kidney Disease Via Targeting Smad7. *Biomed. Pharmacother.* **2023**, *168*, 115747. [CrossRef]
196. Peerapen, P.; Boonmark, W.; Thongboonkerd, V. Trigonelline Prevents Kidney Stone Formation Processes by Inhibiting Calcium Oxalate Crystallization, Growth and Crystal-Cell Adhesion, and Downregulating Crystal Receptors. *Biomed. Pharmacother.* **2022**, *149*, 112876. [CrossRef]
197. Zhou, L.; Wu, K.; Gao, Y.; Qiao, R.; Tang, N.; Dong, D.; Li, X.Q.; Nong, Q.; Luo, D.Q.; Xiao, Q.; et al. Piperlonguminine Attenuates Renal Fibrosis by Inhibiting Trpc6. *J. Ethnopharmacol.* **2023**, *313*, 116561. [CrossRef] [PubMed]
198. Yuan, L.; Yang, J.; Li, Y.; Yuan, L.; Liu, F.; Yuan, Y.; Tang, X. Matrine Alleviates Cisplatin-Induced Acute Kidney Injury by Inhibiting Mitochondrial Dysfunction and Inflammation Via Sirt3/Opa1 Pathway. *J. Cell Mol. Med.* **2022**, *26*, 3702–3715. [CrossRef] [PubMed]
199. Kang, S.; Chen, T.; Hao, Z.; Yang, X.; Wang, M.; Zhang, Z.; Hao, S.; Lang, F.; Hao, H. Oxymatrine Alleviates Gentamicin-Induced Renal Injury in Rats. *Molecules* **2022**, *27*, 6209. [CrossRef] [PubMed]
200. Jiang, G.; Liu, X.; Wang, M.; Chen, H.; Chen, Z.; Qiu, T. Oxymatrine Ameliorates Renal Ischemia-Reperfusion Injury from Oxidative Stress through Nrf2/Ho-1 Pathway. *Acta Cir. Bras.* **2015**, *30*, 422–429. [CrossRef]
201. Yao, M.; Lian, D.; Wu, M.; Zhou, Y.; Fang, Y.; Zhang, S.; Zhang, W.; Yang, Y.; Li, R.; Chen, H.; et al. Isoliensinine Attenuates Renal Fibrosis and Inhibits Tgf-B1/Smad2/3 Signaling Pathway in Spontaneously Hypertensive Rats. *Drug Des. Devel Ther.* **2023**, *17*, 2749–2762. [CrossRef]
202. Zhang, W.; Chen, H.; Xu, Z.; Zhang, X.; Tan, X.; He, N.; Shen, J.; Dong, J. Liensinine Pretreatment Reduces Inflammation, Oxidative Stress, Apoptosis, and Autophagy to Alleviate Sepsis Acute Kidney Injury. *Int. Immunopharmacol.* **2023**, *122*, 110563. [CrossRef]
203. Xiong, Y.; Zhong, J.; Chen, W.; Li, X.; Liu, H.; Li, Y.; Xiong, W.; Li, H. Neferine Alleviates Acute Kidney Injury by Regulating the Ppar-A/Nf-Kb Pathway. *Clin. Exp. Nephrol.* **2024**, 1–19. [CrossRef]
204. Li, H.; Chen, W.; Chen, Y.; Zhou, Q.; Xiao, P.; Tang, R.; Xue, J. Neferine Attenuates Acute Kidney Injury by Inhibiting Nf-Kb Signaling and Upregulating Klotho Expression. *Front. Pharmacol.* **2019**, *10*, 1197. [CrossRef]
205. Hongmei, H.; Maojun, Y.; Ting, L.I.; Dandan, W.; Ying, L.I.; Xiaochi, T.; Lu, Y.; Shi, G.U.; Yong, X.U. Neferine Inhibits the Progression of Diabetic Nephropathy by Modulating the Mir-17-5p/Nuclear Factor E2-Related Factor 2 Axis. *J. Tradit. Chin. Med.* **2024**, *44*, 44–53.
206. Li, H.; Ge, H.; Song, X.; Tan, X.; Xiong, Q.; Gong, Y.; Zhang, L.; He, Y.; Zhang, W.; Zhu, P.; et al. Neferine Mitigates Cisplatin-Induced Acute Kidney Injury in Mice by Regulating Autophagy and Apoptosis. *Clin. Exp. Nephrol.* **2023**, *27*, 122–131. [CrossRef]
207. Li, H.; Tang, Y.; Wen, L.; Kong, X.; Chen, X.; Liu, P.; Zhou, Z.; Chen, W.; Xiao, C.; Xiao, P.; et al. Neferine Reduces Cisplatin-Induced Nephrotoxicity by Enhancing Autophagy Via the Ampk/Mtor Signaling Pathway. *Biochem. Biophys. Res. Commun.* **2017**, *484*, 694–701. [CrossRef]
208. Yin, W.; Wang, J.H.; Liang, Y.M.; Liu, K.H.; Chen, Y.; Chen, Y. Neferine Targeted the Nlrc5/Nlrp3 Pathway to Inhibit M1-Type Polarization and Pyroptosis of Macrophages to Improve Hyperuricemic Nephropathy. *Curr. Mol. Med.* 2024; *online ahead of print*. [CrossRef]
209. Wang, M.X.; Zhao, X.J.; Chen, T.Y.; Liu, Y.L.; Jiao, R.Q.; Zhang, J.H.; Ma, C.H.; Liu, J.H.; Pan, Y.; Kong, L.D. Nuciferine Alleviates Renal Injury by Inhibiting Inflammatory Responses in Fructose-Fed Rats. *J. Agric. Food Chem.* **2016**, *64*, 7899–7910. [CrossRef] [PubMed]
210. Li, D.; Liu, B.; Fan, Y.; Liu, M.; Han, B.; Meng, Y.; Xu, X.; Song, Z.; Liu, X.; Hao, Q.; et al. Nuciferine Protects against Folic Acid-Induced Acute Kidney Injury by Inhibiting Ferroptosis. *Br. J. Pharmacol.* **2021**, *178*, 1182–1199. [CrossRef] [PubMed]
211. Zhai, J.; Chen, Z.; Zhu, Q.; Guo, Z.; Sun, X.; Jiang, L.; Li, J.; Wang, N.; Yao, X.; Zhang, C.; et al. Curcumin Inhibits Pat-Induced Renal Ferroptosis Via the P62/Keap1/Nrf2 Signalling Pathway. *Toxicology* **2024**, *506*, 153863. [CrossRef]
212. Yang, H.; Zhang, H.; Tian, L.; Guo, P.; Liu, S.; Chen, H.; Sun, L. Curcumin Attenuates Lupus Nephritis by Inhibiting Neutrophil Migration Via Pi3k/Akt/Nf-Kb Signalling Pathway. *Lupus Sci. Med.* **2024**, *11*, e001220. [CrossRef] [PubMed]

213. Ghasemzadeh Rahbardar, M.; Hosseinzadeh, H. The Ameliorative Effect of Turmeric (*Curcuma longa* Linn) Extract and Its Major Constituent, Curcumin, and Its Analogs on Ethanol Toxicity. *Phytother. Res.* **2024**, *38*, 2165–2181. [CrossRef]
214. Zhang, H.; Dong, Q.Q.; Shu, H.P.; Tu, Y.C.; Liao, Q.Q.; Yao, L.J. Curcumin Ameliorates Focal Segmental Glomerulosclerosis by Inhibiting Apoptosis and Oxidative Stress in Podocytes. *Arch. Biochem. Biophys.* **2023**, *746*, 109728. [CrossRef]
215. Altamimi, J.Z.; AlFaris, N.A.; Al-Farga, A.M.; Alshammari, G.M.; BinMowyna, M.N.; Yahya, M.A. Curcumin Reverses Diabetic Nephropathy in Streptozotocin-Induced Diabetes in Rats by Inhibition of Pkcβ/P(66)Shc Axis and Activation of Foxo-3a. *J. Nutr. Biochem.* **2021**, *87*, 108515. [CrossRef]
216. Feng, L.; Lin, Z.; Tang, Z.; Zhu, L.; Xu, S.; Tan, X.; Wang, X.; Mai, J.; Tan, Q. Emodin Improves Renal Fibrosis in Chronic Kidney Disease by Regulating Mitochondrial Homeostasis through the Mediation of Peroxisome Proliferator-Activated Receptor-Gamma Coactivator-1 Alpha (Pgc-1α). *Eur. J. Histochem.* **2024**, *68*, 3917. [CrossRef]
217. Dong, X.; Wen, R.; Xiong, Y.; Jia, X.; Zhang, X.; Li, X.; Zhang, L.; Li, Z.; Zhang, S.; Yu, Y.; et al. Emodin Alleviates Crs4-Induced Mitochondrial Damage Via Activation of the Pgc1α Signaling. *Phytother. Res.* **2024**, *38*, 1345–1357. [CrossRef]
218. Wang, L.; Wang, X.; Li, G.; Zhou, S.; Wang, R.; Long, Q.; Wang, M.; Li, L.; Huang, H.; Ba, Y. Emodin Ameliorates Renal Injury and Fibrosis Via Regulating the Mir-490-3p/Hmga2 Axis. *Front. Pharmacol.* **2023**, *14*, 1042093. [CrossRef] [PubMed]
219. Yang, F.; Deng, L.; Li, J.; Chen, M.; Liu, Y.; Hu, Y.; Zhong, W. Emodin Retarded Renal Fibrosis through Regulating Hgf and Tgfβ-Smad Signaling Pathway. *Drug Des. Devel Ther.* **2020**, *14*, 3567–3575. [CrossRef] [PubMed]
220. Tian, N.; Gao, Y.; Wang, X.; Wu, X.; Zou, D.; Zhu, Z.; Han, Z.; Wang, T.; Shi, Y. Emodin Mitigates Podocytes Apoptosis Induced by Endoplasmic Reticulum Stress through the Inhibition of the Perk Pathway in Diabetic Nephropathy. *Drug Des. Devel Ther.* **2018**, *12*, 2195–2211. [CrossRef] [PubMed]
221. Kuang, B.C.; Wang, Z.H.; Hou, S.H.; Zhang, J.; Wang, M.Q.; Zhang, J.S.; Sun, K.L.; Ni, H.Q.; Gong, N.Q. Methyl Eugenol Protects the Kidney from Oxidative Damage in Mice by Blocking the Nrf2 Nuclear Export Signal through Activation of the Ampk/Gsk3β Axis. *Acta Pharmacol. Sin.* **2023**, *44*, 367–380. [CrossRef] [PubMed]
222. Fathy, M.; Abdel-Latif, R.; Abdelgwad, Y.M.; Othman, O.A.; Abdel-Razik, A.H.; Dandekar, T.; Othman, E.M. Nephroprotective Potential of Eugenol in a Rat Experimental Model of Chronic Kidney Injury; Targeting Nox, Tgf-B, and Akt Signaling. *Life Sci.* **2022**, *308*, 120957. [CrossRef]
223. Oikawa, D.; Yamashita, S.; Takahashi, S.; Waki, T.; Kikuchi, K.; Abe, T.; Katayama, T.; Nakayama, T. (+)-Sesamin, a Sesame Lignan, Is a Potent Inhibitor of Gut Bacterial Tryptophan Indole-Lyase That Is a Key Enzyme in Chronic Kidney Disease Pathogenesis. *Biochem. Biophys. Res. Commun.* **2022**, *590*, 158–162. [CrossRef]
224. Altyar, A.E.; Albadrani, G.M.; Farouk, S.M.; Alamoudi, M.K.; Sayed, A.A.; Mohammedsaleh, Z.M.; Al-Ghadi, M.Q.; Saleem, R.M.; Sakr, H.I.; Abdel-Daim, M.M. The Antioxidant, Anti-Inflammatory, and Anti-Apoptotic Effects of Sesamin against Cisplatin-Induced Renal and Testicular Toxicity in Rats. *Ren. Fail.* **2024**, *46*, 2378212. [CrossRef]
225. Rousta, A.M.; Mirahmadi, S.M.; Shahmohammadi, A.; Nourabadi, D.; Khajevand-Khazaei, M.R.; Baluchnejadmojarad, T.; Roghani, M. Protective Effect of Sesamin in Lipopolysaccharide-Induced Mouse Model of Acute Kidney Injury Via Attenuation of Oxidative Stress, Inflammation, and Apoptosis. *Immunopharmacol. Immunotoxicol.* **2018**, *40*, 423–429. [CrossRef]
226. Zhang, R.; Yu, Y.; Deng, J.; Zhang, C.; Zhang, J.; Cheng, Y.; Luo, X.; Han, B.; Yang, H. Sesamin Ameliorates High-Fat Diet-Induced Dyslipidemia and Kidney Injury by Reducing Oxidative Stress. *Nutrients* **2016**, *8*, 276. [CrossRef]
227. Zhang, N.; Zhou, J.; Zhao, L.; Zhao, Z.; Wang, S.; Zhang, L.; Zhou, F. Ferulic Acid Supplementation Alleviates Hyperuricemia in High-Fructose/Fat Diet-Fed Rats Via Promoting Uric Acid Excretion and Mediating the Gut Microbiota. *Food Funct.* **2023**, *14*, 1710–1725. [CrossRef]
228. Zhou, X.; Zhang, B.; Zhao, X.; Lin, Y.; Zhuang, Y.; Guo, J.; Wang, S. Chlorogenic Acid Prevents Hyperuricemia Nephropathy Via Regulating Tmao-Related Gut Microbes and Inhibiting the Pi3k/Akt/Mtor Pathway. *J. Agric. Food Chem.* **2022**, *70*, 10182–10193. [CrossRef] [PubMed]
229. Zhou, X.; Zhang, B.; Zhao, X.; Lin, Y.; Wang, J.; Wang, X.; Hu, N.; Wang, S. Chlorogenic Acid Supplementation Ameliorates Hyperuricemia, Relieves Renal Inflammation, and Modulates Intestinal Homeostasis. *Food Funct.* **2021**, *12*, 5637–5649. [CrossRef] [PubMed]
230. Qu, S.; Dai, C.; Hao, Z.; Tang, Q.; Wang, H.; Wang, J.; Zhao, H. Chlorogenic Acid Prevents Vancomycin-Induced Nephrotoxicity without Compromising Vancomycin Antibacterial Properties. *Phytother. Res.* **2020**, *34*, 3189–3199. [CrossRef] [PubMed]
231. Li, H.-Y.; Yi, Y.-L.; Guo, S.; Zhang, F.; Yan, H.; Zhan, Z.-L.; Zhu, Y.; Duan, J.-A. Isolation, Structural Characterization and Bioactivities of Polysaccharides from Laminaria Japonica: A Review. *Food Chem.* **2022**, *370*, 131010. [CrossRef]
232. Lu, J.; Yao, J.; Pu, J.; Wang, D.; Liu, J.; Zhang, Y.; Zha, L. Transcriptome Analysis of Three Medicinal Plants of the Genus Polygonatum: Identification of Genes Involved in Polysaccharide and Steroidal Saponins Biosynthesis. *Front. Plant Sci.* **2023**, *14*, 1293411. [CrossRef]
233. Ge, J.; Liu, Z.; Zhong, Z.; Wang, L.; Zhuo, X.; Li, J.; Jiang, X.; Ye, X.-Y.; Xie, T.; Bai, R. Natural Terpenoids with Anti-Inflammatory Activities: Potential Leads for Anti-Inflammatory Drug Discovery. *Bioorganic Chem.* **2022**, *124*, 105817. [CrossRef] [PubMed]
234. Galappaththi, M.C.A.; Patabendige, N.M.; Premarathne, B.M.; Hapuarachchi, K.K.; Tibpromma, S.; Dai, D.-Q.; Suwannarach, N.; Rapior, S.; Karunarathna, S.C. A Review of Ganoderma Triterpenoids and Their Bioactivities. *Biomolecules* **2022**, *13*, 24. [CrossRef]
235. Lu, D.; Yang, Y.; Du, Y.; Zhang, L.; Yang, Y.; Tibenda, J.J.; Nan, Y.; Yuan, L. The Potential of Glycyrrhiza from "Medicine Food Homology" in the Fight against Digestive System Tumors. *Molecules* **2023**, *28*, 7719. [CrossRef]
236. Wu, Y.; Wang, X.; Yang, L.; Kang, S.; Yan, G.; Han, Y.; Fang, H.; Sun, H. Potential of Alisols as Cancer Therapeutic Agents: Investigating Molecular Mechanisms, Pharmacokinetics and Metabolism. *Biomed. Pharmacother.* **2023**, *168*, 115722. [CrossRef]

237. Lee, C.H.; Kim, J.H. A Review on the Medicinal Potentials of Ginseng and Ginsenosides on Cardiovascular Diseases. *J. Ginseng Res.* **2014**, *38*, 161–166. [CrossRef]
238. Yokozawa, T.; Liu, Z.W.; Dong, E. A Study of Ginsenoside-Rd in a Renal Ischemia-Reperfusion Model. *Nephron* **1998**, *78*, 201–206. [CrossRef] [PubMed]
239. Kouda, R.; Yakushiji, F. Recent Advances in Iridoid Chemistry: Biosynthesis and Chemical Synthesis. *Chem.—Asian J.* **2020**, *15*, 3771–3783. [CrossRef] [PubMed]
240. Danielewski, M.; Matuszewska, A.; Nowak, B.; Kucharska, A.Z.; Sozański, T. The Effects of Natural Iridoids and Anthocyanins on Selected Parameters of Liver and Cardiovascular System Functions. *Oxid. Med. Cell Longev.* **2020**, *2020*, 2735790. [CrossRef]
241. Bridi, R.; von Poser, G.L.; de Carvalho Meirelles, G. Iridoids as a Potential Hepatoprotective Class: A Review. *Mini Rev. Med. Chem.* **2023**, *23*, 452–479. [PubMed]
242. Zhou, T.Y.; Tian, N.; Li, L.; Yu, R. Iridoids Modulate Inflammation in Diabetic Kidney Disease: A Review. *J. Integr. Med.* **2024**, *22*, 210–222. [CrossRef]
243. Kou, Y.; Li, Z.; Yang, T.; Shen, X.; Wang, X.; Li, H.; Zhou, K.; Li, L.; Xia, Z.; Zheng, X.; et al. Therapeutic Potential of Plant Iridoids in Depression: A Review. *Pharm. Biol.* **2022**, *60*, 2167–2181. [CrossRef]
244. Zhang, F.; Yan, Y.; Xu, J.K.; Zhang, L.M.; Li, L.; Chen, X.; Li, D.X.; Peng, Y.; Yang, H.; Li, L.Z.; et al. Simultaneous Determination of Thirteen Iridoid Glycosides in Crude and Processed Fructus Corni from Different Areas by Uplc-Ms/Ms Method. *J. Chromatogr. Sci.* **2024**, *62*, 562–569. [CrossRef]
245. Cheng, C.; Li, Z.; Zhao, X.; Liao, C.; Quan, J.; Bode, A.M.; Cao, Y.; Luo, X. Natural Alkaloid and Polyphenol Compounds Targeting Lipid Metabolism: Treatment Implications in Metabolic Diseases. *Eur. J. Pharmacol.* **2020**, *870*, 172922. [CrossRef]
246. Li, J.; Gong, X. Tetramethylpyrazine: An Active Ingredient of Chinese Herbal Medicine W Ith Therapeutic Potential in Acute Kidney Injury and Renal Fibrosis. *Front. Pharmacol.* **2022**, *13*, 820071. [CrossRef]
247. Wu, D.; Wen, W.; Qi, C.L.; Zhao, R.X.; Lü, J.H.; Zhong, C.Y.; Chen, Y.Y. Ameliorative Effect of Berberine on Renal Damage in Rats with Diabetes Induced by High-Fat Diet and Streptozotocin. *Phytomedicine* **2012**, *19*, 712–718. [CrossRef]
248. Tang, L.; Lv, F.; Liu, S.; Zhang, S. Effect of Berberine on Expression of Transforming Growth Factor-Beta1 and Type Iv Collagen Proteins in Mesangial Cells of Diabetic Rats with Nephropathy. *Zhongguo Zhong Yao Za Zhi = Zhongguo Zhongyao Zazhi = China J. Chin. Mater. Medica* **2011**, *36*, 3494–3497.
249. Chen, Q.; Li, D.; Wu, F.; He, X.; Zhou, Y.; Sun, C.; Wang, H.; Liu, Y. Berberine Regulates the Metabolism of Uric Acid and Modulates Intestinal Flora in Hyperuricemia Rats Model. *Comb. Chem. High. Throughput Screen.* **2023**, *26*, 2057–2066. [CrossRef] [PubMed]
250. Shan, B.; Wu, M.; Chen, T.; Tang, W.; Li, P.; Chen, J. Berberine Attenuates Hyperuricemia by Regulating Urate Transporters and Gut Microbiota. *Am. J. Chin. Med.* **2022**, *50*, 2199–2221. [CrossRef] [PubMed]
251. Pan, L.; Han, P.; Ma, S.; Peng, R.; Wang, C.; Kong, W.; Cong, L.; Fu, J.; Zhang, Z.; Yu, H.; et al. Abnormal Metabolism of Gut Microbiota Reveals the Possible Molecular Mechanism of Nephropathy Induced by Hyperuricemia. *Acta Pharm. Sin. B* **2020**, *10*, 249–261. [CrossRef] [PubMed]
252. Wang, T.; Zhang, J.; Wei, H.; Wang, X.; Xie, M.; Jiang, Y.; Zhou, J. Matrine-Induced Nephrotoxicity Via Gsk-3β/Nrf2-Mediated Mitochondria-Dependent Apoptosis. *Chem. Biol. Interact.* **2023**, *378*, 110492. [CrossRef]
253. Wang, X.; Lin, Z.; Li, T.; Zhu, W.; Huang, H.; Hu, J.; Zhou, J. Sodium Selenite Prevents Matrine-Induced Nephrotoxicity by Suppressing Ferroptosis Via the Gsh-Gpx4 Antioxidant System. *Biol. Trace Element Res.* **2024**, *202*, 4674–4686. [CrossRef]
254. Wang, H.-W.; Shi, L.; Xu, Y.-P.; Qin, X.-Y.; Wang, Q.-Z. Oxymatrine Inhibits Renal Fibrosis of Obstructive Nephropathy by Downregulating the Tgf-B1-Smad3 Pathway. *Ren. Fail.* **2016**, *38*, 945–951. [CrossRef]
255. Zhu, Z.; Chen, R.; Zhang, L.; Zhu, Z. Simple Phenylpropanoids: Recent Advances in Biological Activities, Biosynthetic Pathways, and Microbial Production. *Nat. Prod. Rep.* **2024**, *41*, 6–24. [CrossRef]
256. Zhu, X.; Quan, Y.-Y.; Yin, Z.-J.; Li, M.; Wang, T.; Zheng, L.-Y.; Feng, S.-Q.; Zhao, J.-N.; Li, L. Sources, Morphology, Phytochemistry, Pharmacology of Curcumae Longae Rhizoma, Curcumae Radix, and Curcumae Rhizoma: A Review of the Literature. *Front. Pharmacol.* **2023**, *14*, 1229963. [CrossRef]
257. Pivari, F.; Mingione, A.; Piazzini, G.; Ceccarani, C.; Ottaviano, E.; Brasacchio, C.; Cas, M.D.; Vischi, M.; Cozzolino, M.G.; Fogagnolo, P.; et al. Curcumin Supplementation (Meriva®) Modulates Inflammation, Lipid Peroxidation and Gut Microbiota Composition in Chronic Kidney Disease. *Nutrients* **2022**, *14*, 231. [CrossRef]
258. Xu, X.; Wang, H.; Guo, D.; Man, X.; Liu, J.; Li, J.; Luo, C.; Zhang, M.; Zhen, L.; Liu, X. Curcumin Modulates Gut Microbiota and Improves Renal Function in Rats with Uric Acid Nephropathy. *Ren. Fail.* **2021**, *43*, 1063–1075. [CrossRef] [PubMed]
259. Mohtashami, L.; Amiri, M.S.; Ayati, Z.; Ramezani, M.; Jamialahmadi, T.; Emami, S.A.; Sahebkar, A. Ethnobotanical Uses, Phytochemistry and Pharmacology of Different Rheum Species (Polygonaceae): A Review. *Adv. Exp. Med. Biol.* **2021**, *1308*, 309–352.
260. Zeng, Y.Q.; Dai, Z.; Lu, F.; Lu, Z.; Liu, X.; Chen, C.; Qu, P.; Li, D.; Hua, Z.; Qu, Y.; et al. Emodin Via Colonic Irrigation Modulates Gut Microbiota and Reduces Uremic Toxins in Rats with Chronic Kidney Disease. *Oncotarget* **2016**, *7*, 17468–17478. [CrossRef]
261. Tucker, P.S.; Scanlan, A.T.; Dalbo, V.J. Chronic Kidney Disease Influences Multiple Systems: Describing the Relationship between Oxidative Stress, Inflammation, Kidney Damage, and Concomitant Disease. *Oxidative Med. Cell. Longev.* **2015**, *2015*, 1–8. [CrossRef]

262. Tain, Y.-L.; Hsu, C.-N. Perinatal Oxidative Stress and Kidney Health: Bridging the Gap between Animal Models and Clinical Reality. *Antioxidants* **2023**, *12*, 13. [CrossRef] [PubMed]
263. Mapuskar, K.A.; Pulliam, C.F.; Zepeda-Orozco, D.; Griffin, B.R.; Furqan, M.; Spitz, D.R.; Allen, B.G. Redox Regulation of Nrf2 in Cisplatin-Induced Kidney Injury. *Antioxidants* **2023**, *12*, 1728. [CrossRef]
264. Honda, T.; Hirakawa, Y.; Nangaku, M. The Role of Oxidative Stress and Hypoxia in Renal Disease. *Kidney Res. Clin. Pract.* **2019**, *38*, 414–426. [CrossRef] [PubMed]
265. Allameh, H.; Fatemi, I.; Malayeri, A.R.; Nesari, A.; Mehrzadi, S.; Goudarzi, M. Pretreatment with Berberine Protects against Cisplatin-Induced Renal Injury in Male Wistar Rats. *Naunyn-Schmiedebergs Arch. Pharmacol.* **2020**, *393*, 1825–1833. [CrossRef]
266. Verma, V.K.; Malik, S.; Mutneja, E.; Sahu, A.K.; Rupashi, K.; Dinda, A.K.; Arya, D.S.; Bhatia, J. Mechanism Involved in Fortification by Berberine in Cddp-Induced Nephrotoxicity. *Curr. Mol. Pharmacol.* **2020**, *13*, 342–352. [CrossRef]
267. El-Horany, H.E.-S.; Gaballah, H.H.; Helal, D.S. Berberine Ameliorates Renal Injury in a Rat Model of D-Galactose-Induced Aging through a Pten/Akt-Dependent Mechanism. *Arch. Physiol. Biochem.* **2020**, *126*, 157–165. [CrossRef]
268. Hasanein, P.; Riahi, H. Preventive Use of Berberine in Inhibition of Lead-Induced Renal Injury in Rats. *Environ. Sci. Pollut. Res.* **2018**, *25*, 4896–4903. [CrossRef] [PubMed]
269. Basile, D.P.; Anderson, M.D.; Sutton, T.A. Pathophysiology of Acute Kidney Injury. *Compr. Physiol.* **2012**, *2*, 1303–1353. [PubMed]
270. Fu, Y.; Xiang, Y.; Li, H.; Chen, A.; Dong, Z. Inflammation in Kidney Repair: Mechanism and Therapeutic Potential. *Pharmacol. Ther.* **2022**, *237*, 108240. [CrossRef] [PubMed]
271. Mosquera-Sulbaran, J.A.; Pedreañez, A.; Vargas, R.; Hernandez-Fonseca, J.P. Apoptosis in Post-Streptococcal Glomerulonephritis and Mechanisms for Failed of Inflammation Resolution. *Pediatr. Nephrol.* **2024**, *39*, 1709–1724. [CrossRef] [PubMed]
272. Zhang, H.; Deng, Z.; Wang, Y. Molecular Insight in Intrarenal Inflammation Affecting Four Main Types of Cells in Nephrons in Iga Nephropathy. *Front. Med.* **2023**, *10*, 1128393. [CrossRef]
273. Vallés, P.G.; Lorenzo, A.F.G.; Garcia, R.D.; Cacciamani, V.; Benardon, M.E.; Costantino, V.V. Toll-Like Receptor 4 in Acute Kidney Injury. *Int. J. Mol. Sci.* **2023**, *24*, 1415. [CrossRef]
274. Yeh, T.H.; Tu, K.C.; Wang, H.Y.; Chen, J.Y. From Acute to Chronic: Unraveling the Pathophysiological Mechanisms of the Progression from Acute Kidney Injury to Acute Kidney Disease to Chronic Kidney Disease. *Int. J. Mol. Sci.* **2024**, *25*, 1755. [CrossRef]
275. Lovisa, S.; Zeisberg, M.; Kalluri, R. Partial Epithelial-to-Mesenchymal Transition and Other New Mechanisms of Kidney Fibrosis. *Trends Endocrinol. Metab.* **2016**, *27*, 681–695. [CrossRef]
276. La Russa, A.; Serra, R.; Faga, T.; Crugliano, G.; Bonelli, A.; Coppolino, G.; Bolignano, D.; Battaglia, Y.; Ielapi, N.; Costa, D.; et al. Kidney Fibrosis and Matrix Metalloproteinases (Mmps). *Front. Biosci.-Landmark* **2024**, *29*, 192. [CrossRef]
277. Evenepoel, P.; Poesen, R.; Meijers, B. The Gut-Kidney Axis. *Pediatr. Nephrol.* **2017**, *32*, 2005–2014. [CrossRef]
278. Ramya Ranjan Nayak, S.P.; Boopathi, S.; Haridevamuthu, B.; Arockiaraj, J. Toxic Ties: Unraveling the Complex Relationship between Endocrine Disrupting Chemicals and Chronic Kidney Disease. *Environ. Pollut.* **2023**, *338*, 122686. [CrossRef] [PubMed]
279. Hayeeawaema, F.; Muangnil, P.; Jiangsakul, J.; Tipbunjong, C.; Huipao, N.; Khuituan, P. A Novel Model of Adenine-Induced Chronic Kidney Disease-Associated Gastrointestinal Dysfunction in Mice: The Gut-Kidney Axis. *Saudi J. Biol. Sci.* **2023**, *30*, 103660. [CrossRef] [PubMed]
280. Lu, X.; Ma, J.; Li, R. Alterations of Gut Microbiota in Biopsy-Proven Diabetic Nephropathy and a Long History of Diabetes without Kidney Damage. *Sci. Rep.* **2023**, *13*, 12150. [CrossRef] [PubMed]
281. Jiang, S.; Xie, S.; Lv, D.; Zhang, Y.; Deng, J.; Zeng, L.; Chen, Y. A Reduction in the Butyrate Producing Species *Roseburia* Spp. and *Faecalibacterium prausnitzii* Is Associated with Chronic Kidney Disease Progression. *Antonie Van Leeuwenhoek* **2016**, *109*, 1389–1396. [CrossRef]
282. Wong, J.; Piceno, Y.M.; DeSantis, T.Z.; Pahl, M.; Andersen, G.L.; Vaziri, N.D. Expansion of Urease- and Uricase-Containing, Indole- and P-Cresol-Forming and Contraction of Short-Chain Fatty Acid-Producing Intestinal Microbiota in Esrd. *Am. J. Nephrol.* **2014**, *39*, 230–237. [CrossRef]
283. Marques, F.Z.; Nelson, E.; Chu, P.Y.; Horlock, D.; Fiedler, A.; Ziemann, M.; Tan, J.K.; Kuruppu, S.; Rajapakse, N.W.; El-Osta, A.; et al. High-Fiber Diet and Acetate Supplementation Change the Gut Microbiota and Prevent the Development of Hypertension and Heart Failure in Hypertensive Mice. *Circulation* **2017**, *135*, 964–977. [CrossRef] [PubMed]
284. Liang, Z.; Tang, Z.; Zhu, C.; Li, F.; Chen, S.; Han, X.; Zheng, R.; Hu, X.; Lin, R.; Pei, Q.; et al. Intestinal Cxcr6+ Ilc3s Migrate to the Kidney and Exacerbate Renal Fibrosis Via Il-23 Receptor Signaling Enhanced by Pd-1 Expression. *Immunity* **2024**, *57*, 1306–1323. [CrossRef]
285. Yan, J.; Herzog, J.W.; Tsang, K.; Brennan, C.A.; Bower, M.A.; Garrett, W.S.; Sartor, B.R.; Aliprantis, A.O.; Charles, J.F. Gut Microbiota Induce Igf-1 and Promote Bone Formation and Growth. *Proc. Natl. Acad. Sci. USA* **2016**, *113*, E7554–E7563. [CrossRef]
286. Gleeson, P.J.; Benech, N.; Chemouny, J.; Metallinou, E.; Berthelot, L.; da Silva, J.; Bex-Coudrat, J.; Boedec, E.; Canesi, F.; Bounaix, C.; et al. The Gut Microbiota Posttranslationally Modifies Iga1 in Autoimmune Glomerulonephritis. *Sci. Transl. Med.* **2024**, *16*, eadl6149. [CrossRef]
287. Lan, T.; Tang, T.; Li, Y.; Duan, Y.; Yuan, Q.; Liu, W.; Ren, Y.; Li, N.; Liu, X.; Zhang, Y.; et al. Ftz Polysaccharides Ameliorate Kidney Injury in Diabetic Mice by Regulating Gut-Kidney Axis. *Phytomedicine* **2023**, *118*, 154935. [CrossRef]
288. Kunter, U.; Seikrit, C.; Floege, J. Novel Agents for Treating Iga Nephropathy. *Curr. Opin. Nephrol. Hypertens.* **2023**, *32*, 418–426. [CrossRef] [PubMed]

289. Zhang, Z.-W.; Han, P.; Fu, J.; Yu, H.; Xu, H.; Hu, J.-C.; Lu, J.-Y.; Yang, X.-Y.; Zhang, H.-J.; Bu, M.-M.; et al. Gut microbiota-based metabolites of Xiaoyao Pills (a typical Traditional Chinese medicine) ameliorate depression by inhibiting fatty acid amide hydrolase levels in brain. *J. Ethnopharmacol.* **2023**, *313*, 116555. [CrossRef] [PubMed]
290. Zhang, Z.-W.; Gao, C.-S.; Zhang, H.; Yang, J.; Wang, Y.-P.; Pan, L.-B.; Yu, H.; He, C.-Y.; Luo, H.-B.; Zhao, Z.-X.; et al. Morinda officinalis oligosaccharides increase serotonin in the brain and ameliorate depression via promoting 5-hydroxytryptophan production in the gut microbiota. *Acta Pharm. Sin. B* **2022**, *12*, 3298–3312. [CrossRef] [PubMed]
291. Wang, Y.; Tong, Q.; Ma, S.-R.; Zhao, Z.-X.; Pan, L.-B.; Cong, L.; Han, P.; Peng, R.; Yu, H.; Lin, Y.; et al. Oral berberine improves brain dopa/dopamine levels to ameliorate Parkinson's disease by regulating gut microbiota. *Signal Transduct. Target. Ther.* **2021**, *6*, 77. [CrossRef]
292. Feng, R.; Shou, J.-W.; Zhao, Z.-X.; He, C.-Y.; Ma, C.; Huang, M.; Fu, J.; Tan, X.-S.; Li, X.-Y.; Wen, B.-Y.; et al. Transforming berberine into its intestine-absorbable form by the gut microbiota. *Sci. Rep.* **2015**, *5*, 12155. [CrossRef]
293. Wu, G.D.; Chen, J.; Hoffmann, C.; Bittinger, K.; Chen, Y.-Y.; Keilbaugh, S.A.; Bewtra, M.; Knights, D.; Walters, W.A.; Knight, R.; et al. Linking Long-Term Dietary Patterns with Gut Microbial Enterotypes. *Science* **2011**, *334*, 105–108. [CrossRef]
294. Turnbaugh, P.J.; Ridaura, V.K.; Faith, J.J.; Rey, F.E.; Knight, R.; Gordon, J.I. The Effect of Diet on the Human Gut Microbiome: A Metagenomic Analysis in Humanized Gnotobiotic Mice. *Sci. Transl. Med.* **2009**, *1*, 6ra14. [CrossRef]

MDPI AG
Grosspeteranlage 5
4052 Basel
Switzerland
Tel.: +41 61 683 77 34

Nutrients Editorial Office
E-mail: nutrients@mdpi.com
www.mdpi.com/journal/nutrients

www.ingramcontent.com/pod-product-compliance
Lightning Source LLC
Chambersburg PA
CBHW062054220926
51850CB00010B/2764
9783725850457